Hepatology Update: Current Management and New Therapies

Guest Editor

DAVID A. SASS, MD

GASTROENTEROLOGY CLINICS OF NORTH AMERICA

www.gastro.theclinics.com

September 2011 • Volume 40 • Number 3

SAUNDERS an imprint of ELSEVIER, Inc.

W.B. SAUNDERS COMPANY
A Division of Elsevier Inc.

Elsevier Inc. • 1600 John F. Kennedy Blvd., Suite 1800 • Philadelphia, Pennsylvania 19103-2899

http://www.theclinics.com

GASTROENTEROLOGY CLINICS OF NORTH AMERICA Volume 40, Number 3
September 2011 ISSN 0889-8553, ISBN-13: 978-1-4557-1096-6

Editor: Kerry Holland
Developmental Editor: Donald Mumford

Gastroenterology Clinics of North America (ISSN 0889-8553) is published quarterly by Elsevier Inc., 360 Park Avenue South, New York, NY 10010-1710. Months of issue are March, June, September, and December. Business and Editorial Offices: 1600 John F. Kennedy Blvd., Suite 1800, Philadelphia, PA 19103-2899. Customer Service Office: 6277 Sea Harbor Drive, Orlando, FL 32887-4800. Periodicals postage paid at New York, NY and additional mailing offices. Subscription prices are $282.00 per year (US individuals), $142.00 per year (US students), $458.00 per year (US institutions), $310.00 per year (Canadian individuals), $558.00 per year (Canadian institutions), $392.00 per year (international individuals), $195.00 per year (international students), and $558.00 per year (international institutions). Foreign air speed delivery is included in all *Clinics* subscription prices. All prices are subject to change without notice. **POSTMASTER:** Send address changes to *Gastroenterology Clinics of North America*, Elsevier Health Sciences Division, Subscription Customer Service, 3251 Riverport Lane, Maryland Heights, MO 63043. Telephone: 1-800-654-2452 (U.S. and Canada); 314-447-8871 (outside U.S. and Canada). Fax: 314-447-8029. E-mail: journalscustomerservice-usa@elsevier.com (for print support); journalsonlinesupport-usa@elsevier.com (for online support).

Reprints. For copies of 100 or more, of articles in this publication, please contact the Commercial Reprints Department, Elsevier Inc., 360 Part Avenue South, New York, New York 10010-1710. Tel. (212) 633-3813, Fax: (212) 462-1935, E-mail: reprints@elsevier.com.

Gastroenterology Clinics of North America is also published in Italian by Il Pensiero Scientifico Editore, Rome, Italy; and in Portuguese by Interlivros Edicoes Ltda., Rua Commandante Coelho 1085, 21250 Cordovil, Rio de Janeiro, Brazil.

Gastroenterology Clinics of North America is covered in *MEDLINE/PubMed (Index Medicus)*, *Excerpta Medica*, *Current Contents/Clinical Medicine*, *Science Citation Index*, *ISI/BIOMED*, and *BIOSIS*.

Printed and bound by CPI Group (UK) Ltd, Croydon, CR0 4YY

Transferred to Digital Print 2011

Contributors

GUEST EDITOR

DAVID A. SASS, MD, FACP, FACG, AGAF
Associate Professor of Medicine and Surgery, Chief of Hepatology, Medical Director of Liver Transplantation, Division of Gastroenterology and Hepatology, Drexel University College of Medicine, Philadelphia, Pennsylvania.

AUTHORS

JAWAD AHMAD, MD, FRCP
Associate Professor of Medicine, Division of Liver Diseases, Mount Sinai School of Medicine, New York, New York

CATHERINE FRENETTE, MD
Medical Director of Liver Transplantation and Director of Liver Cancer Program, Department of Liver Transplantation, The Methodist Hospital Center for Liver Disease and Transplantation, Houston, Texas

GUADALUPE GARCIA-TSAO, MD
Professor of Medicine, Section of Digestive Diseases, Yale University School of Medicine, New Haven; Veterans Affairs Connecticut Healthcare System, West Haven, Connecticut

ROBERT GISH, MD
Chief of Clinical Hepatology, Professor of Clinical Medicine, Medical Director, Center for Hepatobiliary Disease and Abdominal Transplantation, Division of Gastroenterology and Hepatology, University of California San Diego Medical Center, San Diego, California

ALISON B. JAZWINSKI, MD
Fellow, Division of Gastroenterology, Duke University School of Medicine, Durham, North Carolina

EMMET B. KEEFFE, MD, MACP, FRCP
Emeritus Professor of Medicine, Division of Gastroenterology and Hepatology, Stanford University Medical Center, Palo Alto, California

MAXIMILIAN LEE, MD, MPH
Fellow in Transplant Hepatology, Division of Gastroenterology and Hepatology, Stanford University Medical Center, Palo Alto, California

WESLEY LEUNG, MD, FRCPC
Division of Gastroenterology, Department of Medicine, Toronto General Hospital, University of Toronto, Toronto, Ontario, Canada

ANDREW J. MUIR, MD, MHS
Director, Gastroenterology and Hepatology Research, Duke Clinical Research Institute, Duke University School of Medicine, Durham, North Carolina

CHRISTOPHER KENNETH OPIO, MD
Research Fellow, Section of Digestive Diseases, Yale University School of Medicine, New Haven; Veterans Affairs Connecticut Healthcare System, West Haven, Connecticut

DAVID H. OUSTECKY, MD
Fellow, Department of Gastroenterology and Hepatology, Drexel University College of Medicine, Philadelphia, Pennsylvania

NEIL PARIKH, MD
Division of Internal Medicine, Mount Sinai School of Medicine, New York, New York

DAVID J. REICH, MD, FACS
Professor of Surgery and Chief, Division of Multiorgan Transplantation and Heptobiliary Surgery, Drexel University College of Medicine, Philadelphia, Pennsylvania

ANDRES R. RIERA, MD
Internal Medicine Resident, Department of Medicine, Division of General Internal Medicine, Drexel University College of Medicine, Philadelphia, Pennsylvania

KENNETH D. ROTHSTEIN, MD
Associate Professor and Chief, Division of Gastroenterology and Hepatology, Department of Gastroenterology and Hepatology, Drexel University College of Medicine, Philadelphia, Pennsylvania

DAVID A. SASS, MD, FACP, FACG, AGAF
Associate Professor of Medicine and Surgery, Chief of Hepatology, Medical Director of Liver Transplantation, Division of Gastroenterology and Hepatology, Drexel University College of Medicine, Philadelphia, Pennsylvania

PAUL A. SCHMELTZER, MD
Instructor of Medicine, Department of Medicine, Division of Gastroenterology and Hepatology, Mayo Clinic, Rochester, Minnesota

VIJAY H. SHAH, MD
Division of Gastroenterology and Hepatology, Mayo Clinic College of Medicine, Rochester, Minnesota

OBAID S. SHAIKH, MD, FRCP
Professor, Department of Medicine, Division of Gastroenterology, Hepatology and Nutrition, University of Pittsburgh School of Medicine, Pittsburgh, Pennsylvania

ASHWANI K. SINGAL, MD
Division of Gastroenterology and Hepatology, Mayo Clinic, Rochester, Minnesota

VINAY SUNDARAM, MD
Instructor, Department of Medicine, Division of Gastroenterology and Hepatology, Beth Israel Deaconess Medical Center, Harvard Medical School, Boston, Massachusetts

JAYANT A. TALWALKAR, MD, MPH
Associate Professor of Medicine, Department of Medicine, Division of Gastroenterology and Hepatology, Mayo Clinic, Rochester, Minnesota

FLORENCE WONG, MBBS, MD, FRACP, FRCPC
Division of Gastroenterology, Department of Medicine, Toronto General Hospital, University of Toronto, Toronto, Ontario, Canada

ROBERT WONG, MD
Gastroenterology Fellow, Division of Gastroenterology and Hepatology, Stanford University Medical Center, Stanford, California

Contents

Preface: Hepatology Update: Current Management and New Therapies   xi

David A. Sass

Emerging Therapies in Hepatitis C: Dawn of the Era of the Direct-Acting Antivirals   481

Alison B. Jazwinski and Andrew J. Muir

Successful new drugs that directly target the hepatitis C virus at various points in the life cycle are currently in development. The NS3/4A protease inhibitors will be the first to be used in clinical practice and the NS5B polymerase inhibitors will soon follow. These new therapies will initially be used with pegylated interferon-α and ribavirin owing to the common development of viral resistance with monotherapy. However, the ultimate goal is to develop a regimen consisting entirely of oral direct-acting antiviral agents, allowing more patients to be effectively treated with fewer adverse events.

Hepatitis B: Modern End Points of Treatment and the Specter of Viral Resistance   495

Maximilian Lee and Emmet B. Keeffe

The goal of antiviral treatment of chronic hepatitis B is to prevent cirrhosis, hepatic decompensation, hepatocellular carcinoma, and death. To determine the efficacy of antiviral treatment in preventing these clinical outcomes, intermediate surrogate biochemical, virologic, serologic, and histologic end points have been used. Taken together, these end points can help to guide the effectiveness of therapy. This article reviews the current end points of chronic hepatitis B treatment, including the development of antiviral resistance as a complication and failure of treatment.

Noninvasive Tools to Assess Hepatic Fibrosis: Ready for Prime Time?   507

Paul A. Schmeltzer and Jayant A. Talwalkar

Often regarded as the gold standard for fibrosis assessment, liver biopsy carries associated risks; however, it is less than ideal. The need for noninvasive assessment of hepatic fibrosis for disease staging, prognosis, progression, and treatment response is clear. Advances in serologic testing and conventional imaging techniques have reduced the need for liver biopsy. Areas of research include defining cutoff values for specific diseases, further head-to-head comparisons of noninvasive modalities, examination of algorithms using both serum markers and imaging, and the cost-effectiveness of these various tests for diagnostic as well as screening purposes.

Acute Liver Failure: Current Practice and Recent Advances   523

Vinay Sundaram and Obaid S. Shaikh

> Acute liver failure (ALF) is a rare syndrome characterized by rapid onset of severe hepatic dysfunction in the absence of prior liver disease. Cerebral edema is common in patients with advanced hepatic encephalopathy. Advances in critical care (monitoring and management of intracranial hypertension and cerebral oxygen delivery and consumption, and of systemic inflammatory response syndrome and multiorgan dysfunction) have helped improve outcomes. Liver transplantation plays a critical role; therefore, patients with ALF are assigned highest prioritization for donor allografts. Detoxification and bioartificial liver support devices hold promise as bridges to transplantation or spontaneous recovery. Hepatocyte and stem cell transplantation are novel restorative modalities in development.

Nonalcoholic Fatty Liver Disease: Pharmacologic and Surgical Options   541

Neil Parikh and Jawad Ahmad

> Non-alcoholic fatty liver disease (NAFLD) encompasses a spectrum of hepatic steatosis, inflammation and fibrosis that can lead to cirrhosis and the need for liver transplant. NAFLD can be considered as part of the metabolic syndrome as it typically occurs in obese subjects with insulin resistance. Pharmacologic approaches to NAFLD therapy include improving insulin resistance and decreasing oxidative stress, while conservative and surgical weight loss strategies have also shown some promise. However, further well designed prospective studies are required to determine the optimal therapy in NAFLD.

Managing Varices: Drugs, Bands, and Shunts   561

Christopher Kenneth Opio and Guadalupe Garcia-Tsao

> Up to 50% of patients with cirrhosis have esophageal varices at initial endoscopy. Without treatment, varices rupture in about one-third of the patients. Drugs, bands, and shunts have been used in the treatment of varices and variceal hemorrhage, resulting in improved outcomes. The specific use of each therapy depends on the setting and patient characteristics. This article updates the current use of drugs, bands, and shunts in the settings of primary prophylaxis, secondary prophylaxis, and treatment of acute variceal hemorrhage, and shows how they have altered the natural history of varices and variceal hemorrhage.

Hepatorenal Syndrome: Do the Vasoconstrictors Work?   581

Wesley Leung and Florence Wong

> The development of hepatorenal syndrome (HRS) is related to many changes associated with advanced cirrhosis. Because vasoconstrictors correct systemic and splanchnic hemodynamic abnormalities, they are effective treatments for HRS, although only in approximately 40% of HRS patients. Emerging data show that combination

treatment with vasoconstrictors and TIPS may yield better outcomes than either alone. All HRS patients should be assessed for liver transplantation. Reversing HRS before transplantation is associated with better long-term survival. Combined liver–kidney transplantation is indicated for those with irreversible kidney injury. Otherwise, there is some merit in performing a liver transplant first and only considering a kidney transplant later.

Hepatocellular Carcinoma: Locoregional and Targeted Therapies   599

Robert Wong, Catherine Frenette, and Robert Gish

Hepatocellular carcinoma (HCC) is a leading cause of morbidity and mortality worldwide. Advances in cancer screening and surveillance have led to earlier detection and greater treatment options. Although surgical interventions traditionally form the mainstay of curative approaches to HCC, the advent of locoregional and targeted molecular therapies offer patients and practitioners greater options in the management of HCC. This review explores the realm of locoregional therapies in treating HCC with an emphasis on novel developments in localized chemoembolization and systemic molecular-based targeted therapies.

Alcoholic Hepatitis: Prognostic Models and Treatment   611

Ashwani K. Singal and Vijay H. Shah

Alcoholic hepatitis is a distinct subset of alcoholic liver disease. Inflammation and oxidative stress are the two main pathogenetic mechanisms involved in its pathogenesis. Patients with mild disease usually improve with conservative management. However, about 30-50% of those with severe disease succumb to their illness within about 1 month. Therefore, assessment of disease severity is important and practical issue. Currently, hepatologists do not have an ideal scoring system available. With survival benefit of only about 50% with corticosteroids and pentoxifylline, there is need to develop newer and better treatment options to manage these patients. This article also deals with controversies surrounding the role and use of liver transplantation in patients with alcoholic hepatitis.

Liver Transplantation in the 21st Century: Expanding the Donor Options   641

David A. Sass and David J. Reich

The large imbalance between the growing pool of potential liver transplant recipients and the scarcity of donor organs has fueled efforts to maximize existing donors and identify new sources. This article reviews the current state of liver transplantation using allografts from extended criteria donors and from donation after cardiac death, as well as the use of partial allografts (split liver and living-donor liver transplantation). The authors explore the innovation in transplantation geared toward increasing the donor pool and the issues pertaining to matching of these grafts to suitable recipients.

Long-Term Management of the Liver Transplant Recipient: Pearls for the Practicing Gastroenterologist   659

David H. Oustecky, Andres R. Riera, and Kenneth D. Rothstein

Orthotopic liver transplantation is becoming more common, and patients are surviving longer posttransplantation. Special care must be paid to the long-term management of these patients because they are at increased risk for medical problems, malignancies, and adverse effects from immunosuppression. This article addresses the importance of medical care, as well as the complications that may arise, while caring for a liver transplant recipient. A stable and continuing relationship must be developed between the physician and the patient to optimize the long-term outcomes for these individuals.

Index   683

FORTHCOMING ISSUES

December 2011
The Motility Consultation: Challenges in
Gastrointestinal Motility in Everyday
Clinical Practice
Eammon M. M. Quigley, MD,
Guest Editor

March 2012
Modern Management of Benign and
Malignant Pancreatic Disease
Jacques Van Dam, MD, PhD,
Guest Editor

June 2012
Chronic Diarrhea
Heinz Hammer, MD,
Guest Editor

RECENT ISSUES

June 2011
Women's Issues in Gastroenterology
Asyia Ahmad, MD, MPH,
and Barbara B. Frank, MD,
Guest Editors

March 2011
Irritable Bowel Syndrome
William D. Chey, MD,
Guest Editor

December 2010
Advanced Imaging in Gastroenterology
Ralf Kiesslich, MD, PhD,
Guest Editor

ISSUES OF RELATED INTEREST

Clinics in Liver Disease, February 2011 (Volume 15, Issue 1)
Hepatobiliary Manifestations of Diseases Involving Other Organ Systems
Ke-Qin Hu, MD, *Guest Editor*

THE CLINICS ARE NOW AVAILABLE ONLINE!
Access your subscription at:
www.theclinics.com

Preface

Hepatology Update: Current Management and New Therapies

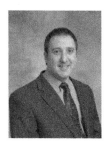

David A. Sass, MD, AGAF
Guest Editor

It is my distinct privilege to be the guest editor of the September 2011 issue of *Gastroenterology Clinics of North America* entitled, "Hepatology Update: Current Management and New Therapies." It has been seven years since an issue of *Gastroenterology Clinics* has been exclusively dedicated to the field of hepatology. The scope of practice of a busy gastroenterologist includes managing patients with complex liver diseases. This issue offers comprehensive reviews by many of the world's leading authorities on a potpourri of topics in hepatology and liver transplantation. As is evident from the titles of each of these articles, the focus of this issue is on "*management*" and the goal is to deliver an authoritative, up-to-date, and evidence-based text to the practicing gastroenterologist to allow them to be at the cutting edge of this rapidly advancing field.

In the first article, Dr Andrew Muir discusses the new advances in hepatitis C therapy with the introduction of the exciting direct-acting antiviral agents that were introduced this summer. We will now be able to offer our genotype 1 patients a cocktail of drugs that may allow for a greater chance at achieving the holy grail of an sustained virologic response. Dr Emmet Keeffe then follows with a discussion of the plethora of oral agents that are now available to combat hepatitis B infection. He delves into current treatment endpoints and offers an approach to the early detection and management of viral resistance. In recent years there has been a major research effort to discover new, noninvasive ways to determine hepatic fibrosis without resorting to the needle biopsy. Dr Jayant A. Talwalkar discusses the diagnostic performance of various serum biomarkers and innovative imaging modalities that have emerged and provides suggestions on how these may be incorporated into clinical practice. In his article on acute liver failure, Dr Obaid Shaikh summarizes a comprehensive management approach to this deadly disease and comments on advances in the field of bioartificial liver support devices to aid the failing liver and provide a bridge to transplantation. As clinicians, we are all acutely aware of the

Gastroenterol Clin N Am 40 (2011) xi–xii
doi:10.1016/j.gtc.2011.06.012
0889-8553/11/$ – see front matter © 2011 Elsevier Inc. All rights reserved.

growing epidemic of obesity and the metabolic syndrome in the United States. It is felt by many that NASH will soon surpass hepatitis C as the leading indication for liver transplantation. It is thus timely for Dr Jawad Ahmad to present pharmacologic and surgical treatment options for this highly prevalent disease.

The next three articles deal with specific complications of cirrhosis. An understanding on how to manage these is imperative in order to afford our patients the opportunity to survive to transplantation. Dr Garcia-Tsao provides a detailed evidence-based approach to the pharmacologic, endoscopic, radiologic, and surgical management of varices, while Dr Florence Wong addresses the ominous hepatorenal syndrome and the current application of vasoconstrictor agents to combat this disease. Hepatocellular carcinoma is a leading cause of morbidity and mortality worldwide and progressive disease poses a constant threat to patients being removed from the liver transplant waitlist. Dr Robert Gish's review explores the realm of locoregional therapies in treating HCC with an emphasis on novel developments in localized chemoembolization and systemic molecular-based targeted therapies. With the exceptionally high short-term mortality facing individuals with severe alcoholic hepatitis, an accurate assessment of disease severity is an important and practical issue for the gastroenterologist. Dr Vijay Shah describes the various prognostic scoring systems and discusses our rather limited treatment options. The final two articles specifically address liver transplantation. In today's climate of organ donor scarcity, Drs Sass and Reich explore the innovation in transplantation geared toward increasing the donor pool and the issues pertaining to matching of these grafts to suitable recipients. Finally, because of the improved long-term survival of liver transplant recipients, many of whom are being followed by community gastroenterologists, Dr Kenneth Rothstein and colleagues offer a detailed management approach to this patient cohort and, in so doing, provide important pearls of wisdom to the practicing clinician.

In summary, readers of this issue of *Gastroenterology Clinics* will not only find new concepts and strategies to apply to their patients with liver disease but also gain a glimpse into what the future holds with regard to emerging therapies. I am greatly indebted to each of the authors and their respective coauthors for their truly invaluable contributions and it is our collective intent to provide a practical, stimulating resource that will be of value in your daily practice. I would like to extend my sincere gratitude to Kerry Holland and her editorial staff at Elsevier for their assistance in compiling this issue. Finally, my love and heartfelt appreciation go to my wife and best friend, Allison, and children, Lauren and Aaron, for their unwavering support and in selflessly allowing me the time to devote many hours so that this project could reach fruition.

David A. Sass, MD, AGAF
Department of Medicine and Surgery
Division of Gastroenterology and Hepatology
Drexel University College of Medicine
245 North 15th Street, 12th Floor
New College Building, Suite 12324
Philadelphia, PA 19102, USA

E-mail address:
dsass@drexelmed.edu

Emerging Therapies in Hepatitis C: Dawn of the Era of the Direct-Acting Antivirals

Alison B. Jazwinski, MD[a], Andrew J. Muir, MD, MHS[b],*

KEYWORDS

- Chronic hepatitis C treatment • Direct-acting antiviral
- Telaprevir • Boceprevir • Mericitabine

Infection with hepatitis C virus (HCV) is a worldwide epidemic affecting up to 3% of the world's population.[1,2] Approximately 80% of people infected with HCV will go on to develop chronic disease. Of these individuals, approximately 25% develop cirrhosis and are vulnerable to its complications, including hepatocellular carcinoma.[3] Treatment for HCV can be curative, and successful treatment improves the quality of life of HCV infected individuals as well as prevents progression of liver disease and its associated morbidity and mortality.[4]

For the last decade, the standard of care treatment for HCV has been pegylated interferon-α (pegIFNα) plus ribavirin (RBV) for 24 to 48 weeks depending on viral genotype.[5] Therapy is expensive, difficult to tolerate, and associated with a variety of quality-of-life–limiting side effects. Furthermore, the response rates to treatment are not optimal; only about 40% of genotype 1–infected patients respond to treatment.[6] Patients infected with genotypes 2 and 3 have a higher rate of treatment response, which approximates 80%.[7]

A major goal within the fields of hepatology and infectious diseases is to improve the rate of response to HCV treatment. Novel discoveries over the past few years, such as the finding of a polymorphism near the *IL28B* gene, have helped identify those patients that are most likely to respond to HCV treatment with pegIFNα and RBV.[8] Additionally, new therapies have been developed, and some of the most promising new drugs are those that act to directly inhibit the virus. These direct-acting antiviral (DAA) drugs are currently in various stages of development, and are described in detail in this review.

[a] Division of Gastroenterology, Duke University Medical Center, 2400 Pratt Street, Terrace Level, Room 0311, Durham, NC 27710, USA
[b] Division of Gastroenterology and Hepatology Research, Duke Clinical Research Institute, Duke University Medical Center, 2400 Pratt Street, Terrace Level, Room 0311, Durham, NC 27710, USA
* Corresponding author.
E-mail address: muir0002@mc.duke.edu

Gastroenterol Clin N Am 40 (2011) 481–494
doi:10.1016/j.gtc.2011.06.005
0889-8553/11/$ – see front matter © 2011 Elsevier Inc. All rights reserved.

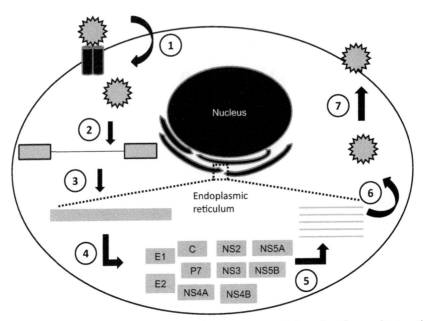

Fig. 1. Viral life cycle. (*1*) The HCV virus attaches to receptors at the cell surface and enters the cell via receptor-mediated endocytosis. (*2*) Positive-strand RNA is released into the cytoplasm and (*3*) translated into a single polypeptide on the ribosome. (*4*) Polypeptide cleaving occurs in the endoplasmic reticulum resulting in 10 viral proteins that form the structural components of the virus and participate in viral replication and other viral functions. (*5*) A replication complex forms on the membrane of the endoplasmic reticulum and RNA replication then occurs. A negative-strand RNA intermediate generates many copies of positive strand RNA. (*6*) Viral RNA is then packaged into a particle and (*7*) released from the hepatocyte.

VIRAL STRUCTURE AND LIFE CYCLE

A basic understanding of the viral structure and life cycle (**Fig. 1**) is important to understand the targets of the new drugs in development. The HCV is a positive single-strand RNA virus with 9.5 kilobases. The virus enters the hepatocyte via a variety of receptors (including glycosaminoglycans, CD81, SR-BI, Claudin-1) by receptor mediated endocytosis. Once in the hepatocyte, the virus is translated into a single long polypeptide on the ribosome then cleaved by both host and viral proteases into 10 functional proteins. A replication complex is formed using viral and host proteins and results in a double-stranded RNA intermediate that includes a positive-strand RNA and a negative-strand RNA. The negative strand serves as a template for the synthesis of positive-strand RNA, which is then packaged and released from the hepatocyte. The synthesis of positive-strand RNA is disproportionate to the negative strand and is transcribed in a 5- to 10-fold excess of negative-strand RNA.[9]

HCV is fairly unique in that there is not a DNA intermediate in the life cycle. Thus, the virus does not incorporate itself into the host DNA. The result is the ability to effectively cure the infection indefinitely. This is in contrast with the hepatitis B virus or HIV, where suppression is the major goal of therapy.[10]

The viral RNA produces 10 functional proteins. These proteins are composed of structural and nonstructural proteins.[9] The nonstructural proteins are involved in viral replication and processing and are the target of most DAAs. These are described in more detail herein.

VIRAL RESISTANCE

An important barrier in the development of antiviral agents is the emergence of virus resistance. There are several qualities of HCV that make it particularly prone to developing drug-resistant strains. The virus has a high rate of replication with 10^{12} virions produced daily.[11] The viral protein that mediates viral replication is NS5B, or RNA-dependent RNA-polymerase. This protein lacks proofreading ability and has a high error rate, thus leading to a variety of genetic strains of virus.[12] In general, viruses that are mutated versions of the wild type have less replication fitness than wild-type virus, and so are present in the blood at lower quantities.[13,14] Some of these mutated viruses result in a change to the viral protein structure; thus, if this occurs at the site where a DAA acts, it may not be effective in inhibiting the action of the protein. Often these drug-resistant strains of virus are present at low levels in the blood at baseline, but when subjected to selection pressure, such as the addition of a DAA, the wild-type virus decreases and the mutated virus increases and ultimately renders the DAA ineffective (**Fig. 2**).[15]

NS3/4A PROTEASE INHIBITORS

The NS3/4A protease acts to cleave the polyprotein into its various functional proteins.[9] First-generation agents that target this protease—boceprevir and telaprevir—are the furthest along in development. Several phase II and III study results are available and are summarized. The primary end point of HCV clinical trials is achievement of sustained virologic response (SVR), which is absence of HCV RNA in the blood 6 months after the completion of treatment.

Boceprevir

Early phase studies of boceprevir revealed that viral load reductions were greater, and the development of resistance lower, when boceprevir was given in combination with pegIFNα.[15] Subsequent early phase studies showed that the highest rates of viral load reductions were seen in patients who received boceprevir 800 mg 3 times daily in combination with both pegIFNα and RBV and served as the basis for the study designs of phase II and III studies.[16] Boceprevir trials have largely used a lead in phase of 4 weeks of pegIFNα and RBV followed by varying courses of triple therapy with boceprevir, pegIFNα, and RBV.

Boceprevir phase II studies
The goal of the Serine Protease Inhibitor Therapy (SPRINT)-1 trial was to determine the effectiveness of boceprevir in combination with pegIFNα and RBV in genotype 1 treatment-naïve patients, and to determine whether a lead in phase of pegIFNα/RBV for weeks before boceprevir therapy improved response rates. A second part of the study evaluated whether lower dose RBV is as effective as standard dose RBV.[17]

Table 1 details the treatment groups and results, including achievement of SVR and relapse. The highest rates of SVR with the lowest relapse rates were seen in the groups that received a total of 48 weeks of therapy (SVR 75% and 67% in lead in group and 48 week treatment group, respectively). The groups that received a total of 28 weeks of therapy had better rates of SVR than the control group (SVR 54% and 56% vs 38%), but had relatively high relapse rates (30% and 24%). The control group had no viral breakthrough, defined as a persistent 2-log_{10} or greater increase from

Virus population pre-treatment   Virus population after the addition of an antiviral drug

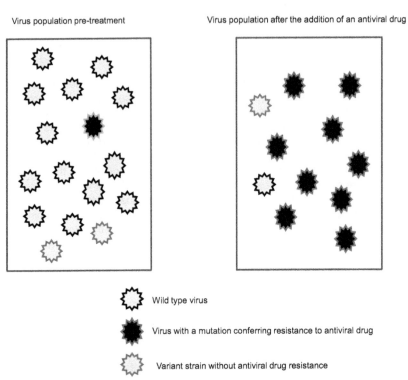

Wild type virus

Virus with a mutation conferring resistance to antiviral drug

Variant strain without antiviral drug resistance

Fig. 2. Viral resistance. In an HCV-infected individual, there are multiple variants of the virus present at baseline. The wild-type virus predominates and has high replicative fitness. Often, variants are present that confer resistance to the action of an antiviral drug; other variants are present that do not confer resistance to antiviral drugs. These variants generally have lower replicative fitness. When selection pressure is applied by adding an antiviral drug, wild-type viruses and viruses with mutations that do not affect antiviral drug action decrease in response to the drug. However, those viral particles that had resistance to the protease inhibitor now have improved replicative fitness and become the dominant strain.

nadir and 50,000 IU/mL or higher. The lead-in groups had less viral breakthrough than the groups with no lead in (4% vs 9%), although this did not reach significance ($P = .057$). Phase III studies were designed using a lead in strategy for all boceprevir groups to minimize viral breakthrough.

In the second part of the trial, a "low-dose" RBV group (400–1000 mg) was compared with a "standard dose" RBV group (800–1400 mg). The low-dose RBV group had lower SVR (36% vs 67%) and higher relapse (22% vs 7%) than the standard dose RBV group. Rates of viral breakthrough were high in both of these groups (27% in low dose and 25% in standard dose). The results of SPRINT-1 suggest that low-dose RBV is not an adequate treatment option.

Boceprevir phase III studies
Table 1 details the treatment groups studied in phase III trials and summarizes the results. The goal of SPRINT-2 was to evaluate the effectiveness of response-guided treatment (RGT) with boceprevir in genotype 1, treatment-naïve patients in 2 cohorts: Non-black patients and black patients.[18] In the RGT group, patients who achieved

Table 1
Boceprevir phase II and III trials

Study/Treatment Group	SVR (%)				Relapse (%)	
SPRINT-1						
B/P/R 28w	54				30	
B/P/R 48w	67				7	
P/R 4w, B/P/R 24w	56				24	
P/R 4w, B/P/R 44w	75				3	
P/R 48w	38				24	
B/P/R 48w – Standard dose R	67				7	
B/P/R 48w – Low dose R	36				22	
	Nonblack	Black			Nonblack	Black
SPRINT-2						
P/R 4w, RGT	67	42			23	14
P/R 4w, B/P/R 44w	68	53			8	17
P/R 48w	40	23			23	14
	Overall	Prior Relapse	Prior Partial Response	Overall		
RESPOND-2						
P/R 4w, RGT	59	69	40	32		
P/R 4w, B/P/R 44w	66	75	52	12		
P/R 48w	21	29	7	32		

Abbreviations: B, boceprevir; P, pegylated interferon-α; R, ribavirin; RGT, response-guided therapy.

undetectable HCV RNA by week 8 and remained negative for HCV RNA at week 24 completed 28 weeks of therapy. Those who did not achieve undetectable HCV RNA by week 8 received a total of 48 weeks of therapy. This group was compared with a group that received the full 48 weeks of therapy. All patients received a 4-week lead-in period with pegIFNα and RBV alone.

The RGT group had similar SVR rates as the group that received 44 weeks of boceprevir (67% vs 68% in the non-black cohort and 42% vs 53% in the black cohort). All boceprevir groups had significantly higher SVR rates than the standard therapy groups. Of the nonblack patients in the RGT group, 47% were eligible to receive a shortened course of therapy (28 weeks). The patients who received 28 weeks of therapy had an SVR rate of 97% and the patients who received 48 weeks of therapy had an SVR rate of 98%. Thus, SPRINT 2 provided the data to support 28 weeks of combination therapy in patients that achieve undetectable viral loads at weeks 8 through 24.

The goal of RESPOND-2 was to assess the response of boceprevir therapy in genotype 1 patients who had prior relapse (undetectable HCV RNA at the end of prior therapy without subsequent attainment of SVR) or partial response (decrease in HCV RNA level of $\geq 2 \log_{10}$ IU/mL by week 12 of prior therapy but detectable HCV RNA level throughout the course of therapy, without achievement of SVR) to standard treatment.[19] Patients with prior null response (lack of 2-$\log_{10}$ reduction in HCV RNA at week 12) were excluded from this study. Patient groups were similar to those in SPRINT-2 and included an RGT group in which patients who achieved a negative viral load at week 8 received only 36 weeks of therapy. The RGT group and the group that received 48 weeks of triple therapy had similar results and were both superior to the control group (SVR 59% and 66% vs 21%). Better response rates were seen in patients with prior relapse to treatment than prior partial response. In the RGT group, 46% of patients were eligible to receive a shorter course of therapy, and these patients had similar rates of SVR when they received a total of 36 weeks of treatment compared with those that received a total of 48 weeks of treatment. Thus, RESPOND-2 supports the use of a shorter course of treatment (36 weeks) for patients with prior relapse and partial response if they achieve a negative viral load at week 8 of treatment.

Adverse events with boceprevir

In general, boceprevir is well-tolerated. However, there is a higher rate of treatment discontinuation and dose reductions in patients that receive boceprevir in combination with pegIFNα and RBV than those that receive standard therapy alone (treatment discontinuation 8%–16% vs 3%–16% and dose reduction 29%–40% vs 14%–26%).[17–19] The most common side effects experienced by patients are typical pegIFNα and RBV related side effects such as flu-like symptoms, fatigue, and nausea. Effects that are more prevalent in those who receive boceprevir are anemia and dysgeusia. Anemia developed in 43% to 56% of patients who received boceprevir in combination with pegIFNα and RBV in phase II and III trials. In SPRINT-2, erythropoietin was administered in 24% of the controls and 43% of boceprevir recipients. Another side effect with boceprevir combination therapy is dysgeusia, which occurred in 37% to 43% of patients.

Telaprevir

Telaprevir monotherapy was also determined to have high rates of viral load reduction, but also resistance development in early phase studies; therefore, its development proceeded with concurrent pegIFNα and RBV. The treatment regimens with telaprevir differ from those described for boceprevir. Early phase studies supported using combination therapy for the first 12 weeks followed by pegIFNα and RBV for 12 to 36 additional weeks. This is opposed to boceprevir, where a lead-in with pegIFNα and RBV was followed by use of the combination therapy. The dose of telaprevir studied in phase II and III trials was 750 mg every 8 hours.

Phase II studies

Multiple phase II studies have been reported with telaprevir, including Protease inhibition for Viral Evaluation (PROVE)-1, -2, and -3. **Table 2** details the treatment groups and results for telaprevir phase II studies.

PROVE-1 studied the effectiveness of telaprevir in genotype 1, treatment-naïve patients.[20] All treatment groups in PROVE-1 received telaprevir in addition to pegIFNα/RBV for 12 weeks, but differed in subsequent duration of pegIFNα-2a/RBV (0, 12, or 36 weeks). The lowest rates of SVR were seen in the group that received only 12 weeks of combination therapy (35%). SVR for standard therapy in this study was 41%. The groups that received combination therapy followed by pegIFNα-2a/RBV for 12 and 36 weeks had the highest rates of SVR (61% and 67%, respectively). Among the telaprevir-containing groups, 7% had viral breakthrough (an increase of >1 $\log_{10}$ unit of HCV RNA compared with the lowest value during the treatment period or HCV RNA value of >100 IU/mL in a patient who had become undetectable). Thus, PROVE-1 showed that telaprevir in combination with pegIFNα/RBV is effective, but must be followed by an additional 12 to 36 weeks of pegIFNα/RBV therapy.

| Table 2 | | | | | | |
| Telaprevir phase II trials | | | | | | |
Study/Treatment Group	SVR (%)			Relapse (%)		
PROVE-1						
T/P/R 12w	35			33		
T/P/R 12w, PR 12w	61			2		
T/P/R 12w, PR 36w	67			6		
P/R 48w	41			23		
PROVE-2						
T/P 12w	36			48		
T/P/R 12w	60			30		
T/P/R 12w, P/R 12w	69			14		
P/R 48w	46			22		
	Overall	Prior Relapse	Prior Partial Response	Overall	Prior Relapse	Prior Partial Response
PROVE-3						
T/P/R 12w, P/R 12w	51	69	39	30	18	37
T/P/R 24w, P/R 24w	53	75	38	13	0	4
T/P 24w	24	42	11	53	46	68
P/R 48w	14	20	9	53	62	40

Abbreviations: P, pegylated interferon-α; R, ribavirin; T, telaprevir.

PROVE-2 evaluated the necessity of RBV in the treatment regimen.[21] Patients were genotype 1 and treatment naïve. The lowest rates of SVR were seen in patients with telaprevir and pegIFNα alone (36%). The SVR for standard therapy was 46%. Treatment groups that received triple therapy alone for 12 weeks, and triple therapy followed by pegIFNα-2a/RBV for 12 weeks had the highest rates of SVR (60% and 69%, respectively). Not only were SVR rates the lowest in the group that received telaprevir with pegIFNα alone, but relapse rates and viral breakthrough were the highest as well (relapse 48%, breakthrough 24%). This is in comparison with standard therapy, with a relapse rate of 22% and breakthrough rate of 1%. The group that received a total of 12 weeks of triple therapy alone had a relapse rate of 30% and breakthrough of 1% compared with the group that received 12 weeks of triple therapy followed by 12 additional weeks of pegIFNα and RBV (relapse 14%, breakthrough 5%). In summary, PROVE-2 demonstrated that RBV is important to achieve higher SVR rates and lower relapse and breakthrough rates, and triple therapy for 12 weeks alone had unacceptable relapse rates.

PROVE-3 studied the effectiveness of telaprevir in genotype 1 patients with prior treatment failure, including those with prior partial response and relapse.[22] The standard therapy group had the lowest rates of SVR in this study (14%). The patient group that did not receive RBV had low rates of SVR as well (24%). The group that received 24 weeks of triple therapy followed by 24 more weeks of pegIFNα and RBV had an SVR rate of 53%. The group that received triple therapy for 12 weeks followed by 12 additional weeks of pegIFNα and RBV had an SVR rate of 51%. Higher rates of response in the triple therapy groups were seen in those patients that had previously relapsed compared with those that had prior partial response (SVR of 69% and 75% vs 39% and 38%). Relapse rates were highest in the standard therapy and telaprevir

Table 3
Teleprevir phase III trials

Study/Treatment Group	SVR (%)				Relapse (%)
ADVANCE					
T/P/R 8w	69				9
T/P/R 12w	75				9
P/R 48w	44				28
ILLUMINATE					
eRVR T/P/R 12w, P/R 12w	92				6
eRVR T/P/R 12w, P/R 36w	88				3
T/P/R 12w, P/R 36w	64				
	Prior Relapse	Prior Partial Response	Prior Null Response	Prior Relapse	Prior Partial Response
REALIZE					
T/P/R 12w, P/R 36w	83	41	29	7	23
P/R 4w, T/P/R 12w, P/R 32w	88	41	33	7	25
P/R 48w	24	9	5	65	33

Abbreviations: eRVR, extended rapid virologic response (negative viral load at week 4 that persists through week 12); P, pegylated interferon-α; R, ribavirin; T, teleprevir.

with pegIFNα alone groups (53% each), followed by the group that received a total of 24 weeks of treatment (30%) and the group that received 48 weeks of treatment (13%). Viral breakthrough was highest in the group that received teleprevir and pegIFNα alone (32%), followed by the groups that received 24 weeks and 48 weeks of therapy (13% and 12%, respectively). The standard therapy group had a breakthrough rate of 3%.

Phase III studies
Table 3 outlines the treatment groups and results from teleprevir phase III trials. All studies were performed using a teleprevir dose of 750 mg every 8 hours. The ADVANCE study evaluated the effectiveness of a shorter course of teleprevir combination therapy.[23] This trial evaluated a type of response guided therapy using the extended rapid virologic response (eRVR, negative viral load at 4 and 12 weeks). Patients who achieved eRVR could shorten the duration of subsequent pegIFNα/RBV from 36 to 12 weeks. Those who did not achieve an eRVR received an additional 36 weeks of pegIFNα/RBV. SVR rates were similar in patients that received 8 and 12 weeks of teleprevir (69% and 75%), and both were significantly higher than the standard therapy group (44%). However, virologic failure occurred in 13% of the patients who received 8 weeks of teleprevir versus 8% in the patients that received 12 weeks of teleprevir, suggesting that a longer duration of teleprevir is important to minimize virologic failure.

ILLUMINATE was an open-label study with no placebo control arm that studied genotype 1, treatment-naïve patients and also evaluated whether patients that achieved an eRVR could complete a shorter course of therapy (24 vs 48 weeks).[24] All patients received 12 weeks of teleprevir in combination with pegIFNα/RBV for 12 weeks. At week 20, patients who achieved an eRVR were randomized to continue receiving PR for 24 or 48 weeks of total treatment. Patients who did not achieve an eRVR received 48 weeks of treatment. In this study, of those patients who achieved an eRVR, 92% of patients treated with a total of 24 weeks of treatment achieved an SVR compared with 88% of patients in the group that received 48 weeks. Additionally, more patients discontinued treatment in the group that was randomized to 48 weeks of treatment than those that received 24 weeks of treatment (12.5% vs 0.6%, respectively). Therefore, in patients who achieve an eRVR, treatment with 24 weeks of therapy is similar to treatment with 48 weeks and is associated with fewer treatment-limiting adverse events.

The REALIZE study investigated telaprevir therapy in genotype 1 patients with prior relapse, partial response, or null response.[25] One distinction from the boceprevir phase III study (RESPOND-2) is the inclusion of null responders (failure to achieve a 2-log reduction in viral load by week 12). SVR was higher for all telaprevir groups compared with standard therapy. Patients with prior relapse had the highest rates of SVR (83% in group that received 48 weeks of treatment and 88% in lead-in group vs 24% in standard therapy). Prior nonresponders had SVR rates of 41% in both telaprevir treatment groups versus 9% in the standard therapy group. One major finding of this study was that prior null responders, a notoriously hard patient group to treat, achieved SVR in 29% and 33% of patients, compared with 5% in the standard therapy arm. Thus, telaprevir therapy for 12 weeks followed by pegIFNα/RBV to complete a total of 48 weeks therapy is effective in patients with prior treatment nonresponse and relapse. The lead-in period did not seem to be significantly more effective.

Adverse events/side effects of telaprevir

Telaprevir is well-tolerated overall. However, discontinuation rates were higher in the telaprevir containing groups than standard therapy in phase II studies (9%–26% vs 4%–7%).[20–22] As with boceprevir, the major treatment-limiting side effects were those that are common to interferon-α–based therapy, such as fever, malaise, and fatigue. However, rash, pruritus, nausea, and diarrhea were more common in telaprevir-receiving groups. The rash that occurs with telaprevir therapy is maculopapular and led to treatment discontinuation more frequently in telaprevir groups (5%–7%) than standard therapy groups (0%–1%). This became apparent in PROVE-1 and rash management plans were subsequently implemented in later studies. The implementation of the rash management plans, which included the use of topical anti-allergic agents and topical or systemic antipruritic agents and discontinuation of telaprevir if progression occurred, led to decreased overall treatment discontinuation in phase III studies. Anemia is another significant adverse event with telaprevir therapy and the average hemoglobin decrease is 0.5 to 1 g/dL higher than that seen with standard therapy alone.

Protease Inhibitor Resistance

Protease inhibitors bind to the active site of the NS3/4A enzyme, mimicking the N-terminal side of the viral substrate. Most of the drug-resistance mutations occur around the protease active site. When the drugs do not fit well into the binding site and protrude from the substrate envelope, they interact with the virus, leading to mutations. Molecular changes then occur that weaken inhibitor binding but do not change the binding of viral substrate.[26] Therefore, the ability of the drug to inhibit the action of the enzyme is impaired, whereas the ability of the protease to cleave the viral proteins and continue its life cycle is preserved.

In early trials of telaprevir and boceprevir, viral resistance rapidly occurred with monotherapy. When telaprevir and boceprevir are used in combination with pegIFNα and RBV, the development of resistance is less frequent, although it still occurs and is reflected in the rates of viral breakthrough. Once telaprevir and boceprevir are stopped, the number of wild-type variants increase and resistant variant decrease, resistant variants are less fit in the absence of selection pressure.[27,28] By 3 to 7 months after telaprevir monotherapy, the majority of virus is wild type, although low levels of resistant variants are still present many months after cessation of therapy.[27,29,30] The cross-resistance profile of boceprevir and telaprevir largely overlap, which suggests that the one protease inhibitor cannot be used when resistant variants have developed to the other.

Clinical use of protease inhibitors

Telaprevir and boceprevir will soon be available for use in clinical practice. As described in detail, treatment with protease inhibitors is complex, and best managed by knowledgeable and experienced specialists. Telaprevir and boceprevir were studied using different treatment regimens. Boceprevir was given for 24 to 44 weeks, in combination with pegIFNα and RBV after a lead-in period of 4 weeks of pegIFNα and RBV. Telaprevir was given for 12 weeks in combination with pegIFNα and RBV, followed by 0, 12, or 36 weeks of pegIFNα and RBV alone. The US Food and Drug Administration has not yet described the appropriate dosing regimen of the protease inhibitors, but we summarize potential treatment regimens, based on the clinical trial designs and results.

Treatment-naïve patients who achieve an RVR with boceprevir, which in this case is determined at week 4 of boceprevir therapy, or week 8 of the full treatment course, can likely complete a total of 28 weeks of treatment. Those who do not achieve an RVR will likely require a full 48 weeks of therapy. Patients with prior nonresponse or relapse who achieve an RVR may be able to complete a shorter course of a total of 36 weeks of therapy, whereas those who do not achieve an RVR will likely require a full 48 weeks of treatment. Clinicians should carefully monitor for the development of anemia in boceprevir-treated patients as well. A side effect that is quite common is dysgeusia, and although this did not lead to treatment discontinuation in the majority of patients, patients should be counseled about this side effect.

Treatment-naïve patients who achieve an eRVR with telaprevir may complete a shorter course of pegIFNα and RBV, for a total of 24 weeks. Others require a total of 48 weeks of treatment. Patients with prior relapse, partial response, or null response likely require a full 48 weeks of treatment (12 weeks of triple therapy followed by 36 weeks of pegIFNα/RBV). Clinicians should monitor closely for the development of anemia, and may need to reduce the RBV dose or add erythropoietin. Additionally, because pruritus and rash are common developments with telaprevir, the treating physician should be familiar with the rash management plan. Dermatologists may also be required to diagnose the severity of the rash to guide plans to discontinue therapy.

The need for 3 times daily dosing may be difficult for patients to comply with. Further studies need to be performed to determine whether these therapies can be administered less frequently, and whether patient compliance becomes an issue in clinical practice.

Protease inhibitor effectiveness by IL28B genotype

Patient samples from ADVANCE, REALIZE, SPRINT-2, and RESPOND-2 have been analyzed for IL28B genotype. The number of patients evaluated ranged from 42% in the ADVANCE study to 80% in REALIZE. In general, the CC genotype was most favorable for treatment response, but protease inhibitors are more effective than standard therapy across all IL28B genotypes.[31–33] Based on this, it is unlikely that testing for IL28B genotype will provide much additional data in the decision to initiate treatment; however, *IL28B* genotype may have a role in determining those patients who can receive shorter courses of therapy.

NS5B RNA POLYMERASE INHIBITORS

The nonstructural protein NS5B, or RNA-dependent RNA polymerase, is a protein that mediates viral replication.[9] NS5B has emerged as another important target of therapy and NS5B inhibitors have been developed in 2 forms: Nucleoside inhibitors and non-nucleoside inhibitors. Polymerase inhibitors are considered to have a high genetic barrier to resistance; thus, the development of resistant variants and clinical viral breakthrough is much less common than what is seen with protease inhibitors. There have been polymerase inhibitors isolated in vitro, however.[34]

Nucleoside Inhibitors

Nucleoside analog inhibitors mimic the natural substrate of the polymerase and become incorporated into the growing RNA chain, terminating replication. The nucleoside inhibitor with the most data supporting its use is mericitabine (R7128). Early phase studies showed significant viral load reductions with mericitabine with no resistance development supporting its use in future studies.[35,36] As with the protease inhibitors, mericitabine was studied in combination with pegIFNα/RBV in phase II studies.

The JUMP-C trial evaluated the effectiveness of response-guided therapy with mericitabine at a dose of 1000 mg in combination with pegIFNα/RBV.[37] Patients who achieved an eRVR received a total of 24 weeks of mericitabine/pegIFNα/RBV and those who did not achieve an eRVR received an additional 24 weeks of pegIFNα/RBV. These groups were compared with a standard therapy arm of pegIFNα/RBV for 48 weeks. A week 36 interim analysis showed that in the mericitabine treatment groups, 60% of patients achieved an eRVR. At 12 weeks after treatment completion (SVR12) 76% of the patients in the 24-week arm had achieved an SVR and 24% relapsed. There was no difference in safety and tolerability of mericitabine compared with standard therapy.

OTHER VIRAL TARGETS OF DRUG DEVELOPMENT

A number of drugs that target other viral proteins are in development, but this review is focused on the therapies expected to impact clinical practice in the near future. Non-nucleoside polymerase inhibitors are in development, and these drugs bind to the polymerase enzyme itself to induce a conformational change and render it ineffective. The NS5A viral protein and cyclophilin host protein are also important components of the viral replication complex, and agents that target these proteins are also in development in early stages.[9]

ORAL COMBINATION THERAPY

Although telaprevir and boceprevir have provided huge steps forward in improving the response rates of treatment for HCV, there remains significantly high adverse events and treatment discontinuation. Also, patients who are not candidates for treatment with pegIFNα and RBV are still not candidates for treatment in this new wave of therapy. The ultimate goal for HCV is to create a shorter, more effective treatment regimen of oral medications with a better side effect profile than pegIFNα/RBV. Similar to the treatment paradigm for HIV, targeting multiple viral replication sites will help to reduce resistance and increase efficacy of treatment.

The INFORM-1 study evaluated the effectiveness of protease inhibitor danoprevir in combination with polymerase inhibitor R7128 (mericitabine) in treatment of both treatment-naïve patients and prior nonresponders with genotype 1 HCV.[38] Patients were treated for 2 weeks, and viral load reductions with combination therapy ranged from 3.9 to 5.3 $\log_{10}$ IU/mL. HCV RNA values were undetectable in 88% of treatment-naïve patients at 2 weeks. All patients were then treated with standard of care, because they had only received 2 weeks of therapy. Final SVR results are pending, but preliminary reports showed markedly improved rates of RVR, early virologic response, and end of treatment response (ETR). In fact, the patient group that received the highest doses of each DAA achieved 100% ETR.

The first report of a successful all-oral combination regimen was reported at the EASL meeting in April 2011. The patient population studied was genotype 1 prior treatment null-responders, the most difficult group to treat. The study evaluated the safety and efficacy of a NS5A replication complex inhibitor BMS-790052 and an NS3 protease inhibitor BMS-650032 alone and in combination with pegIFNα/RBV.[39] Of the 11 patients who received the BMS-790052 and BMS-650032 alone, 7 (64%) had undetectable HCV RNA at week 4, 5 remained undetectable at the end of treatment, and 4 achieved an SVR 12 weeks after treatment completion (SVR12). All patients that received the 2 oral medications in combination with pegIFNα/RBV achieved SVR12.

More research is required to evaluate the safety and efficacy of oral combination therapy, but early results are promising. However, it will be another several years before we can expect to use all-oral combination therapy.

SUMMARY

The HCV viral life cycle provides targets for drug development at virtually every step, and many new drugs aimed at these targets are currently being developed. Clinical practice takes a major step forward this year with the arrival of telaprevir and boceprevir, which will be added to the current standard of care of pegIFNα/RBV. Patients will need to be monitored closely and counseled extensively, and clinicians will need to learn the new response-guided therapy algorithms with these therapies. Although there remains work to be done in the field of HCV, these therapies will allow many more patients the opportunity to eradicate HCV infection.

REFERENCES

1. World Health Organization. Hepatitis C, WHO fact sheet no. 164, revised 2000. Available at: http://www.who.int/mediacentre/factsheets/fs164/en/. Accessed June 7, 2011.
2. Alter M. Epidemiology of hepatitis C virus infection. World J Gastroenterol 2007;13: 2436–41.
3. Seeff L. Natural history of chronic hepatitis C. Hepatology 2002;36(Suppl 1):S35–46.
4. Younossi Z, Singer M, McHutchison J, et al. Cost effectiveness of interferon alpha2b combined with ribavirin for the treatment of chronic hepatitis C. Hepatology 1999;30: 1318–24.
5. Ghany M, Strader D, Thomas D, et al. Diagnosis, management, and treatment of hepatitis C: an update. Hepatology 2009;49:1335–74.
6. McHutchison JG, Lawitz EJ, Shiffman ML, et al. Peginterferon alfa-2b or alfa-2a with ribavirin for treatment of hepatitis C infection. N Engl J Med 2009;361:580–93.
7. Zeuzem S, Hultcrantz R, Bourliere M, et al. Peginterferon alfa-2b plus ribavirin for treatment of chronic hepatitis C in previously untreated patients infected with HCV genotypes 2 or 3. J Hepatol 2004;40:993–9.
8. Ge D, Fellay J, Thompson AJ, et al. Genetic variation in IL28B predicts hepatitis C treatment-induced viral clearance. Nature 2009;461:399–401.

9. Pawlotsky J, Chevaliez S, McHutchison J. The hepatitis C virus life cycle as a target for new antiviral therapies. Gastroenterology 2007;132:1979–98.

10. Monto A, Schooley R, Lai J, et al. Lessons from HIV therapy applied to viral hepatitis therapy: summary of a workshop. Am J Gastroenterol 2010;105:989–1004.

11. Neumann A, Lam N, Dahari H, et al. Hepatitis C viral dynamics in vivo and the antiviral efficacy of interferon-alpha therapy. Science 1998;282:103–7.

12. Ogata N, Alter H, Miller R, et al. Nucleotide sequence and mutation rate of the H strain of hepatitis C virus. Proc Natl Acad Sci U S A 1991;88:3392–6.

13. Yi M, Tong X, Skelton A, et al. Mutations conferring resistance to SCH6, a novel hepatitis C virus NS3/4A protease inhibitor. Reduced RNA replication fitness and partial rescue by second-site mutations. J Biol Chem 2006;281:8205–15.

14. Keiffer T, Kwong A, Picchio G. Viral resistance to specifically targeted antiviral therapies for hepatitis C (STAT-Cs). J Antimicrob Chemother 2010;65:202–12.

15. Sarrazin C, Rouzier R, Wagner F, et al. SCH 503034, a novel hepatitis C virus protease inhibitor, plus pegylated interferon alpha-2b for genotype 1 nonresponders. Gastroenterology 2007;132:1270–8.

16. Schiff E, Poordad FF, Jacobson I, et al. Role of interferon response during REtreatment of null responders with boceprevir combination therapy: results of phase II trial. Gastroenterology 2008;134:A755.

17. Kwo P, Lawitz E, McCone J, et al. Efficacy of boceprevir, an NS3 protease inhibitor, in combination with peginterferon alfa-2b and ribavirin in treatment-naïve patients with genotype 1 hepatitis C infection (SPRINT 1): an open-label, randomized, multicentre phase 2 trial. Lancet 2010;376:705–16.

18. Poordad F, McCone J, Bacon B, et al. Boceprevir for untreated chronic HCV genotype 1 infection. N Engl J Med 2011;364:1195–206.

19. Bacon B, Gordon S, Lawitz E, et al. Boceprevir for previously treated chronic HCV genotype 1 infection. N Engl J Med 2011;364:1207–17.

20. McHutchison J, Everson, G, Gordon S, et al. Telaprevir with peginterferon and ribavirin for chronic HCV genotype 1 infection. N Engl J Med 2009;360:1827–38.

21. Hezode C, Forestier N, Dusheiko G, et al. Telaprevir and peginterferon with or without ribavirin for chronic HCV infection. N Engl J Med 2009;360:1839–50.

22. McHutchison J, Manns M, Muir A, et al. Telaprevir for previously treated chronic HCV infection. N Engl J Med 2010;362:1292–303.

23. Jacobson I, McHutchison J, Dusheiko G, et al. Telaprevir in combination with peginterferon and ribavirin in genotype 1 HCV treatment-naïve patients: final results of the phase 3 ADVANCE study. Hepatology 2010;52(Suppl):427A.

24. Sherman K, Flamm S, Adfal N, et al. Telaprevir in combination with peginterferon alfa 2a and ribavirin for 24 or 48 weeks in treatment-naïve genotype 1 HCV patients who achieved an extended rapid virologic response: final results of phase 3 ILLUMINATE study. Hepatology 2010;52(Suppl):401A.

25. Zeuzem S, Andreone P, Pol S, et al. REALIZE trial final results: telaprevir based regimen for genotype 1 hepatitis C virus infection in patients with prior null response, partial response, or relapse to peginterferon/ribavirin. J Hepatol 2011;54(Suppl 1):S3.

26. Romano K, Ali A, Royer W, et al. Drug Resistance against HCV NS3/4A inhibitors is defined by the balance of substrate recognition versus inhibitor binding. Proc Natl Acad Sci U S A 2010;107:20986–91.

27. Sarrazin C, Kieffer T, Bartels D, et al. Dynamic hepatitis C virus genotypic and phenotypic changes in patients treated with the protease inhibitor telaprevir. Gastroenterology 2007;132:1767–77.

28. Susser S, Welsch C, Wang Y, et al. Characterization of resistance to the protease inhibitor boceprevir in hepatitis C virus-infected patients. Hepatology 2009;50: 1709–18.

29. Forestier N, Susser S, Welker M, et al. Long term follow up of patients previously treated with telaprevir. Hepatology 2008;48(Suppl):1135A–6A.

30. Susser S, Forestier N, Welker N, et al. Detection of resistant variants in the hepatitis C virus NS3 protease gene by clonal sequencing at long-term follow up in patients treated with boceprevir. J Hepatol 2009;50:S7.

31. Poordad F, Bronowicki J, Gordon S, et al. IL28B polymorphism predicts virologic response in patients with hepatitis C genotype 1 treatment with boceprevir (BOC) combination therapy. J Hepatol 2011;54(Suppl 1):S6.

32. Jacobson I, Catlett I, Marcellin P, et al. Telaprevir substantially improved SVR rates across all IL28B genotypes in the ADVANCE trial. J Hepatol 2011;54(Suppl 1):S542.

33. Pol S, Aerssens J, Zeuzem S, et al. Similar SVR rates in IL28B CC, CT, or TT prior relapse, partial- or null-responder patients treated with telaprevir/peginterferon/riba- virin: retrospective analysis of the REALIZE study. J Hepatol 2011;54(Suppl 1):S6.

34. Ali S, Leveque V, Le Pogam S, et al. Selected replicon variants with low level in vitro resistance to hepatitis C virus NS5B polymerase inhibitor PSI-6130 lack cross- resistance with R1479. Antimicrob Agents Chemother 2008;52:4356–69.

35. Lalezari J, Rodriguez-Torres M, et al. Potent Antiviral activity of the HCV nucleoside polymerase inhibitor R7128 with peg-IFN and ribavirin: interim results of R7128 500 mg bid for 28 days. J Hepatol 2008;48(Suppl):S29.

36. Le Pogam S, Kosaka A, et al. No evidence of R7128 drug resistance after up to 4 weeks treatment of GT 1, 2, and 3 hepatitis C virus infected individuals. J Hepatol 2009;50(Suppl):S348.

37. Pockros P, Jensen D, Tsai N. First SVR data with the nucleoside analogue polymerase inhibitor mericitabine (RG7128) combined with peginterferon/ribavirin in treatment- naïve HCV G 1 and 4 patients: interim analysis from the JUMP-C trial. J Hepatol 2011;54(Suppl 1):S538.

38. Gane E, Rouzier R, Stedman C, et al. Antiviral activity, safety, and pharmacokinetics of danoprevir/ritonavir plus pegIFN alpha-2a/RBV in hepatitis C patients. J Hepatol 2011 Feb 24 [Epub ahead of print].

39. Lok A, Gardiner D, Lawitz E, et al. Quadruple therapy with BMS-790052, BMS- 650032 and peg-IFN/RBV for 2 weeks results in 100% SVR12 in HCV genotype 1 null responders. J Hepatol 2011;54(Suppl 1):S536.

Hepatitis B: Modern End Points of Treatment and the Specter of Viral Resistance

Maximilian Lee, MD, MPH[a], Emmet B. Keeffe, MD, MACP, FRCP[b],*

KEYWORDS

• Hepatitis B • Treatment • End points • Outcomes
• Antiviral therapy • Viral resistance

The ultimate goal of treating a chronic infectious disease is the eradication of the infectious agent to prevent organ damage or death. The natural history of untreated chronic hepatitis B may result in the development of cirrhosis, followed by hepatic decompensation and death.[1–5] Hepatocellular carcinoma (HCC) can also occur in patients with chronic hepatitis B virus (HBV) infection, with or without the presence of cirrhosis. Antiviral therapy with oral nucleos(t)ide analog (NUC) agents suppress viral replication but do not directly act on the covalently closed circular DNA that resides within infected hepatocytes; thus, current oral therapy rarely eradicates HBV infection.[2–5] Although these oral antiviral agents are well-tolerated with minimal side effects, prolonged viral suppression runs the risk of selecting for antiviral drug–resistant mutations and causing virologic breakthrough; decreased patient adherence with antiviral treatment may also be associated with breakthrough. Therefore, routine "cure" or eradication of HBV infection is unrealistic, at least with current therapy. Nevertheless, preventing the clinical outcomes, or end points, of this disease remains important and are likely achievable with available treatment.

The development of complications of chronic hepatitis B occur over the long natural history of HBV infection, but are not necessarily uniform as demonstrated by the occurrence of HCC in patients without cirrhosis.[2–5] Furthermore, cirrhosis may take from years to decades to develop, and patients with chronic HBV infection are often asymptomatic before these clinical end points of cirrhosis or HCC are discovered. Judging the efficacy of antiviral therapy by waiting to see if these clinical end points are avoided is neither practical nor ethical. To satisfy the need to assess

[a] Division of Gastroenterology and Hepatology, Stanford University Medical Center, 300 Pasteur Drive, Alway Building M211, Palo Alto, CA 94305-5187, USA
[b] Division of Gastroenterology and Hepatology, Stanford University Medical Center, 750 Welch Road, Suite 210, Palo Alto, CA 94304-1509, USA
* Corresponding author.
E-mail address: ekeeffe@stanford.edu

Gastroenterol Clin N Am 40 (2011) 495–505
doi:10.1016/j.gtc.2011.06.004
0889-8553/11/$ – see front matter © 2011 Elsevier Inc. All rights reserved.

Table 1
End points of therapy for chronic hepatitis B

End Point	Criteria
Histologic	Reduction of fibrosis stage (≥2-point decrease in HAI) and no worsening of fibrosis Reduction of inflammatory activity
Biochemical	Normalization of ALT levels
Virologic	Sustained decrease in serum HBV DNA to low levels, ideally to undetectable
Serologic	HBeAg loss, with seroconversion to anti-HBe HBsAg loss, with or without seroconversion to anti-HBs

Abbreviation: anti-HBs, antibody to HBsAg.

the impact of antiviral therapy, reliable intermediate or surrogate end points have been used as therapeutic goals with the treatment of chronic hepatitis B. According to the National Institutes of Health, surrogate end points are "biomarkers intended to substitute for a clinical endpoint."[6] These surrogate end points should occur on the causal pathway of disease, be highly associated with the long-term clinical end point of interest, and be easier to assess than the ultimate outcome. Furthermore, the effect of an intervention upon the surrogate end point should also have a downstream effect on the prevention of the clinical end point.

The National Institutes of Health–proposed surrogate end points for chronic HBV infection include histologic criteria [decrease in histology activity index (HAI) by ≥2 points with no worsening of fibrosis], biochemical changes [normalization of alanine aminotransferase (ALT)] levels, virologic response (maintained suppression of serum HBV DNA to undetectable levels by a sensitive assay), and serologic changes [loss of hepatitis B e antigen (HBeAg), with or without seroconversion to antibody to HBeAg (anti-HBe), and potentially loss of hepatitis B surface antigen (HBsAg); **Table 1**].[1] Although these surrogate end points are used to assess the efficacy of antiviral therapy, particularly during phase III clinical trials of HBV treatment and by regulatory authorities for licensing new treatments, they do not evaluate the various aspects of disease status associated with chronic hepatitis B. Therefore, such end points may not be sufficient in individual patients for determination of the overall course of treatment such that combination of end points may be necessary.[2–5] Given their intermediate status along the causal pathway of disease, these surrogate end points may still require further clarification of their pathogenic role and impact on ultimate outcomes, although much information has been learned from cohort studies involving both treated and untreated patients.[7,8] In addition, these surrogate end points could be subject to confounding owing to undefined interactions between each other. Last, cost-effectiveness analyses of these various end points are currently unavailable.

HISTOLOGIC END POINT: THE ROLE OF LIVER BIOPSY

Traditionally, liver biopsy has been considered the most direct and accurate method of assessing liver inflammation and fibrosis, and liver histology has been used as the main end point of clinical trials evaluating the efficacy of antiviral therapies. Traditionally, regulatory approval required comparison of pretreatment and end-of-treatment liver biopsies showing histologic improvement, as defined by a 2-point or greater decrease in the HAI and no worsening of fibrosis. With respect to NUC therapies that have been approved (including lamivudine, adefovir, telbivudine, entecavir, and tenofovir), the end-of-treatment achievement of histologic improvement has ranged between 49% and 74% for HBeAg-positive patients and 61% and 72% for HBeAg-negative patients after 1 year of antiviral therapy.[9-16] Monotherapy with peginterferon, or combination therapy with peginterferon plus lamivudine, have shown much lower rates of histologic improvement for HBeAg-positive patients, namely, 22% and 33%, respectively.[17,18] Longer follow-up (>3–5 years of treatment) and determination of whether histologic improvement has been sustained is not required for pivotal clinical trials, but a few small studies have shown persistent histologic improvement as well as regression of fibrosis and even early cirrhosis.[19-21]

Although liver biopsies have provided much important information on the course of liver disease, there remain several limitations, such as sampling variability and error. When biopsies are obtained by percutaneous or transjugular access, the operator is unable to identify or target specific areas of the liver, and sampling is based on the assumption that liver disease uniformly affects the whole liver. In addition, liver biopsies that yield tissue samples less than 2.5 cm in size have been shown to underestimate hepatic fibrosis.[22] Once samples are obtained, interobserver and intra-observer variability with regard to assessment of histologic activity and fibrosis may also occur. The development of various scoring systems, including the HAI (also known as the Knodell score) are intended to standardize evaluation of liver biopsies, but interobserver and intra-observer variability can still be quite variable and affect assessment.[23] Last, inherent in this invasive procedure is the small risk of serious complications, including pneumothorax, hemoperitoneum, and death, which may outweigh the benefit of an individual biopsy or serial repeat biopsies.

Thus, although liver biopsies have provided useful and accurate assessment on the disease activity of chronic HBV infection, they are not currently considered a practical end point outside of clinical trials for antiviral therapies. On the other hand, liver biopsies could still be used to provide not only a histologic end point, but also potentially novel virologic end points, such as direct quantification of intrahepatic HBV DNA or covalently closed circular DNA using polymerase chain reaction.[24]

BIOCHEMICAL END POINT: SERUM ALANINE AMINOTRANSFERASE LEVELS

Serum ALT and aspartate aminotransferase are biochemical markers used to indirectly measure the activity of underlying liver disease. During chronic HBV infection, elevated aminotransferase levels reflect ongoing T-cell–directed cytotoxic activity against HBV-infected hepatocytes, and are associated with an increased risk of liver complications and death.[25] Changes in both serum aminotransferase and HBV DNA levels over time can also help to differentiate between the various stages of chronic HBV infection. According to standard guidelines, the presence of an elevated ALT, in association with an elevated HBV DNA level (depending on HBeAg status), is the major indication for antiviral therapy.[3-6] With NUC antiviral treatment, ALT levels can decrease and eventually normalize over time, whereas the sudden increase in ALT while undergoing therapy or after discontinuing treatment may herald viral reactivation with biochemical and possibly clinical relapse. Hence, normalization of ALT has been included as the biochemical end point in clinical trials of HBV treatment.

Because these hepatic biomarkers are inexpensive and easy to obtain, they would seem to be a satisfactory alternative end point to the invasive histologic assessment of liver disease. In combination with other biomarkers, in the form of the aspartate aminotransferase-to-platelet ratio index,[26] these biomarkers can also be used to assess underlying hepatic fibrosis, although this noninvasive approach has only been validated in patients with chronic hepatitis C. Additionally, the "normal" ranges of ALT and aspartate aminotransferase may not only vary with use of different laboratory assays, but also even in the biopsy-proven absence of underlying liver disease.[27,28] Conversely, up to 23% of patients with chronic hepatitis B and serum aminotransferase levels within the so-called normal range may have serious liver disease, including significant hepatic fibrosis and cirrhosis, with or without hepatic decompensation.[29,30] Such major discrepancies between serum aminotransferase levels and underlying liver biopsy findings calls into question whether this biomarker end point should still be utilized.

Although the measurement of serum ALT levels may be a useful component in helping to elucidate underlying disease activity in chronic hepatitis B, this biomarker cannot stand alone, especially without being accompanied by HBV DNA levels. There is some potential for combining this biomarker with others to provide a noninvasive assessment of underlying necroinflammation, but this approach has been primarily validated in patients with chronic hepatitis C. Additionally, there are already accurate models that reliably predict advanced liver disease, such as the Child–Turcotte–Pugh and Model for End-Stage Liver Disease scores. Last, the lack of sensitivity and specificity for chronic hepatitis B limits the utility of ALT levels as both indicators for antiviral treatment and their normalization as a sole end point.

VIROLOGIC END POINT: SERUM HBV DNA LEVELS

During the natural history of chronic HBV infection, serum HBV DNA levels reflects underlying intrahepatic HBV replication and can be quite dynamic, with very high levels ($>2 \times 10^{6-7}$ IU/mL or $>10^{7-8}$ copies/mL) during the immune tolerant phase, lower levels with chronic HBeAg-negative disease ($<10^5$ IU/mL), and even lower levels during the residual inactive carrier phase (generally <2000 IU/mL.[2–5] Although HBV DNA levels vary greatly, during the immune clearance phase or a reactivation flare that follows the immune tolerance phase, the host immune response against the virus will lead to T-cell–directed liver injury. However, despite the absence of obvious liver injury, large (>3600 patients) prospective cohort studies by the community-based Taiwanese Risk Evaluation of Viral Load Elevation and Associated Liver Disease/Cancer–Hepatitis B Virus Study Group have shown that very high HBV DNA levels ($>10^6$ copies/mL) are significantly associated with the development of cirrhosis and HCC, independent of HBeAg status or serum ALT levels.[31,32] Furthermore, there does not seem to be a risk-free threshold, as even low viral loads ($<10^3$ copies/mL) have been found to be associated with cirrhosis or HCC.[33,34] Therefore, suppression of HBV replication to an undetectable serum level by a sensitive polymerase chain reaction assay has been used as an end point in clinical trials of HBV treatment, and high levels in association with elevated ALT are an indication for treatment.[2–5]

On-therapy virologic response has been demonstrated with both peginterferon and NUC agents. Depending on the NUC, loss of serum HBV DNA ranges between 21% and 76% for HBeAg-positive patients, and a higher range of 51% to 93% in HBeAg-negative patients.[9–14] These rates were achieved (in increasing order) by adefovir, lamivudine, telbivudine, entecavir, and tenofovir. Treatment with standard interferon and peginterferon (with or without lamivudine) achieved viral suppression rates of 25% to 69% and 60% to 87% for HBeAg-positive and HBeAg-negative patients, respectively.[17,18] The clinical benefits of antiviral treatment in reducing the risks of cirrhosis and HCC have been clearly demonstrated,[35] including the potential regression of fibrosis and early cirrhosis.[19–21] However, off-treatment viral response may not be sustainable without long-term treatment, particularly in patients with HBeAg-negative disease, whereas long-term treatment may also induce the development of viral resistance. In patients whose antiviral treatment was discontinued

Table 2
Rates of resistance of nucleus(t)ide analogs in treatment-naïve patients with chronic hepatitis B

Treatment Duration (y)	Lamivudine (%)	Adefovir (%)[a]	Telbivudine (%)		Entecavir (%)	Tenofovir (%)
			HBeAg-Negative Patients	HBeAg-Positive Patients		
1	24	0	2	5	0.2	0
2	38	3	11	25	0.5	0
3	49	11	—	—	1.2	0
4	67	18	—	—	1.2	0
5	70	29	—	—	1.2	—
6	—	—	—	—	1.2	—

Data extracted from references.[3–6,42,43]
  [a] HBeAg-negative patients only.

after 1 year of treatment, the viral relapse rate was very rapid (within 6–12 months after discontinuing treatment), with recurrent detectable viral loads in 95% of HBeAg-positive patients and 92% to 97% of HBeAg-negative patients.[36–38] On the other hand, a longer duration of antiviral therapy (5 years) has increased virologic response rates by about 27% in patients receiving entecavir for HBeAg-positive disease.[39] Hence, the high relapse rates after short-term therapy has encouraged extending the duration of therapy to more than 1 year, at least until achieving both undetectable HBV DNA and HBeAg seroconversion in HBeAg-positive chronic hepatitis B (with a consolidation therapy for 6 months after the appearance of anti-HBe), and long-term in patients with HBeAg-negative chronic hepatitis B, until achievement of HBsAg clearance.[3]

Given the long-term therapy necessary to achieve seroconversion of HBeAg or the clearance of HBsAg, the risk of antiviral resistance becomes a serious concern and has shifted clinical practice toward the use of NUCs with a high genetic barrier to resistance. The first NUC, lamivudine, was used widely around the world and demonstrated the development of resistance in just 1 year of therapy at a rate of 24%, which increased to 70% after 5 years of therapy.[9,35,40] Subsequently developed NUC agents showed lower rates of long-term antiviral resistance; adefovir demonstrated a risk of drug resistance of 29% after 5 years of therapy,[19] telbivudine a 25% rate after 2 years of therapy,[41] entecavir a 1.2% rate after 6 years of therapy,[42] and tenofovir so far no resistance after 4 years of therapy[43] (**Table 2**). Therefore, tenofovir or entecavir should be considered first-line oral agents for antiviral treatment of chronic hepatitis B, especially in patients who are naïve to HBV treatment and in those who prolonged or indefinite therapy is anticipated.

Virologic breakthrough on treatment, however, may not necessarily be due to the development antiviral resistance. Patients on chronic antiviral therapy, similar to those on chronic treatment for hypertension and hyperlipidemia, may not be adherent, which has been estimated to occur in 12.2% of patients with chronic hepatitis B treated with oral agents.[44] It is unclear whether medication nonadherence contributes to the different mechanisms involved in drug resistance under the selective pressure of antiviral therapy,[45] but 1 study suggested that given no change in the background resistance rate of patients receiving adefovir, nonadherence may be a more important contributor to virologic breakthrough rather than drug resistance.[46] For these reasons, mutation testing should be performed to assist in the determination if virologic break-through is due to nonadherence versus antiviral drug resistance.[47]

Achieving sustained suppression of serum HBV DNA to undetectable levels is an important end point for antiviral treatment. Newer NUCs, such as entecavir and tenofovir, have shown both greatly improved viral suppression rates and a high genetic barrier to resistance during long-term treatment, compared with older NUCs like lamivudine. However, a sustained virologic response is not often achieved by patients off-treatment, and reactivation is almost universal for HBeAg-negative patients, occasionally with serious consequences including hepatic decompensation. Therefore, to achieve sustained virologic response, viral suppression needs to be accompanied either HBeAg seroconversion in HBeAg-positive patients or the loss of HBsAg, which are reasonable end points.

SEROLOGIC END POINTS: SEROCONVERSION OF HBeAg AND LOSS OF HBsAg
Seroconversion of HBeAg

During the natural history of chronic HBV infection, patients in the immune tolerant phase may enter the immune clearance phase, because HBV provokes a host immune response that is characterized by either continuous inflammation or acute intermittent flares, with serum ALT levels rising to over 5 times the upper limit of normal. This activity may be accompanied by increased fibrosis and the possible development of cirrhosis or hepatic decompensation. However, in some individuals, HBeAg is spontaneously lost, followed by seroconversion to anti-HBe, normalization of serum ALT levels, resolution of necroinflammation, and decrease in HBV DNA to low levels (usually <2000 IU/mL). This spontaneous clearance of HBeAg ranges between 2% and 15% per year, and may be affected by age, ALT level, and HBV genotype.[48] If HBeAg seroconversion is sustained, the long-term prognosis of these patients is very good, with decreased risk of cirrhosis, HCC, and death, compared with those who do not sustain seroconversion, who serorevert to positive HBeAg, or develop chronic HBeAg-negative disease.[49] Furthermore, HBsAg loss and seroconversion may also occur several years after HBeAg seroconversion, with 1 large series of 1965 patients showing an annual HBsAg seroclearance of 1.2% and high cumulative seroclearance with long-term follow-up of 8% at 10 years, 25% at 20 years, and 45% at 25 years.[50] Improved prognosis with HBeAg seroconversion has made this an important end point in HBV clinical trials, and antiviral therapy with either interferon or a NUC has been shown to increase HBeAg seroconversion rates. Current cross-trial data have shown that after 1 year of treatment with peginterferon, HBeAg seroconversion was higher than with NUC therapy, that is, 25% to 27% versus 21% to 23%, except for adefovir with a much lower rate of 12%.[51] Sustained durability of HBeAg seroconversion at 6 and 12 months after the end of treatment with peginterferon also seems higher at 32% to 33% and 48%, respectively, whereas long-term continuous treatment with older NUC agents, specifically, lamivudine, has been generally required to approach these rates of seroconversion, with the concomitant risk of developing antiviral resistance. Newer NUCs have a high genetic barrier to resistance, which may mitigate this concern, and experience has also shown that they may be able to achieve much higher sustained serologic responses off-treatment; telbivudine- and entecavir-treated patients showed sustained serologic responses of 80% and 70%, respectively, 6 months after discontinuation of treatment.[41,52]

Unfortunately, although HBeAg seroconversion is an important end point, relapse of disease in the form of HBeAg seroreversion or the development of active HBeAg-negative disease, owing to the selection of precore or basal core promoter mutations, is still possible for certain patients, at a rate of 2.2% to 3.3% annually, and higher in those who had late seroconversion after age 40, are males, or have HBV genotype C.[53] The long-term cumulative incidence of chronic HBeAg-negative disease was as high as 24% at the end of 4 years.[54] Nevertheless, in patients with HBeAg-positive disease, HBeAg seroconversion is currently considered an adequate end point for discontinuing therapy, and current guidelines for treatment of HBeAg-positive patients have recommended a 6- to 12-month period of consolidation therapy after achieving seroconversion.[2–5]

Loss of HBsAg

Chronic HBV infection is characterized by the presence of HBsAg, and its spontaneous clearance after HBeAg seroconversion indicates resolution of disease. Patients who have lost HBsAg are at much reduced risk of developing cirrhosis and/or HCC, as compared with those who remained positive for HBsAg.[55] Because the loss of HBsAg correlates well with preventing these outcomes, it is a valid surrogate end point for HBV treatment. In clinical trials, 1 year of antiviral therapy with either peginterferon with or without lamivudine, or NUC monotherapy, can increase the rate of HBsAg loss from the natural spontaneous rate of 1.2% per year to 3% to 7.8% and 0% to 3.2%, respectively, for HBeAg-positive patients.[3] By comparison, in HBeAg-negative disease, the rate of HBsAg loss with either peginterferon or NUC treatment is not significantly higher than the spontaneous clearance rate (≤1% with 1-year treatment).

Because HBsAg loss happens so infrequently in either HBeAg-positive or HBeAg-negative disease, it is an impractical end point. However, given newer and more refined assays, the quantitative measurement of HBsAg levels may soon become more widely available, and change in titers on antiviral treatment may be used to help to predict a virologic response.[56] Levels of HBsAg vary according to phase of HBV infection and are also closely correlated with viral load, with increased HBsAg titers associated with both increased disease activity and viral replication, respectively.[57–59] Longitudinal study of HBsAg titers has shown that loss in HBeAg-negative patients is much slower compared with HBeAg-positive patients, and also that decreases in HBsAg titers by more than 1 log IU/mL by the end of an 8-year follow-up portended HBsAg loss, regardless of HBeAg status.[57] Furthermore, among patients who were treated with a 1-year course of peginterferon, with or without lamivudine, the same level of decrease in HBsAg titers at either 24 weeks of treatment in HBeAg-positive patients[60,61] or 48 weeks of treatment in HBeAg-negative patients[62] had a very high predictive value for the achievement of a sustained serologic response with HBsAg loss at 1 to 3 and 5 years after treatment, respectively. Therefore, quantitative HBsAg levels might be used to identify HBV patients who could respond well to peginterferon treatment; similar studies will need to be done to determine if there is predictive value with use of HBsAg titers in patients treated with NUC analogs.

SUMMARY

The goal of antiviral treatment of chronic hepatitis B is to prevent the complications of cirrhosis, hepatic decompensation, HCC, and death. Because these clinical outcomes may take a long period of time to develop, it is important to use intermediate or surrogate end points to evaluate the efficacy and response to antiviral treatment, and to determine whether treatment can be safely stopped, especially given concern for the development of antiviral resistance with NUC therapy. Although normalization of ALT and suppression of HBV DNA viral replication are associated with favorable outcomes, the durability of their response is low, and these end points are insufficient markers for stopping treatment. HBeAg seroconversion is currently used to discontinue NUC treatment in patients with HBeAg-positive chronic hepatitis B, whereas the stopping rule for HBeAg-negative disease relies on HBsAg loss. However, HBsAg loss occurs very infrequently and is not a practical end point for clinical use, although quantitative HBsAg levels may be useful in identifying patients who could achieve a sustained virologic response to treatment.

REFERENCES

1. Sorrell MF, Belongia EA, Costa J, et al. National Institutes of Health consensus development statement: management of hepatitis B. Ann Intern Med 2009;150: 104–10.
2. Lok AS, McMahon BJ. Chronic hepatitis B: update 2009. Hepatology 2009;50: 661–2.
3. European Association for the Study of the Liver. EASL Clinical Practice Guidelines: management of chronic hepatitis B. J Hepatol 2009;50:227–42.
4. Keeffe EB, Dieterich DT, Han SH, et al. A treatment algorithm for the management of chronic hepatitis B virus infection in the United States: 2008 update. Clin Gastroenterol Hepatol 2008;6:1315–41.
5. Liaw YF, Leung N, Kao JH, et al. Asian-Pacific consensus statement on the management of chronic hepatitis B: a 2008 update. Hepatol Int 2008;2:263–83.
6. Cohn JN. Introduction to surrogate markers. Circulation 2004;109(25 Suppl 1): IV20–1.
7. Liaw YF. Impact of hepatitis B therapy on the long-term outcome of liver disease. Liver Int 2011;31(Suppl 1):117–21.
8. Liaw YF. Natural history of chronic hepatitis B virus infection and long-term outcome under treatment. Liver Int 2009;29(Suppl 1):100–7.
9. Lai CL, Chien RN, Leung NW, et al. A one-year trial of lamivudine for chronic hepatitis B. Asia Hepatitis Lamivudine Study Group. N Engl J Med 1998;339:61–8.
10. Dienstag JL, Schiff ER, Wright TL, et al. Lamivudine as initial treatment for chronic hepatitis B in the United States. N Engl J Med 1999;341:1256–63.
11. Marcellin P, Chang TT, Lim SG, et al. Adefovir dipivoxil for the treatment of hepatitis B e antigen-positive chronic hepatitis B. N Engl J Med 2003;348:808–16.
12. Hadziyannis SJ, Tassopoulos NC, Heathcote EJ, et al. Adefovir dipivoxil for the treatment of hepatitis B e antigen-negative chronic hepatitis B. N Engl J Med 2003;348:800–7.
13. Chang TT, Gish RG, de Man R, et al. A comparison of entecavir and lamivudine for HBeAg-positive chronic hepatitis B. N Engl J Med 2006;354:1001–10.
14. Lai CL, Shouval D, Lok AS, et al. Entecavir versus lamivudine for patients with HBeAg-negative chronic hepatitis B. N Engl J Med 2006;354:1011–20.
15. Lai CL, Gane E, Liaw YF, et al. Telbivudine versus lamivudine in patients with chronic hepatitis B. N Engl J Med 2007;357:2576–88.
16. Marcellin P, Heathcote EJ, Buti M, et al. Tenofovir disoproxil fumarate versus adefovir dipivoxil for chronic hepatitis B. N Engl J Med 2008;359:2442–55.
17. Lau GK, Piratvisuth T, Luo KX, et al. Peginterferon alfa-2a, lamivudine, and the combination for HBeAg-positive chronic hepatitis B. N Engl J Med 2005;352: 2682–95.
18. Marcellin P, Lau GK, Bonino F, et al. Peginterferon alfa-2a alone, lamivudine alone, and the two in combination in patients with HBeAg-negative chronic hepatitis B. N Engl J Med 2004;351:1206–17.

19. Hadziyannis SJ, Tassopoulos NC, Heathcote EJ, et al. Long-term therapy with adefovir dipivoxil for HBeAg-negative chronic hepatitis B for up to 5 years. Gastroenterology 2006;131:1743–51.
20. Dienstag JL, Goldin RD, Heathcote EJ, et al. Histological outcome during long-term lamivudine therapy. Gastroenterology 2003;124:105–17.
21. Chang TT, Liaw YF, Wu SS, et al. Long-term entecavir therapy results in the reversal of fibrosis/cirrhosis and continued histological improvement in patients with chronic hepatitis B. Hepatology 2010;52:886–93.
22. Bedossa P, Dargere D, Paradis V. Sampling variability of liver fibrosis in chronic hepatitis C. Hepatology 2003;38:1449–57.
23. Intraobserver and interobserver variations in liver biopsy interpretation in patients with chronic hepatitis C. The French METAVIR Cooperative Study Group. Hepatology 1994;20:15–20.
24. Zoulim F. New insight on hepatitis B virus persistence from the study of intrahepatic viral cccDNA. J Hepatol 2005;42:302–8.
25. Yuen MF, Yuan HJ, Wong DK, et al. Prognostic determinants for chronic hepatitis B in Asians: therapeutic implications. Gut 2005;54:1610–4.
26. Wai CT, Greenson JK, Fontana RJ, et al. A simple noninvasive index can predict both significant fibrosis and cirrhosis in patients with chronic hepatitis C. Hepatology 2003;38:518–26.
27. Prati D, Taioli E, Zanella A, et al. Updated definitions of healthy ranges for serum alanine aminotransferase levels. Ann Intern Med 2002;137:1–10.
28. Lee JK, Shim JH, Lee HC, et al. Estimation of the healthy upper limits for serum alanine aminotransferase in Asian populations with normal liver histology. Hepatology 2010; 51:1577–83.
29. Lim J, Ayoub W, Chao D, et al. Systematic review and meta-analysis: prevalence of significant histologic disease in chronic hepatitis B infection, high HBV DNA and persistently normal ALT (PNALT) [abstract]. J Hepatol 2011;54(Suppl 1):S151.
30. Liaw YF, Sung JJ, Chow WC, et al. Lamivudine for patients with chronic hepatitis B and advanced liver disease. N Engl J Med 2004;351:1521–31.
31. Iloeje UH, Yang HI, Su J, et al. Predicting cirrhosis risk based on the level of circulating hepatitis B viral load. Gastroenterology 2006;130:678–86.
32. Chen CJ, Yang HI, Su J, et al. Risk of hepatocellular carcinoma across a biological gradient of serum hepatitis B virus DNA level. JAMA 2006;295:65–73.
33. Yuan HJ, Yuen MF, Ka-Ho Wong D, et al. The relationship between HBV-DNA levels and cirrhosis-related complications in Chinese with chronic hepatitis B. J Viral Hepat 2005;12:373–9.
34. Fung J, Yuen MF, Yuen JC, et al. Low serum HBV DNA levels and development of hepatocellular carcinoma in patients with chronic hepatitis B: a case-control study. Aliment Pharmacol Ther 2007;26:377–82.
35. Yuen MF, Seto WK, Chow DH, et al. Long-term lamivudine therapy reduces the risk of long-term complications of chronic hepatitis B infection even in patients without advanced disease. Antivir Ther 2007;12:1295–303.
36. Liaw YF, Leung NW, Chang TT, et al. Effects of extended lamivudine therapy in Asian patients with chronic hepatitis B. Asia Hepatitis Lamivudine Study Group. Gastroenterology 2000;119:172–80.
37. Hadziyannis SJ, Tassopoulos NC, Heathcote EJ, et al. Long-term therapy with adefovir dipivoxil for HBeAg-negative chronic hepatitis B. N Engl J Med 2005;352: 2673–81.

38. Shouval D, Lai CL, Chang TT, et al. Relapse of hepatitis B in HBeAg-negative chronic hepatitis B patients who discontinued successful entecavir treatment: the case for continuous antiviral therapy. J Hepatol 2009;50:289–95.
39. Chang TT, Lai CL, Kew Yoon S, et al. Entecavir treatment for up to 5 years in patients with hepatitis B e antigen-positive chronic hepatitis B. Hepatology 2010;51:422–30.
40. Yuen MF, Fung J, Wong DK, et al. Prevention and management of drug resistance for antihepatitis B treatment. Lancet Infect Dis 2009;9:256–64.
41. Liaw YF, Gane E, Leung N, et al. 2-Year GLOBE trial results: telbivudine is superior to lamivudine in patients with chronic hepatitis B. Gastroenterology 2009;136:486–95.
42. Tenney DJ, Pokornowski KA, Rose RE, et al. Entecavir maintains a high genetic barrier to HBV resistance through 6 years in naïve patients [abstract]. J Hepatol 2009; 50(Suppl 1):S10.
43. Heathcote E, Gane EJ, de Man RA, et al. Long-term (4-year) efficacy and safety of tenofovir disoproxil fumarate (TDF) treatment in HBeAg-positive patients (HBeAg+) with chronic hepatitis B (Study 103): preliminary analysis [abstract]. Hepatology 2010;52(Suppl 4):556A.
44. Chotiyaputta W, Peterson C, Ditah FA, et al. Persistence and adherence to nucleos(t)ide analogue treatment for chronic hepatitis B. J Hepatol 2011;54:12–8.
45. Zoulim F, Durantel D, Deny P. Management and prevention of drug resistance in chronic hepatitis B. Liver Int 2009;29(Suppl 1):108–15.
46. Ha NB, Garcia RT, Trinh HN, et al. Medication nonadherence with long-term management of patients with hepatitis B e antigen-negative chronic hepatitis B. Dig Dis Sci 2011. [Epub ahead of print].
47. Lee M, Keeffe EB. Study of adherence comes to the treatment of chronic hepatitis B [editorial]. J Hepatol 2011;54:6–8.
48. Liaw YF. Hepatitis flares and hepatitis B e antigen seroconversion: implication in anti-hepatitis B virus therapy. J Gastroenterol Hepatol 2003;18:246–52.
49. Fattovich G, Rugge M, Brollo L, et al. Clinical, virologic and histologic outcome following seroconversion from HBeAg to anti-HBe in chronic hepatitis type B. Hepatology 1986;6:167–72.
50. Chu CM, Liaw YF. HBsAg seroclearance in asymptomatic carriers of high endemic areas: appreciably high rates during a long-term follow-up. Hepatology 2007;45:1187–92.
51. Liaw YF, Lau GK, Kao JH, et al. Hepatitis B e antigen seroconversion: a critical event in chronic hepatitis B virus infection. Dig Dis Sci 2010;55:2727–34.
52. Gish RG, Lok AS, Chang TT, et al. Entecavir therapy for up to 96 weeks in patients with HBeAg-positive chronic hepatitis B. Gastroenterology 2007;133:1437–44.
53. Hsu YS, Chien RN, Yeh CT, et al. Long-term outcome after spontaneous HBeAg seroconversion in patients with chronic hepatitis B. Hepatology 2002;35:1522–7.
54. Papatheodoridis GV, Chrysanthos N, Hadziyannis E, et al. Longitudinal changes in serum HBV DNA levels and predictors of progression during the natural course of HBeAg-negative chronic hepatitis B virus infection. J Viral Hepat 2008;15:434–41.
55. Chen YC, Sheen IS, Chu CM, et al. Prognosis following spontaneous HBsAg seroclearance in chronic hepatitis B patients with or without concurrent infection. Gastroenterology 2002;123:1084–9.
56. Moucari R, Marcellin P. Quantification of hepatitis B surface antigen: a new concept for the management of chronic hepatitis B. Liver Int 2011;31(Suppl 1):122–8.
57. Chan HL, Wong VW, Wong GL, et al. A longitudinal study on the natural history of serum hepatitis B surface antigen changes in chronic hepatitis B. Hepatology 2010;52:1232–41.

58. Su TH, Hsu CS, Chen CL, et al. Serum hepatitis B surface antigen concentration correlates with HBV DNA level in patients with chronic hepatitis B. Antivir Ther 2010;15:1133–9.
59. Thompson AJ, Nguyen T, Iser D, et al. Serum hepatitis B surface antigen and hepatitis B e antigen titers: disease phase influences correlation with viral load and intrahepatic hepatitis B virus markers. Hepatology 2010;51:1933–44.
60. Chan HL, Wong VW, Chim AM, et al. Serum HBsAg quantification to predict response to peginterferon therapy of e antigen positive chronic hepatitis B. Aliment Pharmacol Ther 2010;32:1323–31.
61. Ma H, Yang RF, Wei L. Quantitative serum HBsAg and HBeAg are strong predictors of sustained HBeAg seroconversion to pegylated interferon alfa-2b in HBeAg-positive patients. J Gastroenterol Hepatol 2010;25:1498–506.
62. Brunetto MR, Moriconi F, Bonino F, et al. Hepatitis B virus surface antigen levels: a guide to sustained response to peginterferon alfa-2a in HBeAg-negative chronic hepatitis B. Hepatology 2009;49:1141–50.

Noninvasive Tools to Assess Hepatic Fibrosis: Ready for Prime Time?

Paul A. Schmeltzer, MD, Jayant A. Talwalkar, MD, MPH*

KEYWORDS
• Hepatic fibrosis • Noninvasive • Liver biopsy

Often regarded as the gold standard for fibrosis assessment, liver biopsy does carry associated risks given its invasive nature. Moreover, liver biopsy is not a true gold standard owing to interobserver and intra-observer variability and the small amount of tissue that is typically obtained with this procedure. Advances in the development of serologic tests and conventional imaging techniques have been shown to reduce the need for liver biopsy for diagnosing hepatic fibrosis. More commonly, it is a tool that is now reserved for evaluating indeterminate noninvasive tests or excluding features of particular diseases (eg, autoimmune hepatitis, steatohepatitis).

The noninvasive assessment of hepatic fibrosis has been a popular topic of discussion over the past decade. The ideal properties of a noninvasive test include widespread availability, ease of use, cost-efficiency, reproducibility, and the ability to detect changes in fibrosis over time. Furthermore, the ability of noninvasive testing to identify intermediate to advanced histologic stages of fibrosis (stage F2 or higher) without liver biopsy is important as this is the usual threshold to start treatment in eligible subjects with chronic hepatitis C (HCV), for example. In addition, the identification of early stage cirrhosis by noninvasive testing allows for the timely implementation of disease management strategies (hepatocellular carcinoma and variceal screening) to reduce the likelihood of complications.

This article reviews the salient aspects of hepatic fibrogenesis as well as the diagnostic performance of serum markers and imaging techniques that are currently available for detecting hepatic fibrosis. Finally, will provide suggestions as to how these noninvasive methods can be incorporated into routine clinical practice.

Supported by Grant No. EB 010393 from the National Institutes of Health.
Department of Medicine, Division of Gastroenterology and Hepatology, Mayo Clinic, 200 First Street SW, Rochester, MN 55905, USA
* Corresponding author.
E-mail address: talwalkar.jayant@mayo.edu

Gastroenterol Clin N Am 40 (2011) 507–521
doi:10.1016/j.gtc.2011.06.010
0889-8553/11/$ – see front matter © 2011 Elsevier Inc. All rights reserved.

PATHOGENESIS OF HEPATIC FIBROSIS

The hepatic stellate cell is thought to play an integral role in hepatic fibrosis. When in a quiescent state, stellate cells serve as storage reservoirs for retinol (a precursor of vitamin A) and other lipid soluble substances. Moreover, they control extracellular matrix (ECM) turnover and regulate sinusoidal blood flow.[1] Additional fibrogenic cells involved with hepatic fibrogenesis are derived from portal fibroblasts, circulating fibrocytes, bone marrow, and epithelial–mesenchymal cell transition. The proportion of fibrogenic cells from these various sources likely depends on the etiology of liver disease. For example, stellate cells are mainly involved when the damage is centered within the hepatic lobule. On the other hand, portal fibroblasts are observed to contribute more in cholestatic liver disease and ischemia.[2]

A variety of mediators have been shown to promote ongoing stellate cell activation and fibrogenesis, with platelet-derived growth factor and transforming growth factor-β described as 2 of the major cytokines involved with this process.[3] Stellate cell activation occurs through several additional pathways as well. Oxidative stress in the form of reactive oxygen species can activate stellate cells. This pathway may be of particular relevance in alcoholic liver injury, nonalcoholic fatty liver disease, and iron overload syndromes. Parenchymal cell apoptotic bodies can induce an inflammatory response that activates stellate cells as well. Bacterial lipopolysaccharide can elicit a fibrogenic response by binding to stellate cells via Toll-like receptor 4. Lastly, paracrine stimuli from adjacent cell types (macrophages, sinusoidal endothelium, and hepatocytes) can also aid in the transformation of stellate cells from a quiescent to an activated state.[4]

Once activated, stellate cells and fibroblasts transform into myofibroblasts, which are cells that contain contractile filaments. Myofibroblasts have the capacity to alter the composition of the ECM. Progressive changes in the ECM include a change from type IV collagen, heparan sulfate proteoglycan, and laminin to types I and III collagen. Subsequently, ECM accumulates owing to its increased synthesis and decreased degradation.[5] Fibrogenesis is further propagated by positive feedback mechanisms that arise from changes in ECM composition. Changes in membrane receptors (eg, integrins), activation of cellular matrix metalloproteases and increasing matrix stiffness serve as stimuli to perpetuate stellate cell activation.[6] It is this dynamic production and turnover of matrix, as well as increases in matrix stiffness, that form the basis for clinical techniques to noninvasively assess the extent of hepatic fibrosis.

CLINICAL IMPLICATIONS OF HEPATIC FIBROSIS

The accurate detection of hepatic fibrosis stage has important clinical decision-making implications for the management of chronic liver disease. For example, the presence of clinically significant hepatic fibrosis (defined as histologic stage ≥2) influences the timing for antiviral treatment for patients with chronic hepatitis B and C. In patients with nonalcoholic fatty liver disease (NAFLD), the presence of fibrosis overall is suggestive of nonalcoholic steatohepatitis (NASH) and thereby identifies a subset of patients who require closer monitoring and follow-up. Perhaps most important, the presence of early stage or compensated cirrhosis necessitates interval screening for disease-related complications, including esophageal varices and hepatocellular carcinoma.

Serial measurements to evaluate for progression or regression of hepatic fibrosis also have clinical utility. The successful medical treatment of various chronic liver diseases, including viral hepatitis, autoimmune hepatitis, and primary biliary cirrhosis, is often associated with histologic regression of fibrosis in addition to clinical and biochemical improvement. Conversely, monitoring for disease progression allows clinicians to implement treatment in eligible individuals as soon as possible to maximize the probability for a complete response.

LIVER BIOPSY

The introduction of a liver biopsy technique proposed by Menghini changed the field of hepatology in the 1960s.[7] Subsequently, liver biopsy has been considered the gold standard for detecting hepatic fibrosis. In recent times, the indications for liver biopsy have shifted from diagnosis of chronic liver disease to staging and monitoring for disease progression owing to improvements in serum laboratory testing.

Despite its widespread availability and use, there has been an increasing focus on the disadvantages of liver biopsy, which call its value into question. As an invasive procedure, procedure-related complications such as pain are reported in an estimated 20% of patients, and major complications including bleeding, hospitalization, and death are higher than 0.5%.[8] The risk for complications increases further among patients with advanced liver disease affected by thrombocytopenia, coagulopathy, or ascites. For these reasons, patients are becoming more reluctant to undergo repeat liver biopsies to assess disease progression as noninvasive test modalities become available.

Sampling error remains a major limitation for liver biopsy, and is difficult to overcome; only 1/50,000 of the liver is analyzed. Even when the specimen size is adequate (25 mm long), the probability for underestimating fibrosis stage remains as high as 25%.[9] It is important to be aware of this concept when determining the accuracy of liver biopsy. Many studies that evaluate the diagnostic accuracy of noninvasive measurements of fibrosis utilize the area under the receiver operating characteristic curve (AUROC) to gauge performance. Unfortunately, even in the best case scenario, an AUROC or more than 0.90 cannot be achieved for the perfect marker because liver biopsy cannot achieve 100% accuracy based on inherent features of the technique.[10]

A variety of histologic scoring systems have been used to stage hepatic fibrosis. Some systems have 5 stages (0–4) whereas others (eg, Ishak fibrosis score) have 7 stages (0–6). Although systems that include additional stages convey more information, the likelihood of having excellent reproducibility declines. The fibrosis stages identified by classification systems are determined by both the quantity and location of the fibrosis. In other words, the numbered stages do not reflect equal units of severity, but represent categories describing the histologic changes. This semiquantitative nature of histologic scoring systems is also an important consideration when comparing liver biopsy with noninvasive measures, which can provide a continuous quantitative assessment of liver fibrosis.[11]

Serum Fibrosis Markers

Indirect serum fibrosis markers
Significant attention has been paid to the development of serum fibrosis markers over the past 2 decades (**Table 1**). Routine serum biochemical tests to assess hepatic fibrosis were first examined given their wide availability. One simple model proposed that an aspartate aminotransferase (AST) to alanine aminotransferase (ALT) ratio of greater than 1 is indicative of cirrhosis. However, the sensitivity (53%) and negative predictive value (NPV; 81%) for detecting cirrhosis is not robust enough for use in clinical practice.[12] The most commonly studied indirect serum marker test using widely available variables is the AST to platelet count ratio index (APRI). The APRI is calculated as AST (U/L)/upper limit of normal $\times$ 100/platelet count (10^9/L).[13] The

Table 1
Diagnostic performance of serum fibrosis marker panels for detecting advanced hepatic
fibrosis compared with the reference standard of liver biopsy

Panel	Liver Disease	Sensitivity (%)	Specificity (%)	PPV (%)	NPV (%)
AST/ALT ratio	AST/ALT	50	100	100	81
Forns test	Platelets, GGT, cholesterol	94	54	40	96
APRI	AST, platelets	41	95	88	64
Fibrotest	GGT, haptoglobin, bilirubin, APO-A, α2-macroglobulin	87	59	63	85
Fibrospect	Hyaluronic acid, TIMP-1, α2-macroglobulin	83	66	72	78
ELF	Numerous ECM protein and proteinases	90	41	35	92

Abbreviations: ALT, alanine aminotransferase; APO-A, apolipoprotein A; APRI, AST to platelet count ratio index; AST, aspartate aminotransferase; GGT, γ-glutamyl transferase; PPV, positive predictive value; NPV, negative predictive value; TIMP, tissue inhibitor of metalloproteinase.
Data from Rockey DC, Bissell DM. Noninvasive measures of liver fibrosis. Hepatology 2006;43: S113–S20.

performance characteristics of the APRI depend on the cutoff value used (<0.5 to >2.0). Many studies have been conducted to externally validate initial results, but they have been conflicting, in part, because of differences in study methodology.

From a systematic review of 22 studies that examined the APRI in patients with chronic HCV, the average prevalence of clinically significant fibrosis (stages F2–F4) was 47%. With an APRI cutoff set at 0.5[13] for detecting clinically significant hepatic fibrosis (stages 2–4), the summary sensitivity and specificity values were 81% and 50%, respectively. The positive predictive value (PPV) and NPV of the 0.5 cutoff were 59% and 75%, respectively. At a higher cutoff of 1.5, the sensitivity and specificity were 35% and 91%, respectively. The 1.5 threshold led to a tradeoff between PPV (77%) and NPV (61%). With regard to cirrhosis, 12 studies were examined using thresholds of 1.0 and 2.0. The NPVs were excellent at 91% and 94%, respectively, for each threshold value. However, the PPVs for these cutoffs were not high enough to allow one to "rule in" cirrhosis with high accuracy. Thus, the use of APRI in different populations seems to have variable performance in detecting clinically significant hepatic fibrosis in patients with chronic HCV.[14] Fewer studies have been performed using APRI in other chronic liver diseases, but are expected in the future.

FibroTest (Biopredictive, Paris, France) is a proprietary panel developed in 2001 that combines several indirect serum fibrosis markers including α2-macroglobulin, haptoglobin, γ-glutamyl transferase (GGT), apolipoprotein A_1, and total bilirubin. Values of FibroTest range from 0 to 1; higher values indicate a greater probability of significant fibrosis. Serum α2-macroglobulin is an acute phase protein present at sites of inflammation. Haptoglobin is negatively associated with fibrosis because its synthesis is decreased by hepatocyte growth factor. GGT production could be caused by early cholestasis or an increase in epidermal growth factor.[15] The initial work by Imbert-Bismut and colleagues[15] identified these 5 variables as the most informative markers for staging fibrosis in patients with chronic HCV. Subsequently, a meta-analysis of 16 publications demonstrated that a Fibrotest diagnostic cutoff value of 0.31 was associated with a NPV of 91% for excluding significant fibrosis.[16]

In the United States, a version of the Fibrotest assay called FibroSURE (Laboratory Corporation of America, Raritan, NJ) is available for use. FibroSURE contains the same markers as Fibrotest in addition to ALT, patient age, and gender. The FibroSURE assay is mainly used for patients with chronic HCV.

Although FibroTest was initially validated in patients with chronic HCV, further studies showed that it is an effective alternative to liver biopsy in populations with chronic hepatitis B, alcoholic liver disease, and NAFLD. With regard to chronic hepatitis B, Sebastiani and colleagues[17] examined 110 consecutive patients who underwent assessment using multiple noninvasive methods including FibroTest and APRI. With a prevalence of 68% for significant fibrosis, FibroTest had a sensitivity of 81% and a specificity of 90%. However, the NPV was only 64%, which severely limits its utility in clinical practice for these patients. The authors concluded that noninvasive serum markers alone may not be good enough to obviate the need for liver biopsy in staging chronic hepatitis B.[17]

Given the epidemic of obesity and the number of patients at risk for NAFLD in developed countries, 1 study evaluated FibroTest in 170 patients from a secondary care center and 97 patients from multiple centers who were at risk for NAFLD. The authors found that FibroTest reliably detected advanced fibrosis (F2–F4) in patients with NAFLD; the AUROC ranged from 0.75 to 0.86 in the 2 study groups.[18]

False-positive results using FibroTest can occur when elevations in total bilirubin owing to hemolysis, Gilbert syndrome, or other causes of cholestasis are present. Furthermore, test results can be impacted by acute hepatic and/or systemic inflammation, which leads to spurious increases in serum α2-macroglobulin and haptoglobin levels. These factors need to be accounted for when deciding to utilize this noninvasive test modality.

Other indirect serum fibrosis tests which have been studied include the Forns index, which incorporates age, GGT, cholesterol, and platelets.[19] This model has mainly been utilized in patients with chronic HCV. Similarly, the Hepascore combines laboratory (bilirubin, GGT, hyaluronic acid, α-macroglobulin) and demographic data (age, gender) to predict fibrosis in chronic HCV.[20] The FIB-4 index, which uses age, ALT, AST, and platelets,[21] has also been evaluated in HIV/HCV-coinfected individuals and found to be accurate in detecting hepatic fibrosis. These scores are likely to be used less often than FibroTest in clinical practice mainly because of comparatively fewer supporting studies.

Direct Serum Fibrosis Markers

In contrast with indirect markers, the combined use of variables representing unique molecular aspects of hepatic fibrogenesis have been termed "direct" serum fibrosis marker panels. Two commonly available methods are the FIBROSpect II and European Liver Fibrosis (ELF) panels. The FIBROSpect II panel (Prometheus Laboratories Inc., San Diego, CA) is a proprietary technique composed of hyaluronic acid, tissue inhibitor of metalloproteinase 1, and α2- macroglobulin. Patel and colleagues[22] evaluated the diagnostic accuracy of FIBROSpect II in 294 patients with chronic HCV and validated the results in an external cohort of 402 patients. The sensitivity, specificity, and AUC in the external cohort was 77%, 73%, and 0.82, respectively.[22] Their results showed relatively good diagnostic accuracy for the detection of moderate-to-severe fibrosis in patients with chronic HCV. A subsequent investigation among 108 patients validated these initial findings with sensitivity, specificity, and AUROC values of 72%, 74%, and 0.826, respectively.[23]

The ELF panel group consists of age, hyaluronic acid, amino-terminal propeptide of type III collagen, and tissue inhibitor of metalloproteinase-1 for the detection of hepatic fibrosis. In a large cohort study examining patients with various chronic liver disease etiologies, the ELF panel also demonstrated good accuracy in detecting clinically significant hepatic fibrosis (stages F2–F4) in patients with alcoholic and NAFLD as well as chronic HCV. By adopting different test thresholds, sensitivities and specificities of over 90% could be obtained allowing the panel to reliably exclude or detect significant fibrosis.[24]

The use of serum fibrosis markers to assess hepatic effects following antiviral treatment response has been a recent area of interest. Within the Hepatitis C Antiviral Long-term Treatment against Cirrhosis (HALT-C) trial, a prospective study of maintenance pegylated interferon in chronic HCV patients with advanced fibrosis who failed prior treatment, a number of serum fibrosis markers were serially measured over the duration of the study. More specifically, serum samples of YKL-40, tissue inhibitor of metalloproteinase-1, amino-terminal peptide of type III procollagen, and hyaluronic acid were assessed at weeks 0, 24, 48, and 72. Among the markers examined, it was shown that a reduced YKL-40 level at baseline was an independent predictor of a virologic response at week 20. Although levels of some markers increased on antiviral treatment, there were significant reductions in all 4 markers noted among patients achieving a sustained virologic response (SVR) at week 72.[25] Patel and colleagues[26] also studied changes in noninvasive serum markers (FibroSURE and FIBROSpect II) in treatment-naïve patients with chronic HCV given albinterferon alfa-2b and ribavirin. Similar to the HALT-C study, patients achieving SVR had lower baseline scores than nonresponders. Moreover, there were significant declines in HCV FibroSURE and FIBROSpect II scores in those patients who achieved a SVR.[26] One drawback to these studies is that a second comparative liver biopsy was not performed after treatment to document fibrosis regression. Future studies are expected to define the minimum change in serum marker panel score that is clinically significant.

Additional studies have evaluated the prognostic value of noninvasive serum biomarkers. A prospective cohort study compared the 5-year prognostic value of FibroTest with liver biopsy for predicting cirrhosis decompensation and survival among 537 HCV-infected patients. FibroTest values were used to classify those with minimal fibrosis (FibroTest < 0.32), moderate fibrosis (FibroTest 0.32–0.58), and severe fibrosis (FibroTest > 0.58). The authors found FibroTest to be a better predictor of both HCV-related complications (AUROC 0.96 vs 0.91) and HCV-related deaths (AUROC 0.96 vs 0.87) compared with liver biopsy.[27] A similar study evaluated the ability of ELF to predict clinical outcomes (liver-related morbidity and mortality) in 457 patients with chronic liver disease of various etiologies. A unit change in ELF score was associated with a doubling of risk of liver-related outcome and ELF predicted outcome at least as well as liver biopsy.[28] Again, future studies are expected to confirm these initial findings and to see if treatment response influencing prognosis can also be measured by serum markers.

IMAGING TECHNIQUES
Ultrasound-Based Transient Elastography

With the deposition of fibrotic tissue in organs such as the liver, the physical properties or stiffness may also change. Historically, this has been appreciated through physical examination where palpation of a hard or stiff liver often denoted the presence of significant disease. Recent advances in technology can now detect the extent of hepatic fibrosis by providing quantitative measurements of liver stiffness.

First described in 2003, ultrasound-based transient elastography (TE) using FibroScan (Echosens, Paris, France) is able to measure liver stiffness using a transducer probe mounted on a vibrating axis. Activation of the hand-held probe leads to vibrations of mild amplitude and low frequency (50 Hz) that generate 1-dimensional mechanical waves that propagate through the liver. Pulse-echo acquisition then follows the propagating wave and measures its velocity, which is directly proportional to tissue stiffness. Therefore, subjects with higher degrees of fibrosis will have faster wave velocities detected by TE that result in higher liver stiffness measurements. Liver stiffness measurement is expressed in kiloPascals (kPa), with ranges between 2.5 and 75 kPa. Advantages of TE include (1) short acquisition time (100 ms), which allows measurements to be made even though the liver moves with respiration, and (2) region of interest analysis within a cylindrical volume approximately 1 cm wide and 4 cm long, which results in a tissue volume over 100 times the size of a typical liver biopsy specimen. Criteria for valid liver stiffness measurement with TE include a success rate (percentage of successful measurements out of total acquisitions) of at least 60% and an interquartile range which should not exceed 30% of the median value.[29]

Similar to the noninvasive serum fibrosis markers, the initial diagnostic evaluation studies using TE focused on patients with chronic HCV. A preliminary study in 2003 showed excellent reproducibility and diagnostic accuracy for detecting clinically significant hepatic fibrosis and cirrhosis in 67 patients.[30] Subsequent work by Ziol and colleagues[31] among 327 patients with chronic HCV infection revealed sensitivity, specificity, and AUROC values of 55%, 84%, and 0.79 for stage 2 or higher and 84%, 94%, and 0.97 for stage 4 (cirrhosis) using cutoff values of 8.8 and 14.6 kPa, respectively. In multivariate analysis, stage of hepatic fibrosis was highly correlated with liver stiffness as opposed to inflammation grade and extent of steatosis. It should be noted that 76 patients (23%) were excluded from the statistical analysis based on unsuitable liver biopsy specimens or TE examinations that failed to meet criteria for a valid result.[31] Castera and colleagues[32] in 2005 also studied 193 patients with chronic HCV infection who underwent liver biopsy as well as TE, APRI, and FibroTest assessments. The diagnostic performance of FibroScan, FibroTest, and APRI was similar for detecting stages F2 to F4 hepatic fibrosis. For various combinations of noninvasive methods, the diagnostic use of FibroScan and FibroTest was most optimal for detecting stages F2 to F4 and F4 alone. Agreement between FibroScan and FibroTest results for the presence of significant fibrosis was 84% when compared with histology from liver biopsy.[32]

Several meta-analyses have confirmed the diagnostic accuracy of TE in various populations with chronic liver disease. Among 9 studies that evaluated the diagnostic accuracy of TE compared with liver biopsy, a pooled sensitivity of 87% and specificity of 91% was observed for the detection of cirrhosis (stage F4). Chronic HCV with or without viral co-infection was the main etiology of liver disease in eight of these studies. For patients with stages F2 to F4 fibrosis, the accuracy of TE was lower and more variable (sensitivity ranged between 53% and 93%; specificity ranged from 70% to 84%) when compared with results for detecting cirrhosis.[33] A second meta-analysis examined the diagnostic performance of TE in 50 studies including work published in abstract form. Once again, TE was found to be excellent at distinguishing cirrhosis versus no cirrhosis, although the diagnosis of clinically significant fibrosis (F2 to F4) was less accurate. Meta-regression analysis identified underlying liver disease, the fibrosis staging system used, and the country in which the study was performed as major causes of heterogeneity in pooled results.[34] In summary, these meta-analyses show that TE is effective for identifying cirrhosis, but various factors leading to heterogeneity make it less accurate to detect stages F2 to F4 fibrosis.

Fewer studies have assessed the use of TE in chronic liver diseases other than HCV. Coco and colleagues[35] studied 228 consecutive patients with chronic hepatitis

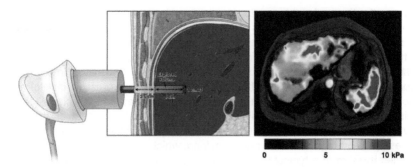

Fig. 1. Representative areas of hepatic parenchyma examined by TE (*left panel*) and MRE (*right panel*) for detecting stage of hepatic fibrosis. A larger region of interest is available for calculating mean liver stiffness with MRE. (*From* Talwalkar JA. Elastography for detecting hepatic fibrosis: options and considerations. Gastroenterology 2008;135:299–302; with permission.)

B (n = 79) and HCV (n = 149). On multivariate analysis, both ALT and fibrosis were the 2 factors independently associated with liver stiffness. Interestingly, 10 patients with ALT flares had up to 3-fold increases in liver stiffness that progressively declined to baseline after resolution of the flare in disease activity. This suggests that TE may not be as reliable for chronic hepatitis B.[35] A small study of 67 patients with NAFLD showed a stepwise increase in liver stiffness with increasing histologic fibrosis. The severity of fibrosis was not affected by grade of activity or amount of steatosis.[36] Patients with chronic cholestatic liver disease have also been examined by TE. Among 69 cases with primary biliary cirrhosis and 26 with primary sclerosing cholangitis, liver stiffness values were found to correlate with histologic stages. The diagnostic performance of TE for detecting stages F2-F4 and F4 fibrosis were excellent with AUROC values above 0.9 for both fibrosis categories.[37] Additional studies in patients with nonviral liver disease are expected to better define the diagnostic accuracy of TE in these populations.

TE is an attractive tool because it is painless, quick (can be performed in <5 minutes), easily reproducible, free of complications, and available at the bedside or on an outpatient basis. In contrast with serum markers, TE is a more direct measure of fibrosis, is not typically affected by extrahepatic disorders, and is applicable to all chronic liver diseases. Limitations for using TE are seen in patients who are obese, have narrow intercostals spaces, have ascites (elastic waves do not propagate through liquids), or experience ALT flares (acute viral hepatitis or acute reactivation of chronic hepatitis B).[38] The impact of obesity on TE seems to be the most critical, because the frequency of incomplete and failed examinations exceeds 20% with body mass index values of 28 kg/m^2 or greater, and continues to rise in frequency with further increases in BMI.[39] Furthermore, strict confinement of the right liver edge for TE measurement may limit the ability to identify the dominant stage of fibrosis if the geographic distribution of fibrosis within an individual patient's liver is heterogeneous (**Fig. 1**).[38]

Magnetic Resonance Elastography

Liver stiffness is also measured using a technique called magnetic resonance elastography (MRE). The initial pioneering work in the 1990s has led to the use of MRE in human subjects for detecting hepatic fibrosis. Using conventional 1.5T magnetic resonance imaging (MRI) scanners, patients are placed in the supine position where a pneumatic driver is placed against the anterior abdominal wall. This driver vibrates at low frequencies (40–120 Hz), which then lead to mechanical wave formation and propagation into the liver. MRE measurements require the patient to hold his breath for 10 to 15 seconds on 4 occasions during the scanning period. A phase-contrast MRI sequence (which can be added to a conventional MRI system) then images the propagating waves. Data from the phase-contrast sequence is then analyzed by specialized computer-based algorithms (which can be added to postprocessing workstations) to create elastograms—quantitative, color-coded images that depict tissue stiffness. Regions of interest are identified on each of the 4 cross-sectional images obtained, and averaged to obtain a mean liver stiffness value measured in kiloPascals. Of note, the numerical results obtained by MRE differ by a factor of 3 when compared with results obtained by TE.[38,40]

Several investigations have been published demonstrating the excellent diagnostic accuracy for MRE in detecting hepatic fibrosis. A pilot study by Huwart and colleagues[41] assessed the feasibility of MRE in a group of 25 consecutive patients with various etiologies of chronic liver disease. The mean liver stiffness was 2.24 ± 0.23 kPa in the 11 patients with minimal fibrosis (F0–F1), 2.56 ± 0.24 kPa in the 4 patients with substantial fibrosis (F2–F3), and 4.68 ± 1.61 kPa in the 10 patients with cirrhosis. There were significant increases in mean liver stiffness with increasing stage of fibrosis.[41] Additional work by Yin and colleagues[42] was performed by examining the performance of MRE in 50 patients with various forms of chronic liver disease and 35 healthy volunteers. In this study, mean liver stiffness also increased systematically with stage of histologic fibrosis. With a cutoff mean liver stiffness value of 2.93 kPa, MRE had a sensitivity of 98% and a specificity of 99% for differentiating any stage of fibrosis from normal liver tissue. For stages F2 to F4, a sensitivity of 86% and specificity of 85% were associated with a mean cutoff value of 4.89 kPa. This study also demonstrated that there was no significant relationship between degree of steatosis and liver stiffness.[42]

An important prospective comparative study was conducted by Huwart and colleagues[43] comparing MRE to TE and APRI in 141 patients with chronic HCV. The success rate of TE was 84%, whereas the rate was 94% for MRE. Further analysis was performed in the 96 patients who had successful histologic and imaging studies. Although MRE, TE, and APRI results increased according to the stage of liver fibrosis, the modality with the highest diagnostic accuracy for stages F2 through F4 and F4 alone was MRE. It should be noted that both MRE and TE had excellent diagnostic performance for the detection of cirrhosis.[43]

Advantages of MRE include that (1) an acoustic window is not required, (2) it is operator independent, (3) it can be performed on obese patients, (4) large cross-sectional areas of hepatic parenchyma can be evaluated (see **Fig. 1**), and (5) a conventional MRI can be obtained at the same time as MRE.[38,40] However, MRE does have some limitations. Standard contraindications for MRI (eg, pacemaker, defibrillator, aneurysm clip) apply when performing MRE. Although obesity is not as detrimental when compared with TE, obese patients still must be able to fit into the magnet bore. At the time of writing, MRE cannot be performed on patients with increased hepatic iron content owing to signal-to-noise limitations that prevent wave visualization. As with TE, liver stiffness measurements can be affected by several other pathologic processes, including hepatic inflammation, or congestion from cardiac disease.[38,40,42]

Emerging Imaging Modalities

Aside from TE and MRE, other noninvasive imaging modalities have been investigated. One such technique is acoustic radiation force imaging (ARFI).

Basically, this is an ultrasound-based method that uses B-mode imaging to locate the region of interest for analysis. Longitudinal, short-duration acoustic pulses cause tissue displacement with generated shear waves moving laterally away from the region of excitation. The speed of these waves are then measured by ultrasound tracking beams.

Friedrich-Rust and colleagues[44] conducted a pilot study of 81 patients with chronic viral hepatitis (64 with HCV and 17 with HBV) that compared ARFI with TE and serologic fibrosis markers (APRI and FibroTest). Two percent of patients had to be excluded from the study owing to failed TE (resulting from obesity). The median velocity in 20 healthy controls was 1.10 m/s (range, 0.85–1.42). The median velocities in the study patients were 1.13 m/s for patients with stage F0, 1.17 m/s for F1, 1.22 m/s for F2, 1.64 for F3, and 2.38 m/s (range, 1.15–3.83) for F4. Of note, there were patients in the healthy control group who had velocities in the cirrhotic range. Despite this, all 3 modalities had similar diagnostic performances. Even though ARFI performed similarly to TE, it does have the advantage of being easily integrated into a standard ultrasound examination. Future studies with larger numbers of subjects are needed to define the role of ARFI.[44]

Diffusion-weighted MRI has been evaluated also for detecting hepatic fibrosis. It allows for qualitative and quantitative assessment of tissue without using gadolinium chelates, thereby eliminating the risk of nephrotoxicity. This technique relies on differences in the mobility of protons (primarily associated with water) between tissues. The degree of diffusion is measured by the apparent diffusion coefficient, where lower values have been described in association with greater degrees of hepatic fibrosis. Other studies, however, have indicated that diminished hepatic perfusion in advanced fibrosis accounts for the change in the apparent diffusion coefficient rather than the restriction of molecular diffusion. Further studies are needed to delineate the exact mechanism behind diffusion changes seen in liver fibrosis. Other limitations of diffusion-weighted MRI include variable apparent diffusion coefficient reproducibility and suboptimal image resolution due to motion artifact.[45]

MR spectroscopy uses[31] phosphorus spectral profiles to provide direct biochemical information on hepatic metabolism. Theoretically, hepatic fibrosis leads to increased turnover of cell membrane synthetic and degradation products. The ratio of phosphomonoesters (PME) to phosphodiesters (PDE) is thought to reflect this process. More specifically, studies have shown that the PME/PDE ratio increases with advanced liver disease. Lim and colleagues[46] enrolled 15 healthy controls and 48 patients with biopsy-proven HCV-related liver disease. Fibrosis and necroinflammatory scores were used to divide the subjects into 3 groups: Mild hepatitis (fibrosis score ≤2/6; necroinflammatory score ≤3/18), moderate-to-severe hepatitis (3 ≤fibrosis score <6 or necroinflammatory score ≥4/18), and cirrhosis (fibrosis score = 6/6). The PME/PDE ratio increased along with disease severity, providing significant differences between the mild hepatitis, moderate hepatitis, and cirrhosis groups. Using a PME/PDE ratio of 0.2 or less, mild hepatitis could be detected with a sensitivity of 76%, and a specificity of 83% (PPV, 72%; NPV, 86%). Similarly, a PME/PDE ratio of 0.3 or greater could identify cirrhosis with a sensitivity of 82% and a specificity of 81% (PPV, 56%; NPV, 93%).[46] MR spectroscopy requires further refinement before it can be assessed more fully in patients with chronic liver disease.

USE OF NONINVASIVE TESTS IN CLINICAL PRACTICE

As described, the majority of studies examining the performance characteristics of serum fibrosis markers and noninvasive imaging were done on patients with chronic viral hepatitis. Both serum tests (FibroTest) and imaging (TE, MRE) modalities can sufficiently identify stages F2 through F4 and F4 alone. With the advent of direct-acting antivirals and IL28 genotyping, the workup and management of HCV will be rapidly changing and the role of noninvasive testing must be evaluated. The expected improvement in genotype 1 SVR rates, for example, may further obviate the need for an initial staging liver biopsy in these patients. Therefore, noninvasive testing could be used as a tool to exclude cirrhosis in those patients who do not have suggestive clinical, laboratory, or imaging findings. Furthermore, noninvasive testing could be performed serially to identify disease progression or regression in patients achieving SVR after therapy.

Recurrent HCV after liver transplantation is a difficult problem, and these patients are often subjected to multiple protocol liver biopsies to stage hepatic fibrosis. Stage 2 fibrosis is the usual threshold for starting HCV treatment posttransplant, as with native liver disease. The use of serum fibrosis markers in this setting may be problematic because immunosuppressive agents can affect some of the variables. Carrion and colleagues[47] evaluated the use of TE in 124 HCV-infected liver transplant recipients. With a liver stiffness cutoff value of 8.5 kPa, the sensitivity, specificity, NPV, and PPV for the diagnosis of grade F2 fibrosis or higher were 90%, 81%, 79%, and 92%, respectively. Furthermore, there was a direct correlation between liver stiffness and hepatic venous pressure gradient for the diagnosis of portal hypertension. This is of potential importance as patients with greater than observed disease severity by liver biopsy may be detected with elastography.[47]

A recent study of 400 US adults showed the prevalence of NAFLD to be 46% with NASH detected in 12.2% of the total cohort.[48,49] These rates are higher than previously estimated, making NAFLD the most common liver disease where noninvasive tests of hepatic fibrosis can be used. The performance characteristics of certain serum markers (FibroTest, ELF) have been validated in patients with NAFLD and seem adequate for the detection of advanced fibrosis. The role of noninvasive imaging in these patients is somewhat more problematic for TE, which can be technically difficult in obese patients compared with MRE.

One interesting niche for noninvasive fibrosis assessment may be in screening patients prescribed methotrexate for chronic inflammatory diseases for clinically significant hepatic fibrosis. Past guidelines, which were based on expert opinion, recommended a liver biopsy after a cumulative methotrexate dose of 1500 mg and repeat biopsies after every additional 1000 to 1500 mg.[50] More recent work has suggested that advanced liver fibrosis is a rare event in patients treated with methotrexate for diseases including Crohn's disease and psoriasis.[51,52] Furthermore, FibroTest and FibroScan have been shown to reliably detect advanced fibrosis in this group of patients. Given the rarity of methotrexate-induced fibrosis and the possible need for serial assessments, the use of these noninvasive tests is attractive in this setting.

In summary, the need for noninvasive assessment of hepatic fibrosis for disease staging, prognosis, progression, and treatment response is clear. The use of serum markers and elastography imaging with TE and MRE is promising, although their role has mainly been within studies in patients with chronic HCV infection (**Table 2**). Additional areas of research include defining cutoff values for specific diseases, further head-to-head comparisons of various noninvasive modalities, and the examination of algorithms using both serum markers and imaging. Moreover, there is a paucity of data analyzing the cost effectiveness of these various tests for diagnostic as well as screening purposes.

Table 2
Advantages and limitations of biopsy and noninvasive tests for detecting hepatic fibrosis

	Liver Biopsy	Serum Markers	TE	MRE
Advantages	Direct observation of fibrosis	Noninvasive	Noninvasive	Noninvasive
	Examines 1/50,000th of hepatic parenchyma	Examines indirect or direct markers of fibrosis	Examines 1 × 4 cm area over right liver edge	Examines multiple areas within right and left liver
	Accurate for detecting cirrhosis	Can be accurate for detecting cirrhosis	Accurate for detecting cirrhosis	Accurate for detecting cirrhosis
Disadvantages	Contraindicated in ascites, coagulopathy	Delays in test result generation with send-out proprietary tests	Failure rate with obesity, narrow rib spaces	Limited by claustrophobia and typical MRI contraindications
	Sampling error and observer variation	False-positive values with hemolysis, inflammation, Gilbert syndrome	False-positive values with inflammation, congestion	False-positive values with inflammation, congestion
	Unsuitable for longitudinal monitoring	Indices may change with disease progression or response to therapy	Liver stiffness does change with disease progression or response to therapy	Liver stiffness does change with disease progression or response to therapy

Data from Castera L, Pinzani M. Biopsy and non-invasive methods for the diagnosis of liver fibrosis: does it take two to tango? Gut 2010;59:861–6.

REFERENCES

1. Geerts A. History, heterogeneity, developmental biology, and functions of quiescent hepatic stellate cells. Semin Liver Dis 2001;21:311–35.
2. Pinzani M, Rombouts K. Liver fibrosis: from the bench to clinical targets. Dig and Liver Dis 2004;36:231–42.
3. Moreira RK. Hepatic stellate cells and liver fibrosis. Arch Pathol Lab Med 2007;131: 1728–34.
4. Friedman SL. Mechanisms of hepatic fibrogenesis. Gastroenterology 2008;134: 1665–9.
5. Bataller R, Brenner DA. Liver fibrosis. J Clin Invest 2005;115:209–18.
6. Schuppan D, Afdhal NH. Liver cirrhosis. Lancet 2008;371:838–51.
7. Menghini G. One-second needle biopsy of the liver. Gastroenterology 1958;35: 190–9.
8. Cadranel JF, Rufat P, Degos F. Practices of liver biopsy in France: results of a prospective nationwide survey. For the Group of Epidemiology of the French Association for the Study of Liver. Hepatology 2000;32:477–81.
9. Bedossa P. Sampling variability of liver fibrosis in chronic hepatitis C. Hepatology 2003;38:1449–57.
10. Mehta SH, Lau B, Afdhal NH, et al. Exceeding the limits of liver histology markers. J Hepatol 2009;50:36–41.
11. Goodman ZD. Grading and staging systems for inflammation and fibrosis in chronic liver diseases. J Hepatol 2007;47:598–607.
12. Sheth SG, Flamm SL, Gordon FD, et al. AST/ALT ratio predicts cirrhosis in patients with chronic hepatitis C virus infection. Am J Gastroenterol 1998;93:44–8.
13. Wai CT, Greenson JK, Fontana RJ, et al. A simple noninvasive index can predict both significant fibrosis and cirrhosis in patients with chronic hepatitis C. Hepatology 2003;38:518–26.
14. Shaheen AA, Myers RP. Diagnostic accuracy of the aspartate aminotransferase-to-platelet ratio index for the prediction of hepatitis C-related fibrosis: a systematic review. Hepatology 2007;46:912–21.
15. Imbert-Bismut F, Ratziu V, Pieroni L, et al. Biochemical markers of liver fibrosis in patients with hepatitis C virus infection: a prospective study. Lancet 2001;357: 1069–75.
16. Poynard T, Imbert-Bismut F, Munteanu M, et al. Overview of the diagnostic value of biochemical markers of liver fibrosis (FibroTest, HCV FibroSure) and necrosis (ActiTest) in patients with chronic hepatitis C. Comparative Hepatology 2004;3:8.
17. Sebastiani G, Vario A, Guido M, et al. Sequential algorithms combining non-invasive markers and biopsy for the assessment of liver fibrosis in chronic hepatitis B. World J Gastroenterol 2007;13:525–31.
18. Ratziu V, Massard J, Charlotte F, et al. Diagnostic value of biochemical markers (FibroTest-FibroSURE) for the prediction of liver fibrosis in patients with non-alcoholic fatty liver disease. BMC Gastroenterol 2006;6:6.
19. Forns X, Ampurdanes S, Llovet JM, et al. Identification of chronic hepatitis C patients without hepatic fibrosis by a simple predictive model. Hepatology 2002;36:986–92.
20. Adams LA, Bulsara M, Rossi E, et al. Hepascore : an accurate validated predictor of liver fibrosis in chronic hepatitis C infection. Clin Chem 2005;51:1867–73.
21. Sterling RK, Lissen E, Clumeck N, et al. Development of a simple noninvasive index to predict significant fibrosis in patients with HIV/HCV coinfection. Hepatology 2006;43: 1317–25.

22. Patel K, Gordon SC, Jacobson I, et al. Evaluation of a panel of non-invasive serum markers to differentiate mild from moderate-to-advanced liver fibrosis in chronic hepatitis C patients. J Hepatol 2004;41: 935–42.
23. Zaman A, Rosen HR, Ingram K, et al. Assessment of FIBROSpect II to detect hepatic fibrosis in chronic hepatitis C patients. Am J Med 2007;120:280,e9–280.
24. Rosenberg WM, Voelker M, Thiel R, et al. Serum markers detect the presence of liver fibrosis: a cohort study. Gastroenterology 2004;127:1704–13.
25. Fontana RJ, Bonkovsky HL, Naishadham D, et al. Serum fibrosis marker levels decrease after successful antiviral treatment in chronic hepatitis C patients with advanced fibrosis. Clin Gastroenterol Hepatol 2009;7:219–26.
26. Patel K, Benhamou Y, Yoshida EM, et al. An independent and prospective comparison of two commercial fibrosi marker panels (HCV FibroSURE and FIBROSpect II) during albinterferon alfa-2b combination therapy for chronic hepatitis C. J Viral Hepat 2009;16:178–86.
27. Ngo Y, Munteanu M, Messous D, et al. A prospective analysis of the prognostic value of biomarkers (Fibrotest) in patients with chronic hepatitis C. Clin Chem 2006;52: 1887–96.
28. Parkes J, Roderick P, Harris S, et al. Enhanced liver fibrosis test can predict clinical outcomes in patients with chronic liver disease. Gut 2010;59:1245–51.
29. Castera L, Forns X, Alberti A. Non-invasive evaluation of liver fibrosis using transient elastography. J Hepatol 2008;48:835–47.
30. Sandrin L, Fourquet B, Hasquenoph JM, et al. Transient elastography: a new noninvasive method for assessment of hepatic fibrosis. Ultrasound Med Biol 2003; 29:1705–13.
31. Ziol M, Handra-Luca A, Kettaneh A, et al. Noninvasive assessment of liver fibrosis by measurement of stiffness in patients with chronic hepatitis c. Hepatology 2005;41: 48–54.
32. Castera L, Vergniol J, Foucher J, et al. Prospective comparison of transient elastography, Fibrotest, APRI, and liver biopsy for the assessment of fibrosis in chronic hepatitis C. Gastroenterology 2005;128:343–50.
33. Talwalkar JA, Kurtz DM, Schoenleber SJ, et al. Ultrasound-based transient elastography for the detection of hepatic fibrosis: systematic review and meta-analysis. Clin Gastroenterol Hepatol 2007;5:1214–20.
34. Friedrich-Rust M, Ong M, Martens S, et al. Performance of transient elastography for the staging of liver fibrosis: a meta-analysis. Gastroenterology 2008;134:960–74.
35. Coco B, Oliveri F, Maina AM, et al. Transient elastography: a new surrogate marker of liver fibrosis influenced by major changes of transaminases. J Viral Hepat 2007;14: 360–9.
36. Yoneda M, Fujita K, Inamori M, et al. Transient elastography in patients with non-alcoholic fatty liver disease (NAFLD). Gut 2007;56;1330–1.
37. Corpechot C, El Naggar A, Poujol-Robert A, et al. assessment of biliary fibrosis by transient elastography in patients with PBC and PSC. Hepatology 2006;43:1118–24.
38. Talwalkar JA. Elastography for detecting hepatic fibrosis: options and considerations. Gastroenterology 2008;135:299–302.
39. Castéra L, Foucher J, Bernard PH, et al. Pitfalls of liver stiffness measurement: a 5-year prospective study of 13,369 examinations. Hepatology 2010;51:828–35.
40. Talwalkar JA, Yin M, Fidler JL, et al. Magnetic resonance imaging of hepatic fibrosis: emerging clinical applications. Hepatology 2008;47:332–42.
41. Huwart L, Peeters F, Sinkus R, et al. Liver fibrosis: non-invasive assessment with MR elastography. NMR Biomed 2006;19:173–9.

42. Yin M, Talwalkar JA, Glaser KJ, et al. Assessment of hepatic fibrosis with magnetic resonance elastography. Clin Gastroenterol Hepatol 2007;5:1207–13.
43. Huwart L, Sempoux C, Vicaut E, et al. Magnetic resonance elastography for the noninvasive staging of liver fibrosis. Gastroenterology 2008;135;32–40.
44. Friedrich-Rust M, Wunder K, Kriener S, et al. Liver fibrosis in viral hepatitis: noninvasive assessment with acoustic radiation force impulse imaging versus transient elastography. Radiology 2009;252:595–604.
45. Taouli B, Koh DM. Diffusion-weighted mr imaging of the liver. Radiology 2010;254: 47–66.
46. Lim AK, Patel N, Hamilton G, et al. The relationship of in vivo 31p mr spectroscopy to histology in chronic hepatitis C. Hepatology 2003;37:788–94.
47. Carrion JA, Navasa M, Bosch, et al. Transient elastography for diagnosis of advanced fibrosis and portal hypertension in patients with hepatitis c recurrence after liver transplantation. Liver Transpl 2006;12:1791–8.
48. Williams CD, Stengel J, Asike MI, et al. Prevalence of nonalcoholic fatty liver disease and nonalcoholic steatohepatitis among a largely middle-aged population utilizing ultrasound and liver biopsy: a prospective study. Gastroenterology 2011; 140:124–31.
49. Charlton M. Fibrosing NASH: on being a blind man in a dark room looking for a black cat (that isn't there). Gastroenterology 2011;140:25–8.
50. Roenigk HH Jr, Auerbach R, Maibach H, et al. Methotrexate in psoriasis: consensus conference. J Am Acad Dermatol 1998;478–85.
51. Laharie D, Zerbib F, Adhoute X, et al. Diagnosis of liver fibrosis by transient elastography (FibroScan) and noninvasive methods in Crohn's disease patients treated with methotrexate. Aliment Pharmacol Ther 2006;23:1621–8.
52. Berends MA, Snoek J, de Jong EM, et al. Biochemical and biophysical assessment of MTX-induced liver fibrosis in psoriasis patients: FibroTest predicts the presence and FibroScan predicts the absence of significant liver fibrosis. Liver Int 2007;27:639–45.

Acute Liver Failure: Current Practice and Recent Advances

Vinay Sundaram, MD[a], Obaid S. Shaikh, MD, FRCP[b],*

KEYWORDS

• Encephalopathy • Brain edema • Liver transplantation

Acute liver failure (ALF), also referred as "fulminant hepatic failure," is a rare syndrome characterized by rapid onset of severe hepatic dysfunction in the absence of preexistent liver disease.[1] The principal manifestations of ALF include jaundice, hepatic encephalopathy, and coagulopathy, often owing to massive or submassive hepatic necrosis.[1,2] An estimated 2000 to 3000 cases of ALF occur in the United States every year.[3] The syndrome has diverse etiologies that manifest wide geographic distribution. In North America and Western Europe, acetaminophen and idiosyncratic drug hepatotoxicity are the predominant causes.[4] In contrast, viral hepatitis B and E are the major causes in Asia.[5,6] Without specialized intensive care management and the availability of liver transplantation, a diagnosis of ALF portends a poor outcome. This article summarizes current practice and recent advances in the management of ALF.

DIAGNOSIS AND INITIAL MANAGEMENT

Early diagnosis of ALF is crucial. Although jaundice and hepatic encephalopathy are the cardinal manifestations of ALF, many patients present with nonspecific symptoms of generalized malaise, nausea, and abdominal discomfort.[7] Thus, concern for severe liver injury is often triggered by abnormal laboratory values. Hepatic encephalopathy develops rapidly in patients with hyperacute failure sometimes preceding jaundice.[7,8] Careful clinical evaluation and laboratory and imaging studies are required to help exclude cirrhosis and to establish the etiology of the disease. The role of liver biopsy is limited and it is often problematic in view of cerebral and hemodynamic instability, and associated coagulopathy.[2]

Patients with ALF are best managed in an intensive care unit. Once diagnostic criteria are met, transfer to a tertiary facility with a liver transplant program is urgent.

[a] Department of Medicine, Division of Gastroenterology and Hepatology, Beth Israel Deaconess Medical Center, Harvard Medical School, 330 Brookline Avenue, Boston, MA 02215, USA
[b] Department of Medicine, Division of Gastroenterology, Hepatology and Nutrition, University of Pittsburgh School of Medicine, Kaufmann Building, Suite 916, 3471 Fifth Avenue, Pittsburgh, PA 15213, USA
* Corresponding author.
E-mail address: obaid@pitt.edu

Gastroenterol Clin N Am 40 (2011) 523–539
doi:10.1016/j.gtc.2011.06.009
0889-8553/11/$ – see front matter Published by Elsevier Inc.

gastro.theclinics.com

Transfer may be considered earlier if a patient with severe acute liver injury is deemed likely to progress to ALF. Worsening coagulopathy and behavioral changes are particularly relevant in this regard. A decision regarding tracheal intubation should be made before transfer. Intubation is particularly recommended for patients with grades III or IV hepatic encephalopathy.[1] Rapid development of hypoglycemia is a concern and should be addressed by a continuous intravenous dextrose infusion and frequent monitoring of blood sugar levels. Encephalopathy in ALF may be associated with agitation and seizures; therefore, a quiet environment is needed to minimize external stimuli.

CEREBRAL EDEMA

Cerebral edema and intracranial hypertension (ICH) are among the most serious complications of ALF.[9] As cerebral edema progresses, fatal uncal herniation may ensue. Residual neurologic deficits have been noted among survivors.[10] Cerebral edema should be suspected in patients with progressive hepatic encephalopathy. Although it is rare among those with grades I or II, its incidence is 25% to 35% with grade III and as high as 65% to 75% with grade IV hepatic encephalopathy.[1] A high index of suspicion is needed because patients may not exhibit classic features including headache, vomiting, bradycardia, hypertension, blurred vision, papilledema, brisk reflexes, and decerebrate rigidity.

The pathogenesis of ICH from ALF is not fully understood; however, hyperammonemia is considered to be a key factor.[11] Once ammonia traverses the blood–brain barrier, astrocytes detoxify it by conversion to glutamine through its reaction with glutamic acid, a process facilitated by the enzyme glutamine synthetase. Glutamine has a direct osmotic effect resulting in astrocyte swelling. In addition, it serves as a "Trojan horse" by releasing ammonia inside the cell that causes mitochondrial dysfunction and oxidative stress, which in turn results in cytotoxicity and cellular edema.[11,12] Furthermore, release of inflammatory cytokines leads to systemic vasodilation and increased intracranial blood volume.[13]

Intracranial Pressure Monitoring

Although leading transplant centers in the United States tend to employ intracranial pressure (ICP) measurement, there are no randomized trials or consensus guidelines to support this practice.[14] ICP is often measured to have an objective parameter to aid in management and prognostication. However, target values are not well-defined and monitor placement is associated with the risk of intracerebral bleeding that may occur in 8% to 10% of cases, although less frequently with an epidural catheter.[15,16] This risk has been shown to be mitigated by the use of recombinant activated factor VII (rFVIIa).[17] Some centers use ICP monitors routinely, whereas others employ it in patients who are at the highest risk of cerebral edema, including those with grades III to IV hepatic encephalopathy, or those receiving vasopressors.[18] Intracranial monitors are more frequently used among patients listed for liver transplantation.[18] The United States Acute Liver Failure Study Group endorses the use of ICP monitors in patients with a high risk of ICH, including nontransplant candidates who have increased likelihood of spontaneous survival.[14]

Cerebral Blood Flow Measurement

ALF is associated with the loss of cerebral blood flow autoregulation.[19] Depending on the cerebral perfusion pressure (CPP), either cerebral hyperemia or hypoxia could develop. Measurement of cerebral blood flow (CBF), in addition to ICP monitoring, may therefore help to manage such patients.[20] Still, CBF-oriented therapies are difficult to implement because the metabolic demands of the brain vary depending on the patient's underlying level of inflammation or sedation, and there is no evidence that CBF monitoring influences outcome.[21] Several tools are available for the indirect measurement of CBF, including the jugular bulb catheter, transcranial Doppler, and xenon-enhanced computed tomography (CT).

Jugular bulb
A jugular bulb catheter may be utilized to assess cerebrovascular autoregulation. This process involves passage of a fine-bore catheter into the internal jugular vein until the tip reaches the jugular bulb, thereby allowing for sampling of blood that drains exclusively from intracranial circulation.[22] Cerebral oxygen uptake is then determined by calculating the arteriojugular oxygen content difference in paired blood samples.[23] During assessment of cerebral autoregulation, it is assumed that cerebral metabolic rate of oxygen remains constant so that the arteriojugular oxygen content difference solely reflects CBF. In reality, the cerebral metabolic rate of oxygen may vary, and that limits the utility of the jugular bulb in the assessment of CBF autoregulation. Jugular bulb placement may also be used to measure brain cytokine production indicative of an inflammatory response that correlates with the severity of ICP.[13]

Transcranial Doppler ultrasonography
Transcranial Doppler ultrasound is a noninvasive method to measure blood flow velocity in the basal intracranial cerebral arteries, thereby indirectly determining CBF via the linear relationship between flow and velocity.[24] Blood flow velocity and CBF measured by transcranial Doppler has been shown to correlate with xenon-enhanced CT determination of CBF.[25] Among patients with ALF, monitoring with transcranial Doppler provides an assessment of cerebral hemodynamics and could be used to predict dynamic changes in CBF and ICP.[26]

Xenon-enhanced CT
CBF measurement with xenon, an inert anesthetic gas, was first described 40 years ago.[27] After the advent of CT, xenon-enhanced scanning was developed to determine regional blood flow.[28] Xenon CT provides both anatomic and functional information that could help to manage patients with ALF.[29] However, there are disadvantages to this modality. For instance, the reproducibility of findings is poor as comparisons of the same region from one study to another are difficult. Furthermore, CBF assessment is restricted to mainly cortical and subcortical regions within the territory of the middle cerebral artery.[21] There is no consensus regarding the use of xenon-enhanced CT in patients with ALF and its application therefore remains limited.

Electroencephalography
Seizure activity is not uncommon among patients with ALF[30]; however, it is often masked by the use of sedatives and paralytic agents. Seizures may acutely elevate ICP,[31] and may also increase cerebral oxygen consumption resulting in ischemia and worsening cerebral edema. Monitoring by continuous electroencephalography would detect subclinical seizure activity that could be treated with anti-epileptic agents.[32] Studies examining the effect of prophylactic anticonvulsants have remained inconclusive.[30,32]

ICH

Normal ICP in a supine healthy adult ranges from 7 to 15 mmHg.[21] The goal of therapy in ALF is to maintain ICP below 20 and 25 mmHg and to preserve CPP, calculated as mean arterial pressure (MAP) – ICP, at 50 to 60 mmHg.[1] Among trauma patients, CPP of 70 mmHg has been noted to be beneficial.[33] However, such goals are not well-defined and are based on the experiences of individual centers.[14] CPP indicates pressure gradient across the cerebral vascular bed.[21] The rationale of increasing the CPP is to enhance CBF to regions of the brain with critically low flow when autoregulation has failed or CPP is below the lower limit of autoregulation.[33]

Initial maneuvers should include elevation of the head of the bed to 30 degrees, maintenance of a neutral neck position and minimizing painful stimuli to reduce patient agitation.[1] Additional modalities include hyperventilation, which rapidly but transiently restores autoregulation of CBF by lowering the partial pressure of carbon dioxide in arterial blood ($PaCO_2$), hypothermia, and medical treatment including mannitol and thiopental.[34,35] Limited evidence also supports the use of hypertonic saline, propofol sedation, and indomethacin.[36,37]

Hyperventilation

Hyperventilation provides a rapid but transient improvement in ICP, with restoration of cerebral autoregulation within several minutes.[38] The goal of hyperventilation is to induce the hypocapnia that causes cerebral vasoconstriction, which in turn reduces CBF leading to a decrease in ICP.[39] In brain-injured patients, both moderate ($PaCO_2$, 31–35 mmHg) and forced ($PaCO_2 \leq 30$ mmHg) hyperventilation have been used to treat ICH.[40] Although hyperventilation effectively reduces ICP, there is concern that the resultant vasoconstriction could worsen cerebral hypoxia and even cause ischemia.[39,40] Careful monitoring of cerebral perfusion and oxygenation is therefore essential. There is no role for prophylactic hyperventilation in patients with ALF.[34] Hyperventilation is likely best used as short-term rescue therapy.[41]

Mannitol

Intravenous mannitol is a potent osmotic agent that does not cross the blood–brain barrier.[42] It reduces ICP by osmotically drawing water from the brain parenchyma into the intravascular space. Although widely accepted as first-line medical therapy for ICH in ALF, there are few published studies to support its use.[35,43] Mannitol is typically administered as a 20% solution in intravenous boluses of 0.25 to 1 g/kg that are repeated every 4 to 6 hours depending on ICP response. Serum osmolality should be measured before each dose, because a serum osmolality greater than 320 mOsm is associated with greater risk of renal tubular toxicity. However, the evidence for this threshold remains obscure.[42] A retrospective study of 605 patients treated with mannitol showed increased mortality only with severe hypernatremia that equated to serum osmolality of 335 to 340 mOsm.[42] Mannitol may thus be used safely, even if higher serum osmolalities are reached, as long as adequate hydration is maintained. Additionally, mannitol fails to normalize ICP once a level of greater than 60 mmHg is reached.

Hypothermia

Hypothermia can transiently reduce ICP in patients with cerebral edema who are refractory to medical therapy. It could thus be used as a bridge to recovery or to liver transplantation. Hypothermia reduces ICP by restoring CBF autoregulation and reactivity to CO_2.[44] The efficacy of moderate hypothermia, as defined by a reduction in core body temperature to 32°C to 33°C, was first noted in brain-injured patients.[45] In subsequent studies among patients with ALF, hypothermia seemed to hasten neurologic recovery.[46] However, the clinical evidence regarding induced hypothermia is limited to small case series.[46,47] A meta-analysis of 5 case series demonstrated that ICP monitoring combined with hypothermia led to improved ICP, CPP, and CBF in 4 of the 5 studies.[48] Hypothermia could be induced by external cooling blankets, intravascular cooling devices, and body suits with monitoring of core body temperatures via a rectal or intravascular thermometer. A paralytic agent or a deep sedative may be needed to prevent reflexive shivering. Moderate hypothermia needs to be used cautiously in view of the potential risks including cardiac arrhythmias, coagulopathy, hypotension, and impaired liver regeneration. Mild hypothermia (core temperature of 34°C–35°C) may also be beneficial with a lesser likelihood of adverse effects.[49] Randomized, controlled trials are needed to confirm the benefits of hypothermia before it is applied routinely.

Hypertonic Saline

Uncontrolled studies of hypertonic saline in patients with traumatic brain injury showed favorable effect on systemic hemodynamics and ICP.[50] Hypertonic saline and dextran solution was noted to be superior to mannitol infusion in another study.[51] However, a recently published, large, randomized trial failed to show a beneficial effect of hypertonic saline on neurologic outcome or survival.[52] The experience in patients with ALF has remained limited. A study of 30 patients with ALF and grades III or IV encephalopathy showed a reduction in the incidence and severity of ICH with hypertonic saline infusion in comparison with the standard of care.[36] Hypertonic saline mitigates ICH through both osmotic and nonosmotic effects. The blood–brain barrier prevents the free flow of water and solutes into and out of the cerebral cells. A high level of circulating sodium creates a gradient that favors the movement of water from the brain tissue into the circulation.[53] It also reduces endothelial swelling that improves CBF through the microcirculation. Hypertonic saline inhibits neutrophil activation and release of proinflammatory cytokines that may help control the systemic inflammatory response syndrome (SIRS) that is often a component of ALF.[54,55]

Hypertonic saline is administered as a continuous infusion or as boluses through a central venous catheter to prevent phlebitis. In addition, potassium and magnesium supplementation may be necessary to avoid the risk of cardiac arrhythmia. Other possible adverse effects include pulmonary edema, central pontine myelinolysis, and hyperchloremic metabolic acidosis.

Barbiturates

Thiopental and pentobarbital are centrally acting hypnotics that reduce brain oxygen utilization. They are considered second-line therapy for severe ICH.[56] Their administration requires continuous electroencephalographic monitoring for dose titration. Because barbiturate infusion may cause systemic hypotension, blood pressure support is often needed to maintain an adequate CPP. Other adverse effects include cardiac arrhythmia and immune suppression that increases the risk of infections and ileus.

COAGULOPATHY

The liver plays a central role in hemostasis as it synthesizes almost all coagulation factors; in addition, it produces many inhibitors of coagulation and proteins involved in fibrinolysis. Coagulopathy [International Normalized Ratio (INR) > 1.5] is therefore considered a key feature of ALF.[1] There are a number of factors involved in the bleeding and clotting diatheses seen in ALF including platelet dysfunction (quantitative and qualitative) and deficiency of clotting factors (II, V, VII, IX, and X) and possibly that of vitamin K.[3] There are reduced levels of fibrinolytic proteins except plasminogen activator inhibitor-1 that is greatly increased, resulting in suppression of fibrinolysis.[57] Anticoagulant factors such as antithrombin III and proteins C and S are also reduced that further helps to rebalance the system.[58] Hemostatic changes in ALF thus incorporate a coagulopathy (measured as prolonged prothrombin and partial thromboplastin time) as well as a tendency to develop thrombotic events such as disseminated intravascular coagulation.[59,60]

In a patient with ALF, correction of the INR to a level that is considered normal is not required for prophylactic purposes and it is likely unobtainable.[61] Any improvement in INR from fresh frozen plasma (FFP) is transient and correction also obscures prothrombin time as a prognostic marker. However, an attempt at improving coagulation parameters is recommended in situations such as clinically significant bleeding, before performing an invasive procedure with high bleeding risk, or before insertion of an ICP monitoring device.[1] There are insufficient data available to support a specific platelet count or INR, although general guidelines include an INR of less than 1.5 and platelet count of more than 50,000/mL.[1] Cryoprecipitate is recommended in patients who have significant hypofibrinogenemia (<100 mg/dL).[14] Administration of vitamin K may be helpful and should be considered in all patients with ALF. However, because of the potential for poor absorption of oral vitamin K, especially in those with bowel wall edema or cholestatic jaundice, intravenous vitamin K is recommended.[62] For patients who do not respond to FFP or who cannot receive FFP owing to volume overload or risk of adverse reactions, rFVIIa may be given.[63] It is advisable to replenish other coagulation factors with FFP and fibrinogen with cryoprecipitate, before rFVIIa is administered.[14] The effect of rFVIIa persists for approximately 2 to 6 hours.[63] Because rFVIIa increases the risk of thrombosis, it should be avoided in patients with prior myocardial infarction, ischemic stroke, or pulmonary embolism, as well as in those with ALF from pregnancy, acute portal vein thrombosis, or Budd–Chiari syndrome.

INFECTIONS AND SIRS

Patients with ALF are highly susceptible to infections. Bacterial infections have been documented in 80% of the cases, most commonly pneumonia (50%), urinary tract infections (22%), intravenous catheter-induced bacteremia (12%), and spontaneous bacteremia (16%).[64] Gram-negative enteric bacilli and gram-positive cocci are most frequently isolated. Fungal infections occur in about one third, largely with candida species.[65] In addition to their propensity to infections, patients with ALF have accentuated hemodynamic, hormonal, and cytokine responses associated with SIRS and septic shock.[66,67] Patients who develop SIRS are more likely to have worsening hepatic encephalopathy and poor outcome.[68] ALF patients may therefore benefit from routine microbiologic surveillance for early detection and treatment of infections. Although evidence supporting the routine use of prophylactic antibiotics is limited to small studies that showed no effect on survival, such a strategy may be beneficial in those with worsening encephalopathy and progression to SIRS.[68–71] Empiric antibiotics are also recommended for patients listed for liver transplantation, because development of infection and sepsis may prompt delisting.[14]

METABOLIC ISSUES AND RENAL FAILURE

Metabolic and electrolyte abnormalities are common in ALF. Patients are prone to develop hypoglycemia because hepatocyte necrosis causes glycogen depletion and defective glycogenolysis and gluconeogenesis.[72] Dextrose infusion would correct the abnormality, but hyponatremia should be avoided because it may exacerbate cerebral edema. Serum phosphate, magnesium, and potassium levels are frequently low and need supplementation. Relative adrenal insufficiency develops in one third of the patients, requiring steroid replacement.[73] Owing to the hypercatabolic state of ALF, nutrition is vital and enteral feedings should be initiated early. If enteral feedings are contraindicated, parenteral nutrition may be utilized.[74]

Renal failure develops in 40% to 50% of patients with ALF.[7,75] A number of factors contribute to the development of renal failure that may present as the hepatorenal syndrome, prerenal azotemia, or acute tubular necrosis. Such factors include toxic agents inducing ALF that are also nephrotoxic (acetaminophen, amanita), other nephrotoxic medications, sepsis, and volume depletion. Management involves withdrawal of nephrotoxic agents, correction of hypovolemia and renal support. The decision to start renal replacement therapy should be based on the level of renal dysfunction, volume overload, and metabolic derangements, such as acidosis and hyperkalemia. Continuous renal replacement therapy is recommended because patients with ALF tolerate intermittent hemodialysis poorly because of hemodynamic instability, fluid shifts and a rise in ICP.[1,76]

CARDIOVASCULAR AND RESPIRATORY SUPPORT

ALF is characterized by a hyperdynamic circulation with high cardiac output, low arterial pressures, and diminished systemic vascular resistance.[77] This results in reduced oxygen delivery and consumption, increasing the risk of tissue hypoxia.[78] Fluid resuscitation is often required and is usually achieved with colloid infusion.[1] After fluid resuscitation, intravenous dopamine or norepinephrine may be initiated to maintain an adequate MAP and CPP.[1] CBF in ALF correlates with arterial pressure owing to loss of autoregulation. It is, therefore, important to maintain cardiovascular stability with well-titrated doses of pressors to avoid worsening cerebral hyperemia and edema.[79] Terlipressin, a vasopressin synthetic analog, has been evaluated in 2 small studies with conflicting results.[80,81] One of the studies raised concern that terlipressin and vasopressin may worsen cerebral hyperemia and ICH.[80]

The development of severe acute lung injury is associated with poor prognosis in ALF.[82] Acute lung injury is characterized by impaired gas exchange and bilateral alveolar or interstitial infiltrates in the absence of congestive cardiac failure.[83] Among patients with ALF, acute lung injury increases the risk of circulatory failure and cerebral edema.[82] Endotracheal intubation is needed in patients with respiratory failure, severe hepatic encephalopathy, or agitation, and before placement of an ICP monitor. There are insufficient data to recommend a standard mode of mechanical ventilation in patients with ALF. Low tidal volume ventilation is beneficial; it is associated with reduced mortality and shorter duration of ventilator use.[84] However, it must be appreciated that decrements in tidal volume decrease minute ventilation and increase the partial pressure of carbon dioxide, which may increase ICP. Respiratory rate should therefore be increased to avoid marked hypercapnia. It is also prudent to maintain the lowest level of positive end-expiratory pressure that achieves adequate oxygenation because high levels may decrease hepatic blood flow.[85]

NONSPECIFIC MEASURES
N-Acetylcysteine

N-acetylcysteine (NAC) is routinely used in acetaminophen induced hepatotoxicity.[86,87] It acts by replenishing glutathione that detoxifies the metabolite, N-acetyl-p-benzo-quinoneimine.[88] In addition, excess NAC also provides substrates for hepatic ATP synthesis, thus supporting mitochondrial energy metabolism.[89] The latter pathway may be particularly important in delayed NAC administration. NAC, when used early, prevents the development of ALF in patients with acetaminophen toxicity; among those who develop ALF, it improves survival.[90]

NAC was also used in non–acetaminophen-induced ALF because it was noted to improve systemic hemodynamics and tissue oxygen delivery and consumption.[91] However, its role remained unclear.[92] A recent randomized, placebo-controlled study showed improved transplant-free survival in patients with non–acetaminophen-induced ALF.[93] This improvement was primarily noted among patients with early (grades I–II) hepatic encephalopathy. No benefit was seen among patients with more advanced encephalopathy. The findings of the study suggested that, for NAC to be effective, it should be initiated early in the disease course. In addition, many patients with ALF of indeterminate etiology may have underlying acetaminophen toxicity, which further supports the use of NAC in all cases.[94]

LIVER-ASSIST DEVICES

Liver-assist devices, if effective, could potentially bridge the patient to liver transplantation or provide vital support during severe functional failure that precedes recovery. Liver-assist devices are either based on blood detoxification or biologic support provided by hepatocytes.

Detoxification Devices

Earlier attempts at extracorporeal liver support involved plasma exchange, whole blood transfusion, hemoperfusion, standard hemodialysis, and high-permeability dialysis.[95,96] Those methods attempted to remove liver toxins, but they lacked efficacy and failed to show significant clinical improvement. In membrane separation methods, toxin removal was largely dependent on the size of the molecules relative to the membrane pore size. Small pore sizes ensured selectivity at the expense of efficacy.[97] The introduction of sorbents (activated charcoal and resins) in hemoperfusion was an improvement because they could preferentially bind toxins without binding nutrients.[98,99] Such devices removed small toxin molecules and larger protein-bound toxins; however, thrombocytopenia, bleeding, and coagulation diatheses and electrolyte imbalances were problematic.

With the realization that most liver toxins are small, hydrophobic molecules that bind to albumin, albumin dialysis methods were introduced. Albumin dialysis attempts to remove molecules, especially albumin-bound toxins, through a dialysis membrane when the dialysate is clean albumin. The system combines the selectivity of a small-pore membrane for molecule transfer with the efficacy of albumin as a molecular adsorbent.[97] It, therefore, has the advantage of removing a wider array of substances compared to hemodialysis. One such system is the molecular adsorbent recirculating system (MARS), which was introduced in 1998 for clinical use.[100] The system is composed of a high-flux hemodialysis membrane separating blood and 5% albumin. Circulating protein-bound liver toxins are transferred from the blood to the albumin dialysate through the membrane. Used dialysate is regenerated by passage through an activated carbon column and an anionic exchange resin column. The MARS device is added to a standard hemodialysis unit in line with the dialyzer; the latter removes small, water-soluble hepatic and renal toxins, such as ammonium and aromatic amino acids. ALF is among the major indications for MARS, particularly among patients with hemodynamic instability. In ALF, MARS causes a rise in systemic vascular resistance and MAP that could result in improved tissue perfusion.[101] A lowering of raised ICP has also been reported.[102] Although there are no controlled studies showing an impact on survival, MARS could be used to stabilize patients while they await a liver allograft. It could potentially enlarge the window for liver transplantation and in some may even help avoid the procedure.[103] Another liver support device is Prometheus, which removes albumin-bound molecules through a modified fractionated plasma separation and adsorption method.[104] It seems to be well-tolerated and may be beneficial, but evidence based on controlled trials is lacking.[105]

Bioartificial Liver Support

Because early detoxification devices failed to show significant clinical promise largely because of their inability to provide physiologic functional support, emphasis shifted to bioartificial liver (BAL). A BAL device is composed of a cartridge (bioreactor) with hollow membrane fibers similar to that used for dialysis.[106] Blood flows through the hollow fibers; the space outside is filled with hepatocytes. The system thus separates circulating blood from hepatocytes by a semipermeable membrane that allows passage of low-molecular-weight molecules. Hepatocytes may remain viable for prolonged periods and provide essential hepatic functions, including protein synthesis, metabolism, conjugation, and detoxification. Several devices have been developed that differ in cell type and design of bioreactor.[107] Currently, a major limitation of BAL is the supply of healthy human hepatocytes. Human embryonic stem cells may provide a more reliable source of hepatocytes that would enable development of robust liver support systems.[108] A selection of BAL devices is described.

Extracorporeal liver assist device

The extracorporeal liver assist device (ELAD) incorporated a hollow fiber bioreactor loaded with human hepatoblastoma (HepG2) cell line.[109] Initial clinical study showed ELAD to provide metabolic support without triggering safety concerns.[110] In a pilot study of patients with ALF, those on ELAD remained hemodynamically stable and were less likely to develop worsening hepatic encephalopathy.[111] The device caused a decline in serum bilirubin and arterial ammonia levels, but there was no effect on survival.

HepatAssist

The HepatAssist device was created as a hybrid liver support system composed of plasma perfusion through a charcoal column and a porous hollow fiber cartridge that contained matrix-attached porcine hepatocytes.[112] Animal studies showed reduction in serum ammonia and lactate levels and an increase in glucose level and blood pressure.[112] In a large, randomized, multicenter, controlled trial of patients with ALF or primary nonfunction of liver allograft, HepatAssist showed no overall benefit in survival.[113] However, a subset analysis of patients with ALF showed survival benefit in those treated with the device.

Academic Medical Center BAL

Developed at the Academic Medical Center of Amsterdam, this devise seeks to bridge patients with ALF to liver transplantation.[114] The system perfused blood through a bioreactor that contained porcine hepatocytes obtained from a specified pathogen free animal. The treatment was well-tolerated and most patients treated in a pilot study were bridged to transplantation.[114] Neurologic and hemodynamic improvement was noted, and there was a decline in serum bilirubin and blood ammonia levels.

BAL Support System

The BAL Support System was developed at the University of Pittsburgh. The device used porcine liver cells housed in a hollow fiber bioreactor.[115] A limited number of patients were treated and all tolerated the treatment well. Moderate biochemical response was noted. Studies in a canine liver failure model showed delay in an increase in blood ammonia, lactate, and prothrombin time.[116]

LIVER TRANSPLANTATION

Liver transplantation is required for all patients with ALF determined to have irreversible liver injury. It is, therefore, mandatory to transfer patients to a liver transplant center in a timely fashion so that the procedure can be applied before contraindications develop. Euglycemia and cardiorespiratory stability have to be ensured during transfer. Contraindications to transplantation include sepsis, severe cardiorespiratory failure, marked ICH with low CPP, and extrahepatic malignancy. Patients with ALF are assigned the highest category for donor allocation in view of the emergent need for transplantation. Prognostic assessment is critical in the decision to list and transplant, because the risks of surgery and long-term immunosuppression have to be weighed against the likelihood of spontaneous recovery.[117] Most centers perform traditional orthotopic liver transplantation, but living donor and auxiliary transplantation have been applied.[118,119] The outcome with all 3 modalities is good, with a 1-year survival rate around 85%. In view of the rarity of the syndrome, ALF remains an uncommon reason for liver transplantation. During 2009 and 2010, 10% of pediatric and 4% of adult liver transplant recipients in the United States were reported to have "acute hepatic necrosis" (Organ Procurement and Transplantation Network; available at: http://optn.transplant.hrsa.gov, updated March 18, 2011).

HEPATOCYTE TRANSPLANTATION

Hepatocyte transplantation involves injection of donor hepatocytes into the liver or spleen.[120] Donor hepatocytes then integrate into the local tissues with the potential to restore hepatic functions in a patient with ALF. Typically, hepatic regeneration follows significant liver injury. Thus, many patients with ALF recover spontaneously without the need for liver transplantation.[121] In view of the difficulty of predicting complete recovery in a patient with ALF, auxiliary liver transplantation has been applied to provide liver support during the phase of severe functional impairment.[119] Once native liver has recovered, immunosuppression is withdrawn, which results in graft atrophy. The procedure eliminates the long-term risks associated with whole liver replacement and immunosuppression. Hepatocyte transplantation is far less invasive than auxiliary transplantation and potentially serves the same purpose. Clinical studies have demonstrated the safety of hepatocyte transplantation.[122] However, several issues need to be resolved before this technique can be widely applied. There remains a shortage of viable donor hepatocytes. Cells are usually obtained from livers deemed unsuitable for transplantation or from unused segments in split-liver transplants.[123] One option is to use livers that are considered suboptimal for transplantation such as "donation after cardiac death" donors.[124] The actual mass of hepatocytes needed to provide optimal support in ALF also remains uncertain.[120] Hepatocytes are often cryopreserved that affects their viability; new cryopreservation protocols are being developed to improve cell survival and function.[125] Embryonic and bone marrow–derived stem cells provide another option to aid hepatic regeneration.[126]

SUMMARY

ALF is an important cause of liver-related morbidity and mortality. Advances in the management of ICH and SIRS, and cardiorespiratory, metabolic, and renal support have improved the outlook of such patients. Early transfer to a liver transplant center is essential. Routine use of NAC is recommended for patients with early hepatic encephalopathy, irrespective of the etiology. The role of hypothermia remains to be determined. Liver transplantation plays a critical role, particularly for those with advanced encephalopathy. Several detoxification and BAL support systems have been developed to serve as a bridge to transplantation or to spontaneous recovery. However, such systems lack sufficient reliability and efficacy to be applied routinely in clinical practice. Hepatocyte and stem cell transplantation may provide valuable adjunctive therapy in the future.

REFERENCES

1. Polson J, Lee WM, American Association for the Study of Liver D. AASLD position paper: the management of acute liver failure. Hepatology 2005;41:1179–97.
2. Shakil AO, Jones BC, Lee RG, et al. Prognostic value of abdominal CT scanning and hepatic histopathology in patients with acute liver failure. Dig Dis Sci 2000;45:334–9.
3. Sass DA, Shakil AO. Fulminant hepatic failure. Liver Transpl 2005;11:594–605.
4. Lee WM, Seremba E. Etiologies of acute liver failure. Curr Opin Crit Care 2008;14: 198–201.
5. Khuroo MS, Kamili S. Aetiology and prognostic factors in acute liver failure in India. J Viral Hepat 2003;10:224–31.
6. Sarwar S, Khan AA, Alam A, et al. Predictors of fatal outcome in fulminant hepatic failure. J Coll Physicians Surg Pak 2006;16:112–6.
7. Shakil AO, Kramer D, Mazariegos GV, et al. Acute liver failure: clinical features, outcome analysis, and applicability of prognostic criteria. Liver Transpl 2000;6: 163–9.
8. O'Grady JG, Schalm SW, Williams R. Acute liver failure: redefining the syndromes. Lancet 1993;342:273–5.
9. Blei AT. Brain edema in acute liver failure. Crit Care Clin 2008;24:99–114.
10. Jackson EW, Zacks S, Zinn S, et al. Delayed neuropsychologic dysfunction after liver transplantation for acute liver failure: a matched, case-controlled study. Liver Transpl 2002;8:932–6.
11. Bjerring PN, Eefsen M, Hansen BA, et al. The brain in acute liver failure. A tortuous path from hyperammonemia to cerebral edema. Metab Brain Dis 2009;24:5–14.
12. Ranjan P, Mishra AM, Kale R, et al. Cytotoxic edema is responsible for raised intracranial pressure in fulminant hepatic failure: in vivo demonstration using diffusion-weighted MRI in human subjects. Metab Brain Dis 2005;20:181–92.
13. Wright G, Shawcross D, Olde Damink SWM, et al. Brain cytokine flux in acute liver failure and its relationship with intracranial hypertension. Metab Brain Dis 2007;22: 375–88.
14. Stravitz RT, Kramer AH, Davern T, et al. Intensive care of patients with acute liver failure: recommendations of the U.S. Acute Liver Failure Study Group. Crit Care Med 2007;35:2498–508.
15. Blei AT, Olafsson S, Webster S, et al. Complications of intracranial pressure monitoring in fulminant hepatic failure. Lancet 1993;341:157–8.

16. Keays RT, Alexander GJ, Williams R. The safety and value of extradural intracranial pressure monitors in fulminant hepatic failure. J Hepatol 1993;18:205–9.

17. Le TV, Rumbak MJ, Liu SS, et al. Insertion of intracranial pressure monitors in fulminant hepatic failure patients: early experience using recombinant factor VII. Neurosurgery 2010;66:455–8.

18. Vaquero J, Fontana RJ, Larson AM, et al. Complications and use of intracranial pressure monitoring in patients with acute liver failure and severe encephalopathy. Liver Transpl 2005;11:1581–9.

19. Larsen FS, Ejlersen E, Hansen BA, et al. Functional loss of cerebral blood flow autoregulation in patients with fulminant hepatic failure. J Hepatol 1995;23:212–7.

20. Czosnyka M, Brady K, Reinhard M, et al. Monitoring of cerebrovascular autoregulation: facts, myths, and missing links. Neurocrit Care 2009;10:373–86.

21. Steiner LA, Andrews PJD. Monitoring the injured brain: ICP and CBF. Br J Anaesth 2006;97:26–38.

22. Goetting MG, Preston G. Jugular bulb catheterization: experience with 123 patients. Crit Care Med 1990;18:1220–3.

23. Steiner LA, Coles JP, Johnston AJ, et al. Assessment of cerebrovascular autoregulation in head-injured patients: a validation study. Stroke 2003;34:2404–9.

24. Newell DW, Aaslid R. Transcranial Doppler: clinical and experimental uses. Cerebrovasc Brain Metab Rev 1992;4:122–43.

25. Kofke WA, Brauer P, Policare R, et al. Middle cerebral artery blood flow velocity and stable xenon-enhanced computed tomographic blood flow during balloon test occlusion of the internal carotid artery. Stroke 1995;26:1603–6.

26. Aggarwal S, Brooks DM, Kang Y, et al. Noninvasive monitoring of cerebral perfusion pressure in patients with acute liver failure using transcranial Doppler ultrasonography. Liver Transpl 2008;14:1048–57.

27. Torizuka K, Hamamoto K, Morita R, et al. Regional cerebral blood flow measurement with xenon 133 and the scinticamera. Am J Roentgenol Radium Ther Nucl Med 1971;112:691–700.

28. Gur D, Wolfson SK Jr, Yonas H, et al. Progress in cerebrovascular disease: local cerebral blood flow by xenon enhanced CT. Stroke 1982;13:750–8.

29. Durham S, Yonas H, Aggarwal S, et al. Regional cerebral blood flow and CO2 reactivity in fulminant hepatic failure. J Cereb Blood Flow Metab 1995;15:329–35.

30. Bhatia V, Batra Y, Acharya SK. Prophylactic phenytoin does not improve cerebral edema or survival in acute liver failure—a controlled clinical trial. J Hepatol 2004;41:89–96.

31. Gabor AJ, Brooks AG, Scobey RP, et al. Intracranial pressure during epileptic seizures. Electroencephalogr Clin Neurophysiol 1984;57:497–506.

32. Ellis AJ, Wendon JA, Williams R. Subclinical seizure activity and prophylactic phenytoin infusion in acute liver failure: a controlled clinical trial. Hepatology 2000;32:536–41.

33. Mascia L, Andrews PJ, McKeating EG, et al. Cerebral blood flow and metabolism in severe brain injury: the role of pressure autoregulation during cerebral perfusion pressure management. Intensive Care Med 2000;26:202–5.

34. Ede RJ, Gimson AE, Bihari D, et al. Controlled hyperventilation in the prevention of cerebral oedema in fulminant hepatic failure. J Hepatol 1986;2:43–51.

35. Canalese J, Gimson AE, Davis C, et al. Controlled trial of dexamethasone and mannitol for the cerebral oedema of fulminant hepatic failure. Gut 1982;23:625–9.

36. Murphy N, Auzinger G, Bernel W, et al. The effect of hypertonic sodium chloride on intracranial pressure in patients with acute liver failure. Hepatology 2004;39:464–70.

37. Tofteng F, Larsen FS. The effect of indomethacin on intracranial pressure, cerebral perfusion and extracellular lactate and glutamate concentrations in patients with fulminant hepatic failure. J Cereb Blood Flow Metab 2004;24:798–804.
38. Strauss G, Hansen BA, Knudsen GM, et al. Hyperventilation restores cerebral blood flow autoregulation in patients with acute liver failure. J Hepatol 1998;28:199–203.
39. Curley G, Kavanagh BP, Laffey JG. Hypocapnia and the injured brain: more harm than benefit. Crit Care Med 2010;38:1348–59.
40. Neumann JO, Chambers IR, Citerio G, et al. The use of hyperventilation therapy after traumatic brain injury in Europe: an analysis of the BrainIT database. Intensive Care Med 2008;34:1676–82.
41. Rabinstein AA. Treatment of brain edema in acute liver failure. Curr Treat Options Neurol 2010;12:129–41.
42. Diringer MN, Zazulia AR. Osmotic therapy: fact and fiction. Neurocrit Care 2004;1: 219–33.
43. Wendon JA, Harrison PM, Keays R, et al. Cerebral blood flow and metabolism in fulminant liver failure. Hepatology 1994;19:1407–13.
44. Jalan R, Olde Damink SW, Deutz NE, et al. Restoration of cerebral blood flow autoregulation and reactivity to carbon dioxide in acute liver failure by moderate hypothermia. Hepatology 2001;34:50–4.
45. Marion DW, Penrod LE, Kelsey SF, et al. Treatment of traumatic brain injury with moderate hypothermia. N Engl J Med 1997;336:540–6.
46. Jalan R, Olde Damink SW, Deutz NE, et al. Moderate hypothermia in patients with acute liver failure and uncontrolled intracranial hypertension. Gastroenterology 2004; 127:1338–46.
47. Jalan R, O Damink SW, Deutz NE, et al. Moderate hypothermia for uncontrolled intracranial hypertension in acute liver failure. Lancet 1999;354:1164–8.
48. Dmello D, Cruz-Flores S, Matuschak GM. Moderate hypothermia with intracranial pressure monitoring as a therapeutic paradigm for the management of acute liver failure: a systematic review. Intensive Care Med 2010;36:210–3.
49. Cordoba J, Crespin J, Gottstein J, et al. Mild hypothermia modifies ammonia-induced brain edema in rats after portacaval anastomosis. Gastroenterology 1999; 116:686–93.
50. Qureshi AI, Suarez JI. Use of hypertonic saline solutions in treatment of cerebral edema and intracranial hypertension. Crit Care Med 2000;28:3301–13.
51. Battison C, Andrews PJD, Graham C, et al. Randomized, controlled trial on the effect of a 20% mannitol solution and a 7.5% saline/6% dextran solution on increased intracranial pressure after brain injury. Crit Care Med 2005;33:196–202.
52. Bulger EM, May S, Brasel KJ, et al. Out-of-hospital hypertonic resuscitation following severe traumatic brain injury: a randomized controlled trial. JAMA 2010;304:1455–64.
53. Toung TJK, Chen C-H, Lin C, et al. Osmotherapy with hypertonic saline attenuates water content in brain and extracerebral organs. Crit Care Med 2007;35:526–31.
54. Jiang W, Desjardins P, Butterworth RF. Cerebral inflammation contributes to encephalopathy and brain edema in acute liver failure: protective effect of minocycline. J Neurochem 2009;109:485–93.
55. Rhind SG, Crnko NT, Baker AJ, et al. Prehospital resuscitation with hypertonic saline-dextran modulates inflammatory, coagulation and endothelial activation marker profiles in severe traumatic brain injured patients. J Neuroinflammation 2010;7:5.

56. Forbes A, Alexander GJ, O'Grady JG, et al. Thiopental infusion in the treatment of intracranial hypertension complicating fulminant hepatic failure. Hepatology 1989; 10:306–10.

57. Pernambuco JR, Langley PG, Hughes RD, et al. Activation of the fibrinolytic system in patients with fulminant liver failure. Hepatology 1993;18:1350–6.

58. Langley PG, Williams R. Physiological inhibitors of coagulation in fulminant hepatic failure. Blood Coagul Fibrinolysis 1992;3:243–7.

59. Langley PG, Forbes A, Hughes RD, et al. Thrombin-antithrombin III complex in fulminant hepatic failure: evidence for disseminated intravascular coagulation and relationship to outcome. Eur J Clin Invest 1990;20:627–31.

60. Lisman T, Caldwell SH, Burroughs AK, et al. Hemostasis and thrombosis in patients with liver disease: the ups and downs. J Hepatol 2010;53:362–71.

61. Gazzard BG, Henderson JM, Williams R. Early changes in coagulation following a paracetamol overdose and a controlled trial of fresh frozen plasma therapy. Gut 1975;16:617–20.

62. Pereira SP, Rowbotham D, Fitt S, et al. Pharmacokinetics and efficacy of oral versus intravenous mixed-micellar phylloquinone (vitamin K1) in severe acute liver disease. J Hepatol 2005;42:365–70.

63. Shami VM, Caldwell SH, Hespenheide EE, et al. Recombinant activated factor VII for coagulopathy in fulminant hepatic failure compared with conventional therapy. Liver Transpl 2003;9:138–43.

64. Rolando N, Philpott-Howard J, Williams R. Bacterial and fungal infection in acute liver failure. Semin Liver Dis 1996;16:389–402.

65. Rolando N, Harvey F, Brahm J, et al. Prospective study of bacterial infection in acute liver failure: an analysis of fifty patients. Hepatology 1990;11:49–53.

66. Rolando N, Wade J, Davalos M, et al. The systemic inflammatory response syndrome in acute liver failure. Hepatology 2000;32:734–9.

67. Tsai M-H, Chen Y-C, Lien J-M, et al. Hemodynamics and metabolic studies on septic shock in patients with acute liver failure. J Crit Care 2008;23:468–72.

68. Vaquero J, Polson J, Chung C, et al. Infection and the progression of hepatic encephalopathy in acute liver failure. Gastroenterology 2003;125:755–64.

69. Rolando N, Gimson A, Wade J, et al. Prospective controlled trial of selective parenteral and enteral antimicrobial regimen in fulminant liver failure. Hepatology 1993;17:196–201.

70. Rolando N, Wade JJ, Stangou A, et al. Prospective study comparing the efficacy of prophylactic parenteral antimicrobials, with or without enteral decontamination, in patients with acute liver failure. Liver Transpl Surg 1996;2:8–13.

71. Salmeron JM, Tito L, Rimola A, et al. Selective intestinal decontamination in the prevention of bacterial infection in patients with acute liver failure. J Hepatol 1992; 14:280–5.

72. Schneeweiss B, Pammer J, Ratheiser K, et al. Energy metabolism in acute hepatic failure. Gastroenterology 1993;105:1515–21.

73. O'Beirne J, Holmes M, Agarwal B, et al. Adrenal insufficiency in liver disease—what is the evidence? J Hepatol 2007;47:418–23.

74. Lee WM, Squires RH Jr, Nyberg SL, et al. Acute liver failure: summary of a workshop. Hepatology 2008;47:1401–15.

75. Ring-Larsen H, Palazzo U. Renal failure in fulminant hepatic failure and terminal cirrhosis: a comparison between incidence, types, and prognosis. Gut 1981;22: 585–91.

76. Davenport A, Will EJ, Davidson AM. Improved cardiovascular stability during continuous modes of renal replacement therapy in critically ill patients with acute hepatic and renal failure. Crit Care Med 1993;21:328–38.
77. Ellis A, Wendon J. Circulatory, respiratory, cerebral, and renal derangements in acute liver failure: pathophysiology and management. Semin Liver Dis 1996;16: 379–88.
78. Wendon JA, Harrison PM, Keays R, et al. Effects of vasopressor agents and epoprostenol on systemic hemodynamics and oxygen transport in fulminant hepatic failure. Hepatology 1992;15:1067–71.
79. Larsen FS, Strauss G, Knudsen GM, et al. Cerebral perfusion, cardiac output, and arterial pressure in patients with fulminant hepatic failure. Crit Care Med 2000;28: 996–1000.
80. Shawcross DL, Davies NA, Mookerjee RP, et al. Worsening of cerebral hyperemia by the administration of terlipressin in acute liver failure with severe encephalopathy. Hepatology 2004;39:471–5.
81. Eefsen M, Dethloff T, Frederiksen H-J, et al. Comparison of terlipressin and noradrenalin on cerebral perfusion, intracranial pressure and cerebral extracellular concentrations of lactate and pyruvate in patients with acute liver failure in need of inotropic support. J Hepatol 2007;47:381–6.
82. Baudouin SV, Howdle P, O'Grady JG, et al. Acute lung injury in fulminant hepatic failure following paracetamol poisoning. Thorax 1995;50:399–402.
83. Bernard GR, Artigas A, Brigham KL, et al. Report of the American-European consensus conference on ARDS: definitions, mechanisms, relevant outcomes and clinical trial coordination. The Consensus Committee. Intensive Care Med 1994;20: 225–32.
84. Anonymous. Ventilation with lower tidal volumes as compared with traditional tidal volumes for acute lung injury and the acute respiratory distress syndrome. The Acute Respiratory Distress Syndrome Network. N Engl J Med 2000;342:1301–8.
85. Bonnet F, Richard C, Glaser P, et al. Changes in hepatic flow induced by continuous positive pressure ventilation in critically ill patients. Crit Care Med 1982;10:703–5.
86. Prescott LF, Illingworth RN, Critchley JA, et al. Intravenous N-acetylcysteine: the treatment of choice for paracetamol poisoning. Br Med J 1979;2:1097–100.
87. Brok J, Buckley N, Gluud C. Interventions for paracetamol (acetaminophen) overdose. Cochrane Database Syst Rev 2006;2:CD003328.
88. Lauterburg BH, Corcoran GB, Mitchell JR. Mechanism of action of N-acetylcysteine in the protection against the hepatotoxicity of acetaminophen in rats in vivo. J Clin Invest 1983;71:980–91.
89. Saito C, Zwingmann C, Jaeschke H. Novel mechanisms of protection against acetaminophen hepatotoxicity in mice by glutathione and N-acetylcysteine. Hepatology 2010;51:246–54.
90. Keays R, Harrison PM, Wendon JA, et al. Intravenous acetylcysteine in paracetamol induced fulminant hepatic failure: a prospective controlled trial. BMJ 1991;303: 1026–9.
91. Harrison PM, Wendon JA, Gimson AE, et al. Improvement by acetylcysteine of hemodynamics and oxygen transport in fulminant hepatic failure. N Engl J Med 1991;324:1852–7.
92. Sklar GE, Subramaniam M. Acetylcysteine treatment for non-acetaminophen-induced acute liver failure. Ann Pharmacother 2004;38:498–500.
93. Lee WM, Hynan LS, Rossaro L, et al. Intravenous N-acetylcysteine improves transplant-free survival in early stage non-acetaminophen acute liver failure. Gastroenterology 2009;137:856–64.

94. Davern TJ 2nd, James LP, Hinson JA, et al. Measurement of serum acetaminophen-protein adducts in patients with acute liver failure. Gastroenterology 2006;130: 687–94.

95. Splendiani G, Tancredi M, Daniele M, et al. Treatment of acute liver failure with hemodetoxification techniques. Int J Artif Organs 1990;13:370–4.

96. Ash SR, Carr DJ, Sullivan TA. Sorbent suspension reactor for extracorporeal detoxification in hepatic failure or drug overdose. ASAIO J 2004;50:lviii–lxv.

97. Mitzner SR, Stange J, Klammt S, et al. Albumin dialysis MARS: knowledge from 10 years of clinical investigation. ASAIO J 2009;55:498–502.

98. O'Grady JG, Gimson AE, O'Brien CJ, et al. Controlled trials of charcoal hemoperfusion and prognostic factors in fulminant hepatic failure. Gastroenterology 1988;94: 1186–92.

99. Bihari D, Hughes RD, Gimson AE, et al. Effects of serial resin hemoperfusion in fulminant hepatic failure. Int J Artif Organs 1983;6:299–302.

100. Stange J, Mitzner SR, Risler T, et al. Molecular adsorbent recycling system (MARS): clinical results of a new membrane-based blood purification system for bioartificial liver support. Artif Organs 1999;23:319–30.

101. Schmidt LE, Wang LP, Hansen BA, et al. Systemic hemodynamic effects of treatment with the molecular adsorbents recirculating system in patients with hyperacute liver failure: a prospective controlled trial. Liver Transpl 2003;9:290–7.

102. Sen S, Rose C, Ytrebo LM, et al. Effect of albumin dialysis on intracranial pressure increase in pigs with acute liver failure: a randomized study. Crit Care Med 2006;34: 158–64.

103. Camus C, Lavoue S, Gacouin A, et al. Liver transplantation avoided in patients with fulminant hepatic failure who received albumin dialysis with the molecular adsorbent recirculating system while on the waiting list: impact of the duration of therapy. Therap Apher Dial 2009;13:549–55.

104. Rifai K, Ernst T, Kretschmer U, et al. Prometheus—a new extracorporeal system for the treatment of liver failure. J Hepatol 2003;39:984–90.

105. Oppert M, Rademacher S, Petrasch K, et al. Extracorporeal liver support therapy with Prometheus in patients with liver failure in the intensive care unit. Therap Apher Dial 2009;13:426–30.

106. Wang Y, Susando T, Lei X, et al. Current development of bioreactors for extracorporeal bioartificial liver (review). Biointerphases 2010;5:FA116–31.

107. Pless G. Bioartificial liver support systems. Methods Mol Biol 2010;640:511–23.

108. Sharma R, Greenhough S, Medine CN, et al. Three-dimensional culture of human embryonic stem cell derived hepatic endoderm and its role in bioartificial liver construction. J Biomed Biotechnol 2010;2010:236147.

109. Sussman NL, Chong MG, Koussayer T, et al. Reversal of fulminant hepatic failure using an extracorporeal liver assist device. Hepatology 1992;16:60–5.

110. Sussman NL, Gislason GT, Conlin CA, et al. The Hepatix extracorporeal liver assist device: initial clinical experience. Artif Organs 1994;18:390–6.

111. Ellis AJ, Hughes RD, Wendon JA, et al. Pilot-controlled trial of the extracorporeal liver assist device in acute liver failure. Hepatology 1996;24:1446–51.

112. Rozga J, Williams F, Ro MS, et al. Development of a bioartificial liver: properties and function of a hollow-fiber module inoculated with liver cells. Hepatology 1993;17: 258–65.

113. Demetriou AA, Brown RS Jr, Busuttil RW, et al. Prospective, randomized, multicenter, controlled trial of a bioartificial liver in treating acute liver failure. Ann Surg 2004;239:660–7.

114. van de Kerkhove MP, Di Florio E, Scuderi V, et al. Phase I clinical trial with the AMC-bioartificial liver. Int J Artif Organs 2002;25:950–9.
115. Mazariegos GV, Kramer DJ, Lopez RC, et al. Safety observations in phase I clinical evaluation of the Excorp Medical Bioartificial Liver Support System after the first four patients. ASAIO J 2001;47:471–5.
116. Patzer JF, 2nd, Mazariegos GV, Lopez R, et al. Preclinical evaluation of the Excorp Medical, Inc, Bioartificial Liver Support System. J Am Coll Surg 2002;195:299–310.
117. Shakil AO. Predicting the outcome of fulminant hepatic failure. Liver Transpl 2005; 11:1028–30.
118. Park SJ, Lim Y-S, Hwang S, et al. Emergency adult-to-adult living-donor liver transplantation for acute liver failure in a hepatitis B virus endemic area. Hepatology 2010;51:903–11.
119. Faraj W, Dar F, Bartlett A, et al. Auxiliary liver transplantation for acute liver failure in children. Ann Surg 2010;251:351–6.
120. Soltys KA, Soto-Gutierrez A, Nagaya M, et al. Barriers to the successful treatment of liver disease by hepatocyte transplantation. J Hepatol 2010;53:769–74.
121. Ostapowicz G, Fontana RJ, Schiodt FV, et al. Results of a prospective study of acute liver failure at 17 tertiary care centers in the United States. Ann Intern Med 2002; 137:947–54.
122. Bilir BM, Guinette D, Karrer F, et al. Hepatocyte transplantation in acute liver failure. Liver Transpl 2000;6:32–40.
123. Mitry RR, Dhawan A, Hughes RD, et al. One liver, three recipients: segment IV from split-liver procedures as a source of hepatocytes for cell transplantation. Transplantation 2004;77:1614–6.
124. Hughes RD, Mitry RR, Dhawan A, et al. Isolation of hepatocytes from livers from non-heart-beating donors for cell transplantation. Liver Transpl 2006;12:713–7.
125. Terry C, Dhawan A, Mitry RR, et al. Optimization of the cryopreservation and thawing protocol for human hepatocytes for use in cell transplantation. Liver Transpl 2010; 16:229–37.
126. Stutchfield BM, Forbes SJ, Wigmore SJ. Prospects for stem cell transplantation in the treatment of hepatic disease. Liver Transpl 2010;16:827–36.

Nonalcoholic Fatty Liver Disease: Pharmacologic and Surgical Options

Neil Parikh, MD[a], Jawad Ahmad, MD, FRCP[b],*

KEYWORDS

- Nonalcoholic fatty liver disease • Nonalcoholic steatohepatitis
- Pioglitazone • Vitamin E • Bariatric surgery

The association of hepatic steatosis with inflammatory changes and fibrosis in obese patients was first described over half a century ago.[1] Although initially thought to be a relatively benign entity, reports began emerging that in some circumstances fat in the liver could lead to cirrhosis or liver failure, as in patients undergoing surgical jejunoileal bypass for morbid obesity.[2]

The histologic features of "fatty liver disease" resemble alcohol-induced liver injury, but because they occur in patients with little or no alcohol consumption, the term nonalcoholic fatty liver disease (NAFLD) was coined. NAFLD is now recognized as one of the most common causes of chronic liver disease in the United States.[3]

NAFLD encompasses a spectrum of diseases that ranges from bland hepatic steatosis, which is generally believed to be a benign condition, to hepatic steatosis with a necroinflammatory component that may or may not have associated fibrosis. This latter condition is termed nonalcoholic steatohepatitis (NASH)[4] and is considered the 'progressive' form of NAFLD.[5]

It is estimated that NAFLD affects up to 25% of the general population[6] or 75 million Americans and that NASH affects approximately 8.6 million Americans, substantially higher than the estimated 1.6% prevalence of hepatitis C viral (HCV) infection.[7] As a result, NASH cirrhosis is projected to surpass HCV as the leading indication for orthotopic liver transplantation (OLT) in the next 10 years.[8]

The natural history and progression of NASH to cirrhosis is unclear with prevalence rates of 3% to 15% in case series[9–11] and small prospective cohorts have shown that NASH may progress to cirrhosis in 9% to 20% of patients.[12–14]

The pathogenesis of fatty liver disease and NASH is yet to be fully elucidated, but the common association with visceral obesity, hyperlipidemia, hypertension, and

[a] Division of Internal Medicine, Mount Sinai School of Medicine, 1 Gustave L. Levy Place, New York, NY 10029, USA
[b] Division of Liver Diseases, Mount Sinai School of Medicine, 1 Gustave L. Levy Place, New York, NY 10029, USA
* Corresponding author.
E-mail address: javbob@hotmail.com

Gastroenterol Clin N Am 40 (2011) 541–559
doi:10.1016/j.gtc.2011.06.001

diabetes mellitus suggests that it is the hepatic manifestation of the metabolic syndrome,[15] with at least 1 of these features present in over 90% of NAFLD patients.

Insulin resistance seems to play a pivotal role in the pathogenesis of NAFLD because it leads to hepatic steatosis. However, only a minority of such patients develops steatohepatitis and progressive liver disease; hence, other insults are required such as apoptosis, oxidative stress, and overexpression of inflammatory cytokines. Similarly, visceral obesity is implicated; it is associated with an increased release of a variety of adipokines [eg, adiponectin, leptin, tumor necrosis factor (TNF)-α], which seem to be important in the creating an environment for increased fibrosis.

Current therapy for NAFLD includes weight loss through diet and exercise and, in more extreme cases, bariatric surgery. Because there is such a strong association between NAFLD and the metabolic syndrome, many treatment options under investigation are aimed at improving insulin sensitivity; other studies have examined the effect of anti-inflammatory or anti-oxidant agents. This article reviews the current literature on pharmacologic and surgical options for NAFLD.

PHARMACOLOGIC TREATMENTS

The need for treatment in NAFLD is based on the concern for progressive liver disease and cirrhosis. Natural history studies indicate this occurs in a minority of patients, but the high prevalence of the disease means an effective treatment could have major economic and health benefits.

Several agents with differing mechanisms of action have been investigated in NAFLD and reflect the different pathways that are thought to be important in pathogenesis. Improving insulin resistance and reducing oxidative stress are the 2 main avenues that have been studied, but several other drugs have been examined.

Thiazolidinediones

Thiazolidinediones (TZDs) function as selective agonists for peroxisome proliferator activated nuclear receptor-γ. Various pathways have been implicated in hypothesizing TZDs actions in NAFLD, but the overriding actions seem to be decreasing hepatic fatty acid levels (by decreasing lipolysis and increasing β-oxidation), redistributing fat content from the liver to peripheral adipose tissue, and promoting insulin sensitivity by facilitating preadipocyte differentiation into insulin-sensitive adipocytes.[16,17] TZDs have also been shown to enhance adiponectin levels, a cytokine whose concentration is decreased in NASH patients and may play a role in decreasing hepatic fat content. Pioglitazone and rosiglitazone have been extensively studied in NAFLD and the trials are summarized in **Tables 1** and **2**. Unfortunately, the majority of trials lacked power and lacked placebo controls. Belfort and colleagues[18] conducted a placebo-controlled trial where they looked at diabetic patients with NASH proven on entry biopsy. Six months of pioglitazone resulted in a significant decrease in steatosis, ballooning injury, and centrilobular inflammation as seen on repeat biopsy. Pioglitazone treatment also significantly improved liver transaminases, markers of insulin sensitivity, and adiponectin levels. However, there was no difference in fibrosis compared with placebo and pioglitazone treatment significantly increased body fat. In another study looking at nondiabetic patients with NASH, 1 year of pioglitazone treatment produced histologic improvement in ballooning injury, Mallory bodies, and fibrosis, but was no better than placebo in terms of steatosis and inflammation. Transaminase levels were once again significantly reduced, but there was no difference in markers of insulin sensitivity; adiponectin levels were increased, but the change was not significant compared with placebo. Significant weight gain was again seen in the TZD group.[16]

Table 1
Summary of trials involving pioglitazone therapy for NAFLD

Author	Year	Design	Patients	Duration (mos)	Liver Enzymes	Steatosis	Necro-inflammation	Fibrosis
Sanyal et al[30]	2004	RCT	20	6	−	+	+	+
Belfort et al[18]	2006	RCT	55	6	+	+	+	−
Aithal et al[16]	2008	RCT	61	12	+	−	+/−	+
Sanyal et al[19]	2010	RCT	80	24	+	+	+	−

Abbreviations: RCT, randomized controlled trial; +, improvement; −, no effect.

In the PIVENS trial, 2 years of pioglitazone therapy in nondiabetic NASH patients resulted in significant improvement in liver transaminases, steatosis, inflammation and overall NAFLD activity score (NAS). Pioglitazone use was also associated with significant resolution of NASH compared with vitamin E or placebo. Ballooning scores improved with pioglitazone but did not reach significance and there was no improvement in fibrosis. Again, significant weight gain was seen despite an improvement in insulin resistance.[19]

Rosiglitazone has been studied in the FLIRT trials. In the original study, 1 year of rosiglitazone treatment resulted in significant improvement in steatosis, transaminase levels, adiponectin levels, and insulin sensitivity. However, there was no improvement in histology based on overall NAS. There was an average weight gain of 1.5 kg in the rosiglitazone arm.[20] An open-label extension of this trial for 2 additional years maintained the significant reductions in steatosis and transaminase levels and, although the NAS improved over the 2 years, the trend was not significant. Among patients who had a greater than 30% reduction in steatosis, significant improvement was shown in necroinflammation and a nonsignificant improvement was seen in ballooning. Weight gain persisted over the 3-year period.[17] In a recent randomized trial comparing rosiglitazone with metformin, rosiglitazone therapy for 1 year significantly reduced transaminase levels, insulin resistance and overall NAS without any change in body mass index (BMI).[21]

Table 2
Summary of trials involving rosiglitazone therapy for NAFLD

Author	Year	Design	Patients	Duration (mos)	Liver Enzymes	Steatosis	Necro-inflammation	Fibrosis
Neuschwander-Tetri et al[88]	2003	Open	30	12	+	n/a	+	+
Ratziu et al[20]	2008	RCT	63	12	+	+	−	−
Ratziu et al[17]	2010	RCT	53	24–36	+	+	−	−
Omer et al[21]	2010	RCT	64	12	+	+	n/a	−

Abbreviations: n/a, not available; RCT, randomized controlled trial; +, improvement; −, no effect.

Table 3
Summary of trials involving vitamin E therapy for NAFLD

Author	Year	Design	Patients	Duration (mos)	Liver Enzymes	Steatosis	Necro-inflammation	Fibrosis
Hasegawa et al[26]	2001	Open	12	12	+	+	+	+
Harrison et al[28]	2003	RCT	49	6	–	n/a	–	+
Sanyal et al[30]	2004	RCT	20	12	n/a	+	–	–
Bugianesi et al[38]	2005	RCT	28	12	+	n/a	n/a	n/a
Sanyal et al[19]	2010	RCT	84	24	+	+	+	–

Abbreviations: n/a, not available; RCT, randomized controlled trial; +, improvement; –, no effect.

Although its effects on ballooning, fibrosis, and adiponectin levels remain controversial, TZD therapy seems to improve insulin sensitivity, liver enzymes, steatosis, and necroinflammation, with pioglitazone being consistently more effective than rosiglitazone.

Discontinuation of TZDs results in a return to pretreatment NASH histology and serum markers, suggesting that TZD therapy would have to be maintained indefinitely for continued treatment response.[22] This is likely to result in weight gain, which is due to increased total body fat and not fluid retention.[23] Because increased total body fat and insulin resistance are the initial triggers in the NAFLD cascade, it is unclear how TZD-induced weight gain would affect NAFLD patients long term and whether the histologic benefits would eventually be reversed. Concerns over cardiovascular events and bone pathology also surround TZD use, but have not been adequately studied in NAFLD patients.

TZD therapy, especially with pioglitazone, seems to be an effective treatment for NASH but needs to be given indefinitely and, given its propensity for weight gain, it needs further study. It can be considered one of the preferred agents in diabetic patients with NASH because these patients already have an indication for TZD therapy.

Vitamin E

Vitamin E (α-tocopherol) is a naturally occurring antioxidant. Its effects in NASH may be secondary to its function as a free radical scavenger or its ability to inhibit cytokines such as transforming growth factor (TGF-β), which plays a role in hepatic stellate cell activity and fibrogenesis as shown in rat models.[24] NASH patients have also been shown to have decreased levels of vitamin E and increased levels of TGF-β as compared with healthy controls,[25,26] and 1 year of vitamin E treatment significantly reduced TGF-β levels in NASH patients.[26] Vitamin E may also have a non-antioxidant mechanism in NASH; it may alter insulin resistance by influencing proliferator activated nuclear receptor-α expression.[27]

Of the multiple open-label and randomized controlled trials (**Table 3**), the largest trial looking at the effects of vitamin E in patients with NASH was the PIVENS trial. A total of 247 nondiabetic patients with NASH were randomized to receive vitamin E, pioglitazone, or placebo daily for 2 years. Vitamin E at 800 U/d resulted in a significant reduction in liver enzymes, steatosis, ballooning, lobular inflammation, and overall

NAS.[19] Although none of the 3 arms had any effect on fibrosis, only vitamin E resulted in a significant improvement in ballooning scores and there was no side effect of weight gain as seen in the pioglitazone arm. Although PIVENS showed no effect on fibrosis, Harrison and colleagues[28] showed that vitamin E at 1000 U/d along with vitamin C 1 g/d significantly improved fibrosis at 6 months.[28] In this trial, which included diabetic patients, vitamin E therapy resulted in significant improvement in fibrosis scores without any changes in inflammation, necrosis, or transaminase levels. Interestingly, the effect on fibrosis was most profound in diabetic patients. Steatosis was not evaluated in the study and minimal improvement in fibrosis scores was also seen in the placebo group. Another open label trial of 300 U/d of vitamin E for 1 year also showed improvement in transaminase levels, steatosis, inflammation, and fibrosis,[26] but was limited by small sample size and lack of paired biopsies.

Vitamin E has also been studied in combination with other NAFLD agents with mixed results. A randomized, controlled trial with ursodeoxycholic acid (UDCA) and vitamin E demonstrated that the combination was more effective than UDCA alone in terms of steatosis and transaminase reduction but there was no significant difference in ballooning, inflammation, or fibrosis.[29] A pilot study looking at vitamin E and pioglitazone versus vitamin E alone in nondiabetic patients showed that the combination was superior to vitamin E alone in terms of NASH histology.[30] Patients receiving both vitamin E and pioglitazone had significant improvements in steatosis, ballooning, inflammation, and fibrosis scores, whereas those on vitamin E alone only significantly reduced their steatosis grade. Not surprisingly, the combination with pioglitazone also demonstrated improved insulin sensitivity compared with vitamin E alone.

Vitamin E treatment seems to be beneficial in NASH, but there is a note of caution. High-dose vitamin E therapy has been associated with increased mortality in other studies,[31] and most NAFLD trials have used doses of vitamin E above the current recommended dose. It is reassuring that the PIVENS trial did not report any increase in mortality from vitamin E use, but may have been underpowered for this end point. It would be prudent until more data emerges to use vitamin E selectively in NASH patients with more severe changes on histology. Combination regimens including vitamin E cannot currently be recommended.

Metformin

Metformin, a biguanide, is traditionally considered first-line treatment for non–insulin-dependent diabetes. Because there is a high prevalence of diabetes in patients with NAFLD, targeting insulin resistance with metformin seems like an appropriate pharmacologic option. Metformin increases the activity of 5'AMP-activated protein kinase, resulting in decreased hepatic glucose production and hepatic insulin resistance.[32] This improvement in insulin sensitivity decreases hepatic lipid accumulation and, therefore, liver steatosis. Moreover, without the steatosis, hepatocytes are theoretically less susceptible to reactive oxygenated species, TGF-β, and other endotoxins that trigger the NASH cascade.[33]

Many trials assessing metformin therapy in NAFLD have been conducted (**Table 4**), but again are hampered by small sample size and poor study design. The first trial using metformin in humans with NAFLD was a small, open-label study that showed that metformin treatment resulted in a significant reduction in transaminase levels, insulin resistance, and liver volume seen on ultrasound compared with a diet-only control group.[34] Another study comparing metformin with diet alone examined histologic end points in a small sample of patients.[35] At the end of 6 months, the metformin group had significant reductions in transaminase levels, insulin resistance, and steatosis as seen on ultrasonography. In terms of histology, however, there was

Table 4
Summary of trials involving metformin therapy for NAFLD

Author	Year	Design	Patients	Duration (mos)	Liver Enzymes	Steatosis	Necro-inflammation	Fibrosis
Marchesini et al[34]	2001	Open	20	4	+	n/a	n/a	n/a
Uygun et al[35]	2004	RCT	36	6	+	+	n/a	n/a
Nair et al[36]	2004	Open	15	12	−	+	−	−
Bugianesi et al[38]	2005	RCT	55	12	+	+	+	+
Loomba et al[37]	2008	Open	28	12	−	+/−	+	−
De Oliveira et al[33]	2008	Open	20	12	+	+	−	+
Haukeland et al[89]	2009	RCT	48	6	−	−	−	−
Garinis et al[39]	2010	RCT	50	6	n/a	+	n/a	n/a
Omer et al[21]	2010	RCT	22	12	−	−	−	−

Abbreviations: n/a, not available; RCT, randomized controlled trial; +, improvement; −, no effect.

no difference between the metformin and diet groups. More patients actually had worsening fibrosis scores in the metformin group compared with the diet-only group, although this trend was not significant. Another open-label trial looked at metformin therapy for 1 year and had a small number of post-treatment liver biopsies.[36] Metformin treatment reduced steatosis in one third, inflammation in one fifth, and fibrosis in just 1 patient. The effect on transaminase levels was mild with an initial decrease and then a return to pretreatment levels by the end of the study. Loomba and colleagues[37] demonstrated a more profound histologic effect in their open-label study. One year of metformin treatment improved the histology in more than 50% of patients and one third of patients showed an impressive 3-point decrease in the NASH activity index. Fibrosis scores decreased minimally, but the changes were not significant. Although insulin sensitivity significantly improved, transaminase levels did not change over the year. However, those patients who histologically responded to metformin had significantly lower transaminase levels as well as a much greater improvement in insulin sensitivity. In another controlled trial, 55 patients were randomized to receive metformin, whereas others received vitamin E or a strict diet regimen.[38] Metformin resulted in significant improvements in insulin sensitivity and the most rapid reduction in transaminase levels. However, at the end of 1 year, the decreased transaminase levels in the metformin group were not significantly different than those reduced levels seen in the diet group. Metformin treatment significantly reduced steatosis, inflammation, and fibrosis, but a very limited number of repeat biopsies were performed.

Recent trials continue to provide mixed results. Omer and colleagues[21] compared metformin with rosiglitazone in a 1-year randomized trial of diabetic NASH patients. Metformin significantly reduced the waist circumference and BMI of patients, but had no effect on transaminase levels or NAS. On the other hand, the combination of metformin with rosiglitazone significantly improved transaminase levels and NAS, suggesting that metformin may have a role in potentiating TZD effects in NAFLD. In another study looking at ultrasound-based assessment of steatosis, metformin was no better than diet in terms of improving steatosis, although it did significantly improve insulin resistance and increase adiponectin levels.[39]

Metformin may improve insulin sensitivity in NAFLD, but its effects on transaminases, steatosis, inflammation, and fibrosis remain unclear. Further trials of longer duration and larger sample sizes that look at histologic outcomes are necessary before metformin can be recommended for use in NAFLD.

Probucol

Probucol is a lipid-lowering agent with potent antioxidant properties, allowing it to function as a free radical scavenger. Moreover, its affinity to accumulate in adipose tissue makes it an attractive candidate for use in NAFLD.

Merat and colleagues[40] have conducted 3 trials of probucol in NAFLD. In their original pilot study, 500 mg of probucol for 6 months significantly reduced transaminase levels as well as total cholesterol. However, most of the reduction in cholesterol was due to a drop in high-density lipoprotein cholesterol (HDL); low-density lipoprotein cholesterol and triglyceride levels did not change significantly. In a subsequent placebo-controlled trial, probucol significantly reduced alanine aminotransferase levels, but there were no changes in aspartate aminotransferase or total cholesterol levels when compared with placebo.[41] HDL levels did decrease in the treatment arm, but the changes were not significant. In the only trial that looked at liver histology, 8 patients received probucol for 1 year and then underwent repeat biopsies.[42] The overall necroinflammatory grade, based on a modified Brunt scoring system that looked at steatosis, ballooning, and inflammation, was significantly improved with probucol treatment. Transaminase levels and steatosis as assessed by ultrasonography were also significantly reduced. There were no changes in the stage of fibrosis, total cholesterol, or HDL levels, but low-density lipoprotein cholesterol levels did decrease significantly. No significant side effects were seen.

Although the trials have been limited by small sample sizes and short durations, they do consistently show a reduction in transaminase levels and the 1 study that evaluated liver histology also demonstrated favorable effects. However, there are concerns over the use of probucol. It is currently not available in many countries, including the United States, because there are more efficacious lipid-lowering alternatives and because of its potential adverse effects. Probucol can lower HDL levels and cardiac arrhythmias have also been seen. Therefore, until randomized, controlled trials show consistent histologic benefits and no adverse effects, probucol cannot be recommended for use in NAFLD.

Pentoxifylline

Pentoxifylline is a phosphodiesterase inhibitor, resulting in decreased activity of TNF-α and TGF-β. TNF-α is a potent inflammatory cytokine that is upregulated in NAFLD and is a mediator of insulin resistance.[43] TGF-β, a primary target of vitamin E therapy in NAFLD, seems to play a role in hepatic stellate cell activity and fibrogenesis.[24] Therefore, pentoxifylline could theoretically function as an antioxidant, antifibrotic, and insulin-sensitizing agent in NAFLD.

The majority of trials evaluating the effects of pentoxifylline in NAFLD have been limited by small sample size, short duration, lack of a placebo control, and no analysis of histologic outcomes (**Table 5**). One of the original pilot studies used 1600 mg/d of

Table 5
Summary of trials involving pentoxifylline therapy for NAFLD

Author	Year	Design	Size	Duration (mos)	Transaminases	Steatosis	Necro-inflammation	Fibrosis
Adams et al[43]	2004	Open	20	12	+	n/a	n/a	n/a
Satapathy et al[44]	2004	Open	18	6	+	n/a	n/a	n/a
Satapathy et al[45]	2007	Open	9	12	+	+	+	+
Lee et al[46]	2008	RCT	20	3	+	n/a	n/a	n/a

Abbreviations: n/a, not available; RCT, randomized controlled trial; +, improvement; −, no effect.

pentoxifylline for 1 year and showed a significant reduction in transaminase levels, but one third of the patients withdrew from the study because of nausea.[43] No changes were seen in fasting glucose, triglyceride, or HDL cholesterol levels. Using 1200 mg/d also significantly decreased transaminase levels and the reduced dose did not cause nausea.[44] Fasting serum insulin, the homeostasis model assessment of insulin resistance (HOMA-IR), and TNF-α levels were also significantly reduced by pentoxifylline in this trial. An extension of this trial was then conducted to look at the histologic effects of pentoxifylline. Of the original 15 patients that received 1200 mg/d for 6 months, 9 continued treatment for a full year and underwent repeat liver biopsies.[45] A majority showed a reduction in steatosis, necroinflammation, and fibrosis. Transaminase levels and insulin sensitivity also significantly improved. There were no significant side effects seen at the 1200 mg/d dose and no patients dropped out of the study. In one of the few placebo-controlled trials, pentoxifylline significantly reduced transaminase levels, but had no effect on TNF-α, IL-6, or hyaluronic acid levels when compared with placebo.[46]

Pentoxifylline at 1200 mg/d is a safe and promising potential agent in NAFLD. However, until a larger placebo-controlled study evaluates histologic end points, pentoxifylline cannot be recommended. Two trials are currently ongoing and the results of these and other future trials will hopefully facilitate a more definite conclusion on the use of pentoxifylline in NAFLD.

Betaine

Betaine is currently approved for use in homocystinuria because it converts homocysteine to methionine. A consequence of this conversion is the production of S-adenosylmethionine (SAM). In mouse NAFLD models, SAM has been shown to prevent fatty infiltration and SAM levels may be reduced in NAFLD.[47] Therefore, betaine should increase SAM levels and may protect against liver injury in NAFLD patients.

Two trials from The Mayo Clinic shed light on this theory. In the original pilot study, 7 patients completed 1 year of betaine treatment and underwent repeat biopsies.[48] Transaminase levels and fibrosis stage were significantly reduced at the end of treatment. Steatosis and necroinflammation also showed improvement, but these changes did not achieve significance. These promising findings led to a recent randomized, placebo-controlled trial where 35 patients received betaine for 1 year.[49] Unfortunately, when compared with placebo, betaine showed no significant improvement in transaminase levels, necroinflammation, or fibrosis. Betaine treatment

Table 6
Summary of trials involving UDCA therapy for NAFLD

Author	Year	Design	Patients	Duration (mos)	Liver Enzymes	Steatosis	Necro-inflammation	Fibrosis
Laurin et al[52]	1996	Open	24	12	+	+	−	−
Lindor et al[53]	2004	RCT	166	24	−	−	−	−
Adams et al[54]	2010	Open	12	6	−	n/a	n/a	n/a
Leuschner et al[55]	2010	RCT	139	18	−	−	+/−	−
Ratziu et al[56]	2010	RCT	126	12	+	n/a	n/a	n/a

Abbreviations: n/a, not available; RCT, randomized controlled trial; +, improvement; −, no effect.

significantly increased SAM levels and reduced steatosis, but the overall NAS did not improve. The major shortcoming of this trial was that one third of the study patients had advanced fibrosis or cirrhosis at baseline; therefore, one could argue that these patients were unlikely to show any histologic improvement.

Despite its ability to increase SAM levels and reduce steatosis, betaine currently has no role in the treatment of NAFLD.

UDCA

UDCA is a secondary bile acid that plays a role in lipid metabolism by regulating intestinal cholesterol uptake. Beyond its role in preventing the formation of cholesterol gallstones, UDCA has also been hypothesized to have anti-apoptotic and anti-oxidant effects.[50,51] This is thought to be because of its ability to modulate intracellular signaling and decrease mitochondrial production of reactive oxygenated species. It is these effects that made UDCA an attractive therapeutic option in NAFLD. Multiple trials have looked at the efficacy of UDCA in NAFLD patients (**Table 6**). However, like most NAFLD studies, the majority of these trials have been small, uncontrolled, and lacking in liver histologic assessment.

One of the original studies was a small pilot study that looked at treatment with UDCA or clofibrate, a lipid-lowering agent, in patients with biopsy-proven NASH.[52] Patients with concomitant gallstones were treated with UDCA, whereas those with high triglycerides were treated with clofibrate. One year of UDCA treatment resulted in a significant reduction in serum transaminase levels and steatosis grades. No significant difference was seen in necroinflammation or fibrosis. Given these initial findings, a large, randomized, controlled trial looked at 166 patients for 2 years.[53] In this study, UDCA significantly reduced transaminase levels and steatosis as in the pilot study. However, similar improvements were also seen in the placebo arm; therefore, overall, there was no difference between UDCA and placebo in terms of transaminases or liver histology. Although the study had a large sample size at the start of the trial, there were a significant number of subject withdrawals with much fewer repeat biopsies and no intention-to-treat analysis. Moreover, the improvement seen in the placebo arm was unusually high. Although these considerations question the validity of the study to a certain extent, it was concluded that UDCA was no better than placebo.

Given these disappointing results and the fact that higher doses of UDCA have been more effective in other liver diseases, high-dose UDCA was then studied in the treatment of NASH. The pilot study used approximately double the original 15 mg/kg per day dosing and concluded that 6 months of high-dose UDCA had no significant effect on transaminase levels.[54] Histology was not a primary end point and the study included mostly patients with severe NASH. Two recent randomized, controlled trials have provided conflicting results on the efficacy of high-dose UDCA. Leuschner and colleagues[55] looked at 139 patients for 18 months. The study, which used an intention-to-treat analysis and was conducted at 25 different medical centers in Germany and Greece, concluded that high-dose UDCA only significantly improves necroinflammation compared with placebo. No difference was seen in transaminase activity, steatosis, ballooning, fibrosis, or the overall NAS. In the second trial, 126 patients were randomized to high-dose UDCA or placebo for 12 months.[56] There was a 30% reduction in transaminase levels as compared with placebo as well as significant reduction in serum fibrosis markers. Actual histology, however, was not analyzed.

UDCA at both low and high doses has a relatively benign side effect profile. It is readily available and frequently used for various hepatobiliary conditions. However, despite the promise shown in early pilot trials, UDCA has not consistently shown any superiority over placebo in multiple large trials and until convincing histologic evidence is presented, UDCA cannot be recommended as a first-line agent for NAFLD.

WEIGHT LOSS STRATEGIES
Pharmacologic Treatment

The epidemic of obesity in the Western World over the last couple of decades has been well chronicled and it has led to a rise in other features of the metabolic syndrome, including NAFLD.

Several studies have shown improvement in liver enzymes in NAFLD patients after dietary and exercise weight loss programs,[57,58] and this seems to correlate with histologic changes.[59] Typically, weight loss in these situations is not sustainable over the long term and a more permanent surgical solution to obesity would seem to provide a more reliable alternative.

In the last few years, several drugs have been approved in the United States that promote weight loss. In fatty liver disease, the best studied drug is orlistat, which inhibits lipase and leads to fat maldigestion. In obese patients with NASH, orlistat leads to improvement in histology. As with other weight loss agents, this effect is mediated through the weight loss rather than any direct effect of the drug.[60]

The conclusion from dietary and drug-mediated weight loss studies is that this approach can work, but typically requires strict adherence and is difficult to maintain. Thus, there is a need for permanent therapy.

Endoscopic Treatment

A central tenet of obesity surgery techniques is to decrease the gastric volume, thereby promoting early satiety. This result can also be achieved endoscopically.

Weight loss can be induced by inflating an intragastric balloon at endoscopy, which can remain in situ typically for 6 months. Many of these studies have been performed in Europe but suffer from the heterogeneity of balloons available and the lack of a control group. They are often the prelude to bariatric surgery. However, the morbidity associated with these balloons is very low and they can be inserted in the ambulatory setting.

The Bioenterics intragastric balloon has been the most widely studied. This device is placed in the stomach at endoscopy and then inflated with 600 to 700 mL of saline (usually with methylene blue). The balloon is left inflated for 6 months and then removed. Several studies have concluded that it is very effective in inducing weight loss with a recent Spanish study in 714 consecutive patients demonstrating a decrease in mean BMI of 6.5 kg/m^2 (from 37.6 to 31.1 kg/m^2).[61]

In comparison with surgery, such as laparoscopic sleeve gastrectomy, intragastric balloon placement is equally effective in inducing weight loss and has less morbidity, but lacks the ability to maintain weight loss when the balloon is removed.[62]

Similarly, in NAFLD patients (defined by the presence of fat on ultrasonography), the Bioenterics balloon leads to weight loss, with those patients who noted a decrease in BMI of more than 10% improving their liver enzymes (alanine amino-transferase, 30 down to 21 IU/L) and insulin resistance as measured by the HOMA-IR (from 4.95 to 2.69).[63] In fact, in obese patients with the metabolic syndrome, the presence of severe steatosis and insulin resistance defined by the HOMA-IR was predictive of a response to the Bioenterics balloon in a series of 130 Italian patients.[64] It remains to be seen whether endoscopic therapy will start to compete with bariatric surgery as a treatment for obesity in the United States.

SURGICAL OPTIONS
Bariatric Surgery

Surgical weight loss procedures have been employed for several decades, but it was only in 1991 that the National Institutes of Health issued a consensus statement that bariatric surgery was an appropriate indication for patients with a BMI over 40 kg/m^2 (or >35 kg/m^2 with comorbidities).[65]

Even at this time, surgery was limited by postoperative complications, often due to the open technique employed. The advent of laparoscopy meant that the same surgery could be performed with less perioperative morbidity and the last 20 years have seen an exponential growth in laparoscopic bariatric surgery such that it is among the most common operative procedures performed in the United States with more than 200,000 procedures in 2009.[66]

Multiple operative techniques fall under the banner of bariatric surgery, but they either cause gastric volume restriction or intestinal malabsorption, or a combination of the two. Gastric banding procedures such as vertical banded gastroplasty and laparoscopic adjustable gastric banding (LAGB) are examples of restrictive surgeries, whereas jejunoileal bypass and the duodenal switch operation lead to malabsorption. The commonest procedure, however, is a Roux-en-Y gastric bypass (RYGB), which is a combination approach; as is a biliopancreatic diversion (BPD) and BPD with duodenal switch (BPD/duodenal switch operation). It is beyond the scope of this paper to discuss these individual techniques in detail, but suffice it to say they are all effective. The most popular is the RYGB, which typically leads to the greatest and most durable decrease in BMI.[67]

The effect of bariatric surgery on NAFLD has been reported in multiple studies, but is limited by heterogeneity of design and lack of postoperative histology in many patients. Despite this, there are compelling data that weight loss after bariatric surgery improves NASH (**Table 7**).

Mattar and colleagues[68] observed a decrease in the prevalence of the metabolic syndrome from 70% to 14% among 70 patients who underwent laparoscopic RYGB after an average 60% loss of excess body weight. All patients underwent repeat liver biopsy a mean of 15 months after surgery and demonstrated dramatic improvements in liver steatosis (88% to 8%), inflammation (23% to 2%), and fibrosis (31% to 13%).[68]

A smaller study with blinded pathology review noted similar results after RYGB. This study was notable for improvement in fibrosis in up to half of patients less than

Table 7
Summary of bariatric surgery trials for NAFLD

Author	Year	Surgery	Patients	Time between biopsies (months)	Metabolic syndrome	Steatosis	Necroinflammation	Fibrosis
Mattar et al[68]	2005	RYGB	70	12	+	+	+	+
Clark et al[69]	2004	RYGB	16	10	n/a	+	+	+
Dixon et al[70]	2004	LAGB	36	26	+	+	+	+
Stratopoulos et al[72]	2005	VBG	51	18	+	+	+	+/−
Kral et al[73]	2004	BPD	104	41	+	+	+	+/−
Mathurin et al[73]	2004	LAGB/BPD/RYGB	381	60	+	+	+/−	−

Abbreviations: n/a, not available; +, improvement; −, no effect.

1 year after surgery, as well as complete resolution of steatosis in almost all patients. However, this may have been due to selection bias, because the repeat biopsy was taken at the time of elective incisional hernia repair, which may have only been performed in the healthiest patients.[69]

Studies of LAGB have shown histologic improvement comparable to RYGB and those patients with the metabolic syndrome had the greatest improvement with weight loss.[70] Interestingly, γ-glutamyl transferase levels and to a lesser extent aspartate aminotransferase seem to be the best serum correlates of histologic changes of NASH, rather than alanine aminotransferase.[71]

Vertical banded gastroplasty seems to lead to similar results as RYGB and LAGB, with the exception of fibrosis. Reduction of BMI in 51 patients with morbid obesity and NASH was associated with improvement in steatosis and inflammation, as well as fasting glucose and lipid levels. However, 40% of patients demonstrated no improvement in fibrosis and 12% actually had an increase on biopsy a mean of 18 months after surgery.[72]

The largest study using BPD noted improvement in the metabolic syndrome, but not all patients had decreased fibrosis associated with weight loss, although this did seem to be the case in the small percentage of patients with cirrhosis at the time of surgery.[73]

A recent review and meta-analysis of 15 studies of bariatric surgery in NAFLD with paired liver biopsy data determined that the vast majority of patients had improvement in steatosis and NASH, with resolution seen in 70% and fibrosis regression in 66%. However, the authors acknowledged that many of the studies were limited by small numbers and did not use standardized biopsy assessment. Publication bias was also a potential problem.[74]

The limited nature of the literature in this area was underscored by a Cochrane review, which found no randomized, controlled studies and even a paucity of appropriate cohort studies. Of the 21 studies included, all showed an improvement in steatosis and inflammation and the majority an improvement in fibrosis, although 4 studies described some deterioration in fibrosis. However, these types of reviews require very strict inclusion criteria and performing such trials in this patient population would be very difficult, an issue appreciated by the authors.[75]

In addition to sustained weight loss, changes in insulin resistance after bariatric surgery persist long term and are reflected in improvement in histology. Mathurin and colleagues[76] prospectively followed 381 severely obese patients after bariatric surgery for 5 years and noted a decrease in steatosis from 37% to 16% and a decrease in NASH from 27% to 14%. In multivariate analysis, the persistence of insulin resistance predicted the persistence of steatosis and ballooning on biopsy, meaning that weight loss alone was not enough to improve the fatty liver disease.[76]

The effectiveness of bariatric surgery in morbidly obese patients is not in doubt, but the safety of the various operative procedures in patients with underlying liver disease remains a concern. The metabolic associations of NAFLD and the possibility of advanced liver disease might lead to an increased risk of postoperative complications and, in some cases, hepatic decompensation. A recent prospective study has demonstrated that these fears may be unfounded, because NAFLD was not associated with increased morbidity after surgery, even among patients with portal hypertension.[77]

However, immediate postoperative complications after bariatric surgery are a concern. In the largest multicenter study examining this issue in 4776 patients, 4.3% of patients had a major adverse event within 30 days, defined by death, reintervention, venous thromboembolism, and failure to be discharged from the hospital. The only predictive factor for an adverse outcome was very high BMI.[78]

Despite the success of bariatric surgery in NAFLD, it should be noted that there are case reports of subacute liver failure occurring months or years later after both RYGB and BPD. The etiology of the liver failure in these cases was unclear, but theories postulated included inflammatory and hormonal responses to the surgery; impaired functional integrity of the intestinal mucosal barrier to toxins and cytokines; nutritional deficiencies; and dramatic weight loss as most patients had a preoperative BMI of greater than 50 kg/m². The pathologic findings in the explanted liver ranged from massive necrosis to intense macrovesicular steatosis and cirrhosis, reinforcing the lack of an obvious etiology. However, it would seem prudent to monitor patients with higher BMIs and more dramatic weight loss and ensure close dietary supervision.[79,80]

LIVER TRANSPLANTATION

Decompensated liver disease in the setting of NASH cirrhosis is a relatively uncommon finding compared with other common causes of liver disease such as HCV, but the sheer scale of the obesity epidemic in the United States has lead to predictions that NASH cirrhosis will become the leading indication for OLT in the next decade.[8]

The speed at which NASH is overtaking the typical indications for OLT is concerning. According to the United Network of Organ Sharing, the first adult OLT for a definitive diagnosis of NASH cirrhosis took place in 1996 and was only a tiny fraction of the total adult OLT performed in that year (0.11%). Since then, the number of OLTs performed for NASH cirrhosis has increased by more than 40-fold in 10 years.[81]

OLT is a major operative procedure and patients with NASH typically have comorbid conditions that may increase the risk of perioperative or postoperative death. Over the last few years, several studies have looked at the outcome after OLT for NASH patients and whether it cures the underlying metabolic abnormalities. The studies have been hampered by the lack of a serum test for NASH; therefore, cryptogenic cirrhosis is often considered to be "burnt out" NASH and is included in the analysis.

The largest study from the University of Pittsburgh examined 98 NASH cirrhosis patients and compared their outcome after OLT with control patients with HCV, alcoholic liver disease, and cholestatic liver disease.[81] This study was unique in requiring all NASH cirrhosis patients to have a histologic diagnosis of NASH and also included a cohort of cryptogenic cirrhosis patients in one of the control arms. The findings were surprising in that outcome after OLT was similar irrespective of diagnosis, even though NASH patients were heavier and were more likely to have diabetes and hypertension. However, closer examination demonstrated that older (age >60 years) and heavier (BMI >30 kg/m²) NASH patients with diabetes and hypertension had prohibitive 50% 1-year mortality. These findings were replicated by other groups suggesting that OLT for NASH cirrhosis has acceptable outcomes despite comorbid conditions.[82]

It remains unclear whether OLT "cures" the underlying metabolic abnormalities in NASH because NASH can recur after OLT. The same group from the University of Pittsburgh looked at their well-characterized NASH cirrhosis cohort and noted that 70% developed fatty liver after transplant and one quarter had recurrent NASH. There was no graft loss owing to recurrent disease because of the relatively short 3-year follow-up period, but 18% of patients still had stage 2 or greater fibrosis, raising concerns for graft loss with longer follow-up. There were no independent predictors of recurrence, although most patients displayed features of the metabolic syndrome.[83] Other investigators have noted recurrent steatosis and NASH after transplant for NASH cirrhosis and cryptogenic cirrhosis but this does not seem to impact long-term survival.[84,85]

Interestingly, even among patients transplanted for other reasons, the metabolic syndrome is significantly more common after OLT. The reasons for this are unclear, but may be related to immunosuppressive drugs, particularly because calcineurin inhibitors are implicated in the increase in diabetes after transplantation,[86] and this phenomenon is only likely to increase in the future.[87] As yet, there are no studies looking at the impact of pharmacologic therapy in preventing or treating recurrent NASH after OLT.

OLT seems to be an acceptable option for patients with end-stage liver disease secondary to NASH, but further studies are required to detail the effect of recurrent disease on long-term outcomes and whether drug therapy or amelioration of the metabolic syndrome may alter the natural history of disease.

SUMMARY

The last decade has seen many studies examining the prevalence and natural history of NAFLD in the United States and it is clear that this disease is likely to be an important cause of liver-related morbidity in the future. Several pharmacologic therapies have shown some promise; currently, vitamin E and insulin-sensitizing agents such as pioglitazone can be considered in appropriate cases. Conservative measures to promote weight loss still have a role to play, but the obesity epidemic in the Western World has reached such proportions that bariatric surgery is proving to be an attractive option for patients with a BMI greater than 35 to 40 kg/m^2. Well-designed prospective studies are required to ensure that all of these therapies are safe and effective in the long term. Newer agents will likely be investigated as the pathogenesis of NAFLD and fibrosis progression in NASH are further elucidated.

REFERENCES

1. Zelman S. The liver in obesity. Arch Intern Med 1958;90:141–56.
2. Peters RL, Gay T, Reynolds TB. Post-jejunoileal-bypass hepatic disease. Its similarity to alcoholic hepatic disease. Am J Clin Pathol 1975;63:318–31.
3. Ong JP, Younossi ZM. Epidemiology and natural history of NAFLD and NASH. Clin Liver Dis 2007;11:1–16.
4. Ludwig J, Viggiano TR, McGill DB, et al. Nonalcoholic steatohepatitis: Mayo Clinic experiences with a hitherto unnamed disease. Mayo Clin Proc 1980;55:434–8.
5. Angulo P. Nonalcoholic fatty liver disease and liver transplantation. Liver Transpl 2006;12:523–34.
6. Angulo P. Nonalcoholic fatty liver disease. N Engl J Med 2002;346:1221–31.
7. Armstrong GL, Wasley A, Simard EP, et al. The prevalence of hepatitis C virus infection in the United States, 1999 through 2002. Ann Intern Med 2006;144:705–14.
8. Charlton M. Nonalcoholic fatty liver disease: a review of current understanding and future impact. Clin Gastro and Hepatol 2004;2:1048–58.
9. Powell EE, Cooksley WG, Hanson R, et al. The natural history of nonalcoholic steatohepatitis: a follow up study of forty-two patients for up to 21 years. Hepatology 1990;11:74–80.
10. Angulo P, Keach JC, Batts, KP, et al. Independent predictors of liver fibrosis in patients with nonalcoholic steatohepatitis. Hepatology 1999;30:1356–62.
11. Evans CD, Oien KA, MacSween RN, et al. Non-alcoholic steatohepatitis: a common cause of progressive chronic liver injury? J Clin Pathol 2002;55:689–92.
12. Ong JP, Younossi ZM. Nonalcoholic fatty liver disease (NAFLD)—two decades later: are we smarter about its natural history? Am J Gastroenterol 2003;98:1915–7.
13. Adams LA, Sanderson S, Lindor KD, et al. The histological course of nonalcoholic fatty liver disease: a longitudinal study of 103 patients with sequential liver biopsies. J Hepatol 2005;42:132–8.

14. Harrison SA, Torgerson S, Hayashi PH. The natural history of nonalcoholic fatty liver disease: a clinical histopathological study. Am J Gastroenterol 2003;98:2042–7.
15. Marchesini G, Brizi M, Bianchi G, et al. Nonalcoholic fatty liver disease: a feature of the metabolic syndrome. Diabetes 2001;50:1844–50.
16. Aithal GP, Thomas JA, Kaye PV, et al. Randomized, placebo-controlled trial of pioglitazone in nondiabetic subjects with nonalcoholic steatohepatitis. Gastroenterology 2008;135:1176–84.
17. Ratziu V, Charlotte F, Bernhardt C, et al. Long-term efficacy of rosiglitazone in nonalcoholic steatohepatitis, results of the Fatty Liver Improvement with Rosiglitazone Therapy (FLIRT 2) extension trial. Hepatology 2010;51:445–53.
18. Belfort R, Harrison SA, Brown K, et al. A placebo-controlled trial of pioglitazone in subjects with nonalcoholic steatohepatitis. N Engl J Med 2006;355:2297–307.
19. Sanyal A, Chalasani N, Kowdley KV, et al. Pioglitazone, vitamin E, or placebo for nonalcoholic steatohepatitis. N Engl J Med 2010;362:1675–85.
20. Ratziu V, Giral P, Jacqueminet S, et al. Rosiglitazone for nonalcoholic steatohepatitis: one-year results of the randomized placebo-controlled Fatty Liver Improvement with Rosiglitazone Therapy (FLIRT) trial. Gastroenterology 2008;135:100–10.
21. Omer Z, Cetinkalp S, Akyildiz M, et al. Efficacy of insulin-sensitizing agents in nonalcoholic fatty liver disease. Eur J Gastroenterol Hepatol 2010;22:18–23.
22. Lutchman G, Modi A, Kleiner DE, et al. The effects of discontinuing pioglitazone in patients with nonalcoholic steatohepatitis. Hepatology 2007;46:424–9.
23. Balas B, Belfort R, Harrison SA, et al. Pioglitazone treatment increases whole body fat but not total body water in patients with nonalcoholic steatohepatitis. J Hepatology 2007;47:565–70.
24. Parola M, Muraca R, Dianzani I, et al. Vitamin E dietary supplementation inhibits transforming growth factor beta 1 gene expression in the rat liver. FEBS Lett 1992;308:267–70.
25. Strauss R. Comparisons of serum concentrations of alpha-tocopherol and beta-carotene in a cross-sectional sample of obese and nonobese children (NHANES III). National Health and Nutrition Examination Survey. J Pediatr 1999;134:160–5.
26. Hasegawa T, Yoneda M, Nakamura K, et al. Plasma transforming growth factor-beta 1 level and efficacy of alpha-tocopherol in patients with nonalcoholic steatohepatitis, a pilot study. Aliment Pharmacol Ther 2001;15:1667–72.
27. Yakaryilmaz F, Guliter S, Savas B, et al. Effects of vitamin E treatment on peroxisome proliferator-activated receptor-alpha expression and insulin resistance in patients with nonalcoholic steatohepatitis, results of a pilot study. Intern Med J 2007;37:229–35.
28. Harrison SA, Torgerson S, Hayashi P, et al. Vitamin E and vitamin C treatment improves fibrosis in patients with nonalcoholic steatohepatitis. Am J Gastroenterol 2003;98:2485–90.
29. Dufour JF, Oneta CM, Gonvers JJ, et al. Randomized placebo-controlled trial of ursodeoxycholic acid with vitamin E in nonalcoholic steatohepatitis. Clin Gastroenterol Hepatol 2006;4:1537–43.
30. Sanyal A, Mofrad P, Contos M, et al. A pilot study of vitamin E versus vitamin E and pioglitazone for the treatment of nonalcoholic steatohepatitis. Clin Gastroenterol Hepatol 2004;2:1107–15.
31. Miller ER III, Pastor-Barriuso R, Dalal D, et al. Meta-analysis: high-dosage vitamin E supplementation may increase all-cause mortality. Ann Intern Med 2005;142:37–46.
32. Zhou G, Myers R, Li Y, et al. Role of AMP-activated protein kinase in mechanism of metformin action. J Clin Invest 2001;108:1167–74.

33. De Oliveira CP, Stefano JD, de Siueira ER, et al. Combination of N-acetylcysteine and metformin improves histological steatosis and fibrosis in patients with nonalcoholic steatohepatitis. Hepatol Res 2008;38:159–65.
34. Marchesini G, Brizi M, Bianchi G, et al. Metformin in nonalcoholic steatohepatitis. Lancet 2001;358:893–4.
35. Uygun A, Kadayifici A, Isik AT, et al. Metformin in the treatment of patients with nonalcoholic steatohepatitis. Aliment Pharmacol Ther 2004;19:537–44.
36. Nair S, Diehl AM, Wiseman M, et al. Metformin in the treatment of nonalcoholic steatohepatitis: a pilot open label trial. Aliment Pharmacol Ther 2004;20:23–8.
37. Loomba R, Lutchman G, Kleiner DE, et al. Pilot study of metformin for the treatment of nonalcoholic steatohepatitis. Aliment Pharmacol Ther 2009;29:172–82.
38. Bugianesi E, Gentilcore E, Manini R, et al. A randomized controlled trial of metformin versus vitamin E or prescriptive diet in nonalcoholic fatty liver disease. Am J Gastroenterol 2005;100:1082–90.
39. Garinis GA, Fruci B, Mazza A, et al. Metformin versus dietary treatment in nonalcoholic hepatic steatosis: a randomized study. Int J Obes 2010;34:1255–64.
40. Merat S, Malekzadeh R, Sohrabi MR, et al. Probucol in the treatment of nonalcoholic steatohepatitis: an open-labeled study. J Clin Gastroenterol 2003;36:266–8.
41. Merat S, Malekzadeh R, Sohrabi MR, et al. Probucol in the treatment of nonalcoholic steatohepatitis: a double-blind randomized controlled study. J Hepatol 2003;38:414–8.
42. Merat S, Aduli M, Kazemi R, et al. Liver histology changes in nonalcoholic steatohepatitis after one year of treatment with probucol. Dig Dis Sci 2008;53:2246–50.
43. Adams LA, Zein CO, Angulo P, et al. A pilot trial of pentoxifylline in nonalcoholic steatohepatitis. Am J Gastroenterol 2004;99:2365–8.
44. Satapathy SK, Garg S, Chauhan, et al. Beneficial effects of tumor necrosis factor-alpha inhibition by pentoxifylline on clinical, biochemical, and metabolic parameters of patients with nonalcoholic steatohepatitis. Am J Gastroenterol 2004;99:1946–52.
45. Satapathy SK, Sakhuja P, Malhotra V, et al. Beneficial effects of pentoxifylline on hepatic steatosis, fibrosis, and necroinflammation in patients with nonalcoholic steatohepatitis. J Gastroenterol Hepatol 2007;22:634–8.
46. Lee YM, Sutedja DS, Wai CT, et al. A randomized controlled pilot study of pentoxifylline in patients with nonalcoholic steatohepatitis. Hepatol Int 2008;2:196–201.
47. Song Z, Deaciuc I, Zhou Z, et al. Involvement of AMP-activated protein kinase in beneficial effects of betaine on high-sucrose diet-induced hepatic steatosis. Am J Physiol Gastrointest Liver Physiol 2007;293:894–902.
48. Abdelmalek MF, Angulo P, Jorgensen RA, et al. Betaine, a promising new agent for patients with nonalcoholic steatohepatitis: results of a pilot study. Am J Gastroenterol 2001;96:2711–17.
49. Abdelmalek MF, Sanderson SO, Angulo P, et al. Betaine for nonalcoholic fatty liver disease, results of a randomized placebo-controlled trial. Hepatology 2009;50:1818–26.
50. Rodrigues CM, Steer CJ. The therapeutic effects of ursodeoxycholic acid as an anti-apoptotic agent. Expert Opin Investig Drugs 2001;10:1243–53.
51. Rodrigues CM, Fan G, Wong PY, et al. Ursodeoxycholic acid may inhibit deoxycholic acid-induced apoptosis by modulating mitochondrial transmembrane potential and reactive oxygen species production. Mol Med 1998;4:165–78.
52. Laurin J, Lindor KD, Crippin JS, et al. Ursodeoxycholic acid or clofibrate in the treatment of nonalcoholic steatohepatitis: a pilot study. Hepatology 1996;23:1464–7.
53. Lindor KD, Kowdley KV, Heathcote EJ, et al. Ursodeoxycholic acid for treatment of nonalcoholic steatohepatitis, results of randomized trial. Hepatology 2004;39:770–8.

54. Adams LA, Angulo P, Petz J, et al. A pilot trial of high-dose ursodeoxycholic acid in nonalcoholic steatohepatitis. Hepatol Int 2010;4:628–33.
55. Leuschner UF, Lindenthal B, Hermann G, et al. High-dose ursodeoxycholic acid therapy for the treatment of nonalcoholic steatohepatitis: a double-blind, randomized, placebo-controlled trial. Hepatology 2010;52:472–9.
56. Ratziu V, de Ledinghen V, Oberti F, et al. A randomized controlled trial of high-dose ursodeoxycholic acid for nonalcoholic steatohepatitis. J Hepatol 2010;54:1011–9.
57. Suzuki A, Lindor K, St Saver J, et al. Effect of changes on body weight and lifestyle in nonalcoholic fatty liver disease. J Hepatol 2005;43:1060–6.
58. Andersen T, Gluud C, Franzmann M, et al. Hepatic effects of dietary weight loss in morbidly obese subjects. J Hepatol 1991;12:224–9.
59. Huang M, Greenson J, Chao C, et al. One-year intense nutritional counseling results in histological improvement in patients with non-alcoholic steatohepatitis: a pilot study. Am J Gastroenterol 2005;100:1072–81.
60. Harrison SA, Fecht W, Brunt EM, et al. Orlistat for overweight subjects with nonalcoholic steatohepatitis: a randomized, prospective trial. Hepatology 2009;49:80–6.
61. Lopez-Nava G, Rubio MA, Prados S, et al. BioEnterics® intragastric balloon (BIB®). Single ambulatory center Spanish experience with 714 consecutive patients treated with one or two consecutive balloons. Obes Surg 2011;21:5–9.
62. Genco A, Cipriano M, Materia A, et al. Laparoscopic sleeve gastrectomy versus intragastric balloon: a case-control study. Surg Endosc 2009;23:1849–53.
63. Ricci G, Bersani G, Rossi A, et al. Bariatric therapy with intragastric balloon improves liver dysfunction and insulin resistance in obese patients. Obes Surg 2008;18:1438–42.
64. Forlano R, Ippolito AM, Iacobellis A, et al. Effect of the BioEnterics intragastric balloon on weight, insulin resistance, and liver steatosis in obese patients. Gastrointest Endosc 2010;71:927–33.
65. NIH conference. Gastrointestinal surgery for severe obesity. Consensus Development Conference Panel. Ann Intern Med 1991;115:956–61.
66. American Society for Metabolic and Bariatric Surgery (2009). Fact sheet: metabolic & bariatric surgery. Available at: www.asbs.org. Accessed June 7, 2011.
67. Tice JA, Karliner L, Walsh J, et al. Gastric banding or bypass? A systematic review comparing the two most popular bariatric procedures. Am J Med 2008;121:885–93.
68. Mattar SG, Velcu LM, Rabinovitz M, et al. Surgically-induced weight loss significantly improves nonalcoholic fatty liver disease and the metabolic syndrome. Ann Surg 2005;242:610–7.
69. Clark JM, Alkhuraishi AR, Solga SF, et al. Roux-en-Y gastric bypass improves liver histology in patients with non-alcoholic fatty liver disease. Obes Res 2005;13:1180–6.
70. Dixon JB, Bhathal PS, Hughes NR, et al. Nonalcoholic fatty liver disease: Improvement in liver histological analysis with weight loss. Hepatology 2004;39:1647–54.
71. Dixon JB, Bhathal PS, O'Brien PE. Weight loss and non-alcoholic fatty liver disease: falls in gamma-glutamyl transferase concentrations are associated with histologic improvement. Obes Surg 2006;16:1278–86.
72. Stratopoulos C, Papakonstantinou A, Terzis I, et al. Changes in liver histology accompanying massive weight loss after gastroplasty for morbid obesity. Obes Surg 2005;15:1154–60.
73. Kral JG, Thung SN, Biron S, et al. Effects of surgical treatment of the metabolic syndrome on liver fibrosis and cirrhosis. Surgery 2004;135:48–58.

74. Mummadi RR, Kasturi KS, Chennareddygari S, et al. Effect of bariatric surgery on nonalcoholic fatty liver disease: systematic review and meta-analysis. Clin Gastroenterol Hepatol 2008;6:1396–402.
75. Chavez-Tapia NC, Tellez-Avila FI, Barrientos-Gutierrez T, et al. Bariatric surgery for non-alcoholic steatohepatitis in obese patients. Cochrane Database Syst Rev 2010; 1:CD007340.
76. Mathurin P, Hollebecque A, Arnalsteen L, et al. Prospective study of the long-term effects of bariatric surgery on liver injury in patients without advanced disease. Gastroenterology 2009;137:532–40.
77. Ribeireiro T, Swain J, Sarr M, et al. NAFLD and insulin resistance do not increase the risk of postoperative complications among patients undergoing bariatric surgery—a prospective analysis. Obes Surg 2011;21:310–5.
78. Longitudinal Assessment of Bariatric Surgery (LABS) Consortium, Flum DR, Belle SH, King WC, et al.Perioperative safety in the longitudinal assessment of bariatric surgery. N Engl J Med 2009;361:445–54.
79. D'Albuquerque LA, Gonzalez AM, Wahle RC, et al. Liver transplantation for subacute hepatocellular failure due to massive steatohepatitis after bariatric surgery. Liver Transpl 2008;14:881–5.
80. Cotler SJ, Vitello JM, Guzman G, et al. Hepatic decompensation after gastric bypass surgery for severe obesity. Dig Dis Sci 2004;49:1563–8.
81. Malik SM, deVera ME, Fontes P, et al. Outcome after liver transplantation for NASH cirrhosis. Am J Transplant 2009;9:782–93.
82. Bhagat V, Mindikoglu AL, Nudo CG, et al. Outcomes of liver transplantation in patients with cirrhosis due to nonalcoholic steatohepatitis versus patients with cirrhosis due to alcoholic liver disease. Liver Transpl 2009;15:1814–20.
83. Malik SM, Devera ME, Fontes P, et al. Recurrent disease following liver transplantation for nonalcoholic steatohepatitis cirrhosis. Liver Transpl 2009;15:1843–51.
84. Yalamanchili K, Saadeh S, Klintmalm GB, et al. Nonalcoholic fatty liver disease after liver transplantation for cryptogenic cirrhosis or nonalcoholic fatty liver disease. Liver Transpl 2010;16:431–9.
85. Dureja P, Mellinger J, Agni R, et al. NAFLD recurrence in liver transplant recipients. Transplantation 2011;91:684–9.
86. Laish I, Braun M, Mor E, et al. Metabolic syndrome in liver transplant recipients: prevalence, risk factors, and association with cardiovascular events. Liver Transpl 2011;17:15–22.
87. Pagadala M, Dasarathy S, Eghtesad B, et al. Posttransplant metabolic syndrome: an epidemic waiting to happen. Liver Transpl 2009;15:1662–70.
88. Neuschwander-Tetri BA, Brunt EM, Wehmeier KR, et al. Improved nonalcoholic steatohepatitis after 48 weeks of treatment with the PPAR-gamma ligand rosiglitazone. Hepatology 2003;38:1008–17.
89. Haukeland JW, Konopski Z, Eggesbo HB, et al. Metformin in patients with nonalcoholic fatty liver disease: a randomized, controlled trial. Scand J Gastroenterol 2009; 44:853–60.

Managing Varices: Drugs, Bands, and Shunts

Christopher Kenneth Opio, MD[a,b], Guadalupe Garcia-Tsao, MD[a,b],*

KEYWORDS

- Varices • Variceal hemorrhage • Portal hypertension
- Ligation • Propranolol • Nadolol • Portosystemic shunt
- TIPS

Up to 50% of patients with cirrhosis have esophageal varices at initial endoscopy,[1,2] and nearly all patients with varices have a high portal pressure, that is, an hepatic venous pressure gradient (HVPG) of 12 mmHg or higher (normal, 3–5).[3] In patients without varices, esophageal varices develop and grow in size at a rate of about 7% per year as a result of ongoing portal hypertension.[4,5] It has been shown that varices develop at a significantly higher rate in patients with a baseline HVPG above 10 mmHg and in patients in whom the HVPG increases by more than 10% in the first year.[4] Without treatment, varices rupture in about one third of patients, with the highest rates observed in patients with large varices, red wale marks. and/or in Child C patients.[6] In the past, and before the use of drugs, bands, and/or shunts, 4 of 10 patients with acute variceal hemorrhage (AVH) died at 6 weeks, one third rebled at 6 weeks, and only about one third survived beyond 1 year.[7]

This article updates the current use of drugs, bands, and shunts in the different settings—primary prophylaxis, secondary prophylaxis, and the treatment of AVH—and shows how they have altered the natural history of varices and variceal hemorrhage.

DRUGS

Most currently used drugs to treat varices and/or variceal hemorrhage cause splanchnic vasoconstriction leading to a reduction in portal venous inflow and consequently to a decrease in portal pressure. Drugs in this category include nonselective β-blockers (NSBB), vasopressin and its analog terlipressin, and somatostatin and its analogs, octreotide and vapreotide. Vasodilators are another type of drugs that can reduce portal pressure through intrahepatic vasodilatation. However,

Supported by grants from the National Institutes of Health (P30 DK34989 and K24 DK02727-02), and from the Yale-Mulago Medical Fellowship Foundation.

[a] Section of Digestive Diseases, Yale University School of Medicine, 333 Cedar Street – 1080 LMP, New Haven, CT 06510, USA

[b] VA Connecticut Healthcare System, 960 Campbell Avenue - 111 H, West Haven, CT 06516, USA

* Corresponding author. 333 Cedar Street – 1080 LMP, New Haven, CT 06510, USA.
E-mail address: guadalupe.garcia-tsao@yale.edu

most of the vasodilators currently available, specifically nitrates (which have been the most widely investigated), act not only on the intrahepatic circulation, but also have a potentially deleterious systemic vasodilating effect and seem to reduce portal pressure through reflex splanchnic vasoconstriction that results from hypotension rather than by causing intrahepatic vasodilatation.[8] In fact, a randomized, controlled trial (RCT) of isosorbide mononitrate (ISMN) versus placebo in the prevention of first variceal hemorrhage showed a higher variceal hemorrhage rate in the ISMN group.[9,10] Therefore, vasodilators used alone are not recommended in the management of portal hypertension, but are used in combination with NSBB when they have a synergistic portal pressure-reducing effect.

NSBB

Propranolol and nadolol are the most commonly used NSBB for the chronic outpatient management of varices/variceal hemorrhage. NSBB act through β-1 and β-2 adrenergic receptor blockade. β-1 Blockade leads to a decrease in portal flow by decreasing cardiac output, whereas β-2 blockade leads to a decrease in portal flow directly by inducing splanchnic vasoconstriction. The latter effect is the most important effect and explains the lack of correlation between the decrease in heart rate induced by NSBB (a β-1 effect) and the decrease in portal pressure.[11] More recently, a role for angiogenesis in the development of portal hypertension in cirrhosis has been described[12,13] and, interestingly, there is evidence that propranolol has an antiangiogenic effect.[14,15]

NSBBs lead to a median reduction in HVPG of approximately 15%,[16] with 37% of the patients being hemodynamic "responders"; that is, their HVPG decreases to levels below 12 mmHg and/or is reduced by more than 20% from baseline.[17] Hemodynamic responders have been shown to have a significantly lower incidence of variceal hemorrhage and a significantly better survival.[18,19] This incidence seems to be similar to that reported for patients treated with shunt therapies [either surgical or transjugular intrahepatic portosystemic shunt (TIPS); **Fig. 1**]. Although it would seem rational to monitor the HVPG response to NSBB and adjust their dose accordingly during the therapy of varices/variceal hemorrhage, HVPG measurements are not standardized or widely used. Therefore, the currently recommended dose of NSBB is the dose that is maximally tolerated by the patient with an ideal heart rate goal of 50 to 55 bpm (**Table 1**).[20,21] It has recently been shown that NSBB dose titration performed in a nurse-led clinic results in higher maintenance doses of NSBB and a very low discontinuation rate (5%), lower than that observed in a RCT setting (~15%).[22]

The most common side effects related to NSBB are lightheadedness, fatigue, and shortness of breath and the prospect of experiencing these side effects detract many patients from electing to take NSBB.[23] Additionally, up to 15% of the patients may have relative contraindications (eg, sinus bradycardia, insulin-dependent diabetes) or absolute contraindications (eg, obstructive pulmonary disease, heart failure, aortic valve disease, heart block, peripheral arterial insufficiency) to NSBB.

A recent study suggests that NSBB are associated with a poorer survival in patients with refractory ascites and that NSBB should be contraindicated in this setting.[24] However, the study is retrospective and the groups were disparate at baseline, with patients on NSBB having more advanced disease as shown by a higher prevalence of varices and variceal hemorrhage. Contrary to this finding, in a meta-analysis of NSBB versus placebo for recurrent variceal hemorrhage, sensitivity analysis showed that NSBB were associated with a significant survival benefit in patients with the most severe liver disease.[25] This survival benefit could be explained, at least partially, by

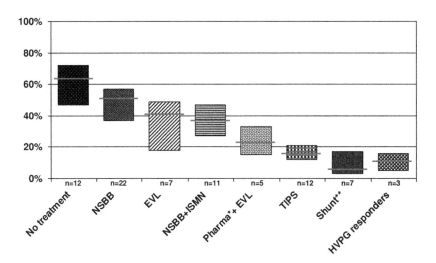

*Pharma= NSBB+ISMN (3) or NSBB (2); **Shunt = DSRS (4) or total shunt (3)
NSBB=non-selective beta-blockers; EVL= endoscopic variceal ligation; ISMN= Isosorbide mononitrate

Fig. 1. Results on rebleeding for different therapies used in patients with cirrhosis and a prior episode of variceal hemorrhage. The figure summarizes fully published RCTs included in several meta-analyses.[10,18,27,37] Results are expressed as median (*red line*) and interquartile ranges (*box*). Differences in inclusion criteria, follow-up, times, and outcome measurements preclude comparisons among groups.

the finding that NSBB may lower the risk of spontaneous bacterial peritonitis in patients with cirrhosis and ascites.[26] At this time, and unless stronger evidence arises, the use of NSBB in patients with refractory ascites should not be contraindicated.

NSBB in the prevention of varices
A large, multicenter, double-blind RCT of timolol, an NSBB, versus placebo in patients with cirrhosis and portal hypertension but without varices showed a similar rate of development of varices in both treatment groups with a higher rate of adverse events in the timolol group.[4] Therefore, NSBB are not recommended for the prevention of varices.

Notably, in this very compensated group of patients, treatment of the underlying cause of cirrhosis (alcohol abstention, antiviral therapy) is the mainstay of therapy, because treating the etiology can potentially reduce portal pressure, thereby reducing variceal development.

NSBB in the prevention of first variceal hemorrhage
Overall, NSBB compared with placebo or no active drug decreases the risk of the first episode of variceal hemorrhage (over 2 years) by about 50%.[27] In patients with medium/large varices, who are at the greatest risk of first variceal hemorrhage, propranolol or nadolol significantly reduce the risk of first variceal hemorrhage, from 30% to 14% at a median follow-up of 2 years.[27] Only 11 patients need to be treated to prevent 1 bleeding episode.

Meta-analyses of trials comparing NSBB versus endoscopic variceal ligation (EVL) show that EVL is more effective in preventing first variceal hemorrhage, without

Table 1
Drugs for the primary or secondary prophylaxis of variceal hemorrhage

Therapy	Starting Dose	Therapy Goals	Maintenance/Follow-up	Comments
Propranolol	20 mg orally twice a day. Adjust every 2–3 days until treatment goal is achieved. Maximal daily dose should not exceed 320 mg.	Maximum tolerated dose. Aim for resting heart rate of 50–55 bpm	At every outpatient visit, make sure that patient is appropriately β-blocked Continue indefinitely. If for primary prophylaxis, no need for follow-up EGD If for secondary prophylaxis, make sure that endoscopic procedures are scheduled.	If for secondary prophylaxis, start in hospital as soon as acute vasoconstrictor (eg, octreotide) is discontinued.
Nadolol	40 mg orally once a day. Adjust every 2–3 days until treatment goal is achieved. Maximal daily dose should not exceed 160 mg.	As for propranolol.	As for propranolol.	As for propranolol.
Isosorbide-5-mononitrate	Only to be used in conjunction with propranolol or nadolol. 10 mg orally at night every day. Adjust every 2–3 days by adding 10 mg in the AM and then in the PM. Maximal dose is 20 mg twice a day.	Maximal tolerated dose. Systolic blood pressure >95 mmHg.	Continue indefinitely.	Started after patients are on a stable maintenance dose of NSBB. Recommended only for secondary prophylaxis.

Abbreviation: EGD, esophagogastroduodenoscopy.

differences in mortality.[28] However, meta-analyses restricted to trials with an adequate design[29] or with a sample size greater than 100[30] show no differences in the rate of first variceal hemorrhage between NSBB and EVL. Therefore, because both therapies seem equal, it has been recommended that the choice should depend on local resources, patient preferences, and presence of contraindications to either therapy.[21]

NSBB have advantages that go beyond the prevention of first variceal hemorrhage. In this setting, reductions in HVPG of only less than 10% to 12% from baseline have been associated with a decrease in the development of ascites, spontaneous bacterial peritonitis, and death.[31,32] This is not surprising; as these complications result at least partially from portal hypertension. Therefore, it is reasonable to start with NSBB and switch to EVL in cases of intolerance to NSBB.

Patients with small varices with red wale marks or that are present in a Child C patient have the same (or an even greater) risk of hemorrhage than patients with large varices and are therefore considered "high risk." Because EVL is not feasible in many of these cases, NSBB are the currently recommended therapy.[21] In other patients with small varices, nadolol was shown to significantly decrease progression to large varices[33] and in these patients NSBB could be administered, although this is considered optional.[21] Once patients are started on NSBB, there is no need to perform follow-up endoscopies.

NSBB in the prevention of recurrent variceal hemorrhage
If patients who have recovered from an episode of AVH receive no therapy, the risk of recurrent variceal hemorrhage is very high at around 65% in 1 to 2 years. NSBB significantly reduce the risk of rebleeding, and prolong survival.[25,27] Only 5 patients need to be treated with a NSBB to prevent 1 rebleeding episode.

The efficacy of NSBB has been shown to correlate with hemodynamic response. In this setting, a reduction in HVPG of more than 20% from the baseline value, or to values of 12 mmHg or lower, is associated with a very low rebleeding rate of approximately 11%,[34] a rate comparable to that associated with shunting therapies (**Fig. 1**). HVPG-guided therapy cannot yet be recommended in daily practice, not only owing to the lack of standardization of HVPG measurements, but also because of uncertain issues such as the best timing (or need) for repeat HVPG measurement and the best treatment for hemodynamic nonresponders.[35]

The combination of pharmacologic therapy (NSBB with or without ISMN) plus EVL seems to be more effective than either therapy alone[36] (**Fig. 1**). NSBB plus EVL remains the recommended first-line treatment to prevent recurrent variceal hemorrhage.[20]

As a rule, NSBB should be initiated once variceal hemorrhage is controlled and acute intravenous vasoactive drugs have been discontinued; that is, between 2 and 5 days after the initiation of intravenous therapy.

NSBB Plus Nitrates
In hemodynamic studies, the association of vasodilators such as ISMN or prazosin with NSBB leads to a greater reduction in HVPG (20%–24%) compared with the reduction observed with NSBB alone.[16,37] However, complications, mainly ascites and/or symptomatic hypotension, occur more frequently with combination therapy. The rate of HVPG responders with NSBB plus ISMN is 44%, a rate that is significantly higher than that observed with NSBB alone (37%).[17] In RCT, a meta-analysis has confirmed a significantly higher number of side effects for NSBB plus ISMN (38%)

compared with NSBB alone (23%), with a higher discontinuation rate (15% vs 6%, respectively).[10] Recommended doses of ISMN are shown in **Table 1**.

NSBB plus ISMN in the prevention of first variceal hemorrhage

The largest, double-blind RCT comparing propranolol plus placebo versus propranolol plus ISMN showed no differences in the rate of first variceal hemorrhage or mortality between groups.[38] These findings have been confirmed in a recent Cochrane meta-analysis.[10] Therefore, the combination of NSBB plus nitrates is not recommended in the primary prophylaxis of variceal hemorrhage.

NSBB plus nitrates in the prevention of recurrent variceal hemorrhage

A single RCT fully published in English compared propranolol alone versus propranolol plus ISMN and showed, at the end of the study, a borderline significant difference in favor of combination therapy regarding prevention of recurrent variceal hemorrhage ($P = .05$). This difference became significant after an additional year of follow-up ($P = .03$), without differences in the incidence of overall rebleeding.[39] A recent Cochrane meta-analysis confirms no differences in the rate of overall bleeding or mortality between these therapies, but a borderline lower rate of recurrent variceal hemorrhage in patients on combination NSBB plus nitrates (relative risk, 0.71; 95% confidence interval, 0.52–0.96) and with a higher rate of side effects.[10]

Compared with endoscopic therapy (sclerotherapy or EVL), NSBB plus ISMN show no differences regarding recurrent hemorrhage, but seem to reduce mortality, although this effect was not confirmed in trial sequential analysis.[10] This effect on mortality is consistent with results from one of the studies included in the meta-analysis that shows that, in the long term (82-month follow-up) propranolol plus ISMN is associated with a better survival compared with EVL.[40]

The combination of NSBB with ISMN has similar rates of recurrent hemorrhage compared with EVL alone, whereas the combination of pharmacologic (NSBB alone or NSBB with ISMN) plus EVL has lower rebleeding rates than either therapy alone, consistent with results of a recent meta-analysis[41] and a recent summary of trials.[36] Therefore, the recommended therapy for prevention of recurrent variceal hemorrhage is EVL plus pharmacologic therapy.[20] Because the combination of NSBB and ISMN has more adverse events than NSBB alone and, until a survival advantage of NSBB and ISMN can be confirmed, the recommended pharmacologic therapy to be associated to EVL is NSBB alone.[20,42]

Parenteral Vasoconstrictors in the Treatment of Acute Variceal Hemorrhage

In the setting of AVH, NSBB are not indicated and have not been tested given their slow action and a potentially deleterious effect blocking the heart rate response to hypovolemia. Intravenously administered splanchnic vasoconstrictors that lower portal pressure acutely are vasopressin (and its analog terlipressin) and somatostatin (and its analogs octreotide and vapreotide). Parenteral vasoconstrictors, particularly if safe, are generally applicable and can be initiated as soon as a diagnosis of variceal hemorrhage is suspected, even before diagnostic esophagogastroduodenoscopy (EGD).[43]

Vasopressin is the most potent splanchnic vasoconstrictor. It reduces blood flow to all splanchnic organs, leading to a decrease in portal venous inflow and a decrease in portal pressure. Unfortunately, the clinical usefulness of vasopressin is limited by its multiple side effects that are related to splanchnic vasoconstriction (eg, bowel ischemia) and to systemic vasoconstriction (eg, hypertension, myocardial ischemia). Combining vasopressin with transdermal glyceryl trinitrate has been shown to reduce some of these side effects. However, because other much safer drugs are now available, vasopressin plus nitroglycerin is only recommended when these are unavailable.

Terlipressin is a synthetic analog of vasopressin that has a longer biological activity and significantly fewer side effects than vasopressin. It is the only vasoconstrictor that has shown a survival benefit when compared with placebo.

Somatostatin and analogs such as octreotide and vapreotide also cause splanchnic vasoconstriction at pharmacologic doses, both through an inhibition of the release of vasodilatory peptides (mainly glucagon) and a local vasoconstrictive effect. Bolus injections of both somatostatin and octreotide cause a marked reduction in portal pressure but, with continuous infusion, only somatostatin seems to maintain a portal hypotensive effect.[44] Somatostatin and its analogs may have an added benefit of decreasing the postprandial (including blood in stomach) elevation in portal pressure.[45,46] The near absence of side effects of somatostatin and analogs represents a major advantage over other vasoconstrictive agents, allowing them to be administered for a longer period of time.

RCTs comparing different pharmacologic agents demonstrate no differences among them regarding control of hemorrhage and early rebleeding, although vasopressin is associated with more adverse events.[27] In practice, the choice of pharmacologic agent is usually based on availability and cost. Octreotide, a somatostatin analog, is the only safe vasoactive drug available in the United States. Doses and schedules for the different vasoconstrictors are shown in **Table 2**.

A meta-analysis of RCTs comparing vasoactive drugs versus sclerotherapy in the control of AVH did not find any differences in control of bleeding, 5-day failure rate, rebleeding or mortality, with a significantly higher rate of adverse events with sclerotherapy.[47] However, another meta-analysis shows that the use of parenteral vasoconstrictors (mostly octreotide) plus endoscopic therapy is more effective than endoscopic therapy alone[48]; therefore, the combination of pharmacologic and endoscopic therapy is the most rational approach in the treatment of AVH.[20,42]

New Drugs

Currently, fewer than half of the patients treated with NSBB and nitrates are hemodynamic responders. If this proportion could be increased with new drugs, outcomes could be improved and the need to measure HVPG to monitor response to therapy would no longer be an issue.

New drugs that have been tested in the treatment of portal hypertension are mainly those that, at least theoretically, decrease intrahepatic vascular resistance either by blocking adrenergic activity or by increasing the delivery of nitric oxide to the intrahepatic circulation. Unfortunately, vasodilators may also produce systemic vasodilatation with aggravation of the hyperdynamic circulatory state, leading to sodium retention and renal vasoconstriction.

Carvedilol is a NSBB with added vasodilatory effect through anti-α_1 adrenergic activity. At a mean dose of 31 mg/d it has a significant portal pressure-reducing effect (19%, with 58% being HVPG responders), but can also decrease arterial pressure and lead to fluid retention.[49] However, a recent RCT on primary prophylaxis of variceal hemorrhage that compared carvedilol at a lower dose (maximum 12.5 mg/d) with EVL showed a significantly lower rate of first variceal hemorrhage with carvedilol (10%) compared with EVL (23%), without differences in mortality or side effects.[50] However, the study has some problems[51] and the hemorrhage rates are within the described rates of first variceal hemorrhage in RCTs of NSBB (7%–46%) or EVL (0%–25%).[28]

Table 2
Drugs for the treatment of AVH

Therapy	Initial Dose	Therapy Goals	Maintenance Dose/Follow-up	Comments
Octreotide	IV bolus of 50 μg. Start upon suspicion of variceal hemorrhage (before endoscopic confirmation).	Control of AVH	IV infusion of 50 μg/h Duration: 2–5 days A repeat bolus of 50 μg can be administered if rebleeding or failure	Only available IV vasoconstrictor in the US (used off label for this indication)
Somatostatin	IV slow bolus of 250 μg. Start upon suspicion of variceal hemorrhage (before endoscopic confirmation).	Control of AVH	IV infusion of 250 μg/h Increase dose to 500 μg/h if rebleeding or failure	Not available in the US
Terlipressin	For the first 48 hours: boluses of 2 mg IV every 4 hours. Start upon suspicion of variceal hemorrhage (before endoscopic confirmation).	Control of AVH	After first 48 hours: 1 mg IV every 4 hours Total duration: 2–5 days	Not available in the US
Vapreotide	Bolus of 50 μg IV bolus. Start upon suspicion of variceal hemorrhage (before endoscopic confirmation).	Control of AVH	IV infusion of 50 μg/h Duration: 2–5 days A repeat bolus of 50 μg can be administered if rebleeding or failure	Not available in the US
Vasopressin plus nitroglycerin	IV infusion at 0.2–0.4 U/min (maximal dose is 0.8 U/min). Always given with IV infusion of nitroglycerin 40 μg/min (maximal dose is 400 μg/min).	Control of AVH	Adjust nitroglycerin systolic blood pressure >90 mmHg Maximal duration 24 hours	Very rarely used because of high rate of side effects Given toxicity should only be initiated once variceal source of hemorrhage is confirmed

Therefore, carvedilol is considered a promising alternative that needs to be further explored before it can be widely recommended.[21]

Another drug that is promising based on proof-of-concept studies but that has not been tested in RCT looking at clinical end points is simvastatin, which acts on portal pressure by improving liver generation of the vasodilator nitric oxide and by improving hepatic endothelial dysfunction in patients with cirrhosis.[52] In a hemodynamic, placebo-controlled study, simvastatin at a dose of 20 to 40 mg/d was shown to reduce HVPG modestly (8% compared with no change in patients randomized to placebo).[53] This effect occurred without changes in portal flow, indicating that the effect was due to a decrease in intrahepatic resistance. Results of ongoing RCTs assessing its effect combined with NSBB on clinical end points are eagerly awaited, but until then its use cannot be widely recommended.

Although angiotensin receptor blockers and angiotensin-converting enzyme inhibitors have been shown to reduce portal pressure, their use is associated with decreased creatinine clearance[54] and they are therefore not recommended. However, a recent meta-analysis of individual patient data of studies that used these drugs shows that, in patients with Child A cirrhosis, angiotensin receptor blockers and angiotensin-converting enzyme inhibitors reduce portal pressure with minimal side effects, with deleterious effects being mostly observed in patients with decompensated cirrhosis.[55]

Other vasodilators that have been tested recently are sildenafil, a phosphodiesterase inhibitor, and NCX-1000 [2(acetyloxy) benzoic acid-3(nitrooxymethyl)phenyl ester], a nitric oxide-releasing derivative of ursodeoxycholic acid. Both had shown selective vasodilatory effect on intrahepatic circulation in animal models of cirrhosis. However, in hemodynamic patient studies, neither reduced HVPG significantly, although both were associated with a significant, potentially deleterious, decrease in blood pressure.[56,57]

Prophylactic antibiotics are non-vasoactive drugs that have been shown to reduce the rate of bacterial infections and to improve survival in patients with AVH.[58] This effect is partially due to a decrease in the early rebleeding rate.[59] Their use in the setting of AVH is considered standard of care.[20,21]

BANDS

Esophagogastroduodenoscopy (EGD) is an essential procedure for the diagnosis, grading, and treatment of varices and variceal hemorrhage. The endoscopic method of choice in the therapy of varices and variceal hemorrhage is EVL, which consists of the placement of rubber bands around varices so that they will undergo necrosis and will eventually disappear.

In expert hands, EVL is highly effective for controlling bleeding and for the eradication of varices. However, because it is a local therapy that has no effect on portal pressure, varices always recur after endoscopic eradication. It is, therefore, necessary to carry out lifelong surveillance and repeat EVL when varices recur.

EVL has essentially replaced the use of endoscopic sclerotherapy based on 2 meta-analysis of RCTs comparing EVL versus sclerotherapy in secondary prophylaxis of variceal hemorrhage, both of which showed a superiority of EVL in preventing recurrent variceal hemorrhage, with fewer complications and a lower number of endoscopic sessions needed to achieve eradication.[60,61] Notably, the combination of EVL and sclerotherapy has been shown to confer no advantages over EVL alone and has a higher complication rate.[62] Therefore, evidence accumulated so far should discourage the use of combination EVL plus sclerotherapy.

The technique of EVL uses multiband devices with application of the bands started at the gastroesophageal junction progressing upward in a spiral manner for approximately 5 to 8 cm. An average of 3 banding sessions (each performed every 1–2 weeks) are required to achieve eradication of varices (disappearance of varices or varices that are too small to be sucked into the banding device). After varices are eradicated, the first surveillance endoscopy should be performed 3 months later and, if negative, surveillance can be lengthened to every 6 months (**Table 2**).

Bands in the Prevention of First Variceal Hemorrhage

The finding that EVL was superior to sclerotherapy in the secondary prophylaxis of variceal hemorrhage prompted the performance of prospective studies to assess its efficacy in preventing first variceal hemorrhage (primary prophylaxis). Initial studies comparing EVL with no treatment were unjustified because they ignored the fact that an effective therapy (NSBB) already existed at the time.

Even though meta-analyses of RCTs comparing EVL versus NSBB show a benefit of EVL in preventing first variceal hemorrhage,[28,63,64] when trials with an appropriate treatment allocation, a longer follow-up, or that include a reasonable number of patients (>100) are analyzed, this borderline benefit of EVL disappears.[29,51] Because both NSBB and EVL seem to be equally effective in preventing first variceal hemorrhage, the side effects of each become an important issue. Although the number of side effects is greater with NSBB than with EVL, it is the quality of side effects that is more important. Whereas no lethal side effects have been reported with the use of NSBB, 3 deaths resulting from EVL-induced bleeding ulcers were reported in these trials.[64] Nevertheless, no differences in mortality between treatment groups have been shown in any of these meta-analyses.[63,64]

This has led to the recommendation that either NSBB or EVL are reasonable options in the primary prophylaxis of variceal hemorrhage. The choice should be based on local resources and expertise, patient preference and characteristics, side effects, and contraindications.[21,65] Despite this recommendation, there are currently centers that perform predominantly EVL; others prefer the more rational approach of starting with NSBB and switching to EVL if there is intolerance to NSBB.

A very recent trial compared EVL plus nadolol versus nadolol alone and reported that the combination treatment did not enhance effectiveness of primary prophylaxis, while increasing adverse events.[66] Therefore, in this setting combination therapy is not currently recommended.

Bands in the Treatment of AVH

Two meta-analyses have shown that EVL and sclerotherapy are equally effective in controlling AVH with control rates of 80% to 90% (**Table 3**).[61,64] However, in a more recent RCT comparing somatostatin plus either sclerotherapy or EVL, the incidence of patients surviving without therapeutic failure was significantly greater in patients randomized to EVL.[67] Serious side effects were also less common with EVL. Therefore, EVL is the recommended form of endoscopic therapy for acute esophageal variceal bleeding, although sclerotherapy may be used in the presence of active hemorrhage if ligation is technically difficult.[68]

EVL should be performed at the time of diagnostic EGD if and when a variceal source of hemorrhage is confirmed and even in the absence of active hemorrhage from a varix. The process should be started at the gastroesophageal junction with placement of approximately 6 bands, particularly on the vessel with stigmata of bleeding. Repeat EVL can be attempted if hemorrhage is not controlled or if the patient has early recurrence of variceal hemorrhage.

Table 3
Bands and shunts in the treatment of varices and variceal hemorrhage

Therapy	Setting	Treatment Goal	Surveillance	Comments
EVL	AVH	Ligation of bleeding varix(ces) with the highest likelihood of having bled	May be repeated if bleeding recurs after initial control	Combined with parenteral vasoactive drugs. If technically difficult, perform endoscopic variceal sclerotherapy.
EVL	Primary or secondary prophylaxis	Repeat every 2–4 weeks until varices are eradicated or are too small to band	First EGD performed 1–3 months after obliteration and every 6–12 mos thereafter.	Proton pump inhibitors can be used to prevent postbanding ulcers.
TIPS	AVH or secondary prophylaxis	Reduction of portosystemic pressure gradient to <12 mmHg	Check for TIPS patency at months 2 and 6, and every 6 months thereafter using Doppler ultrasonography	If evidence of shunt dysfunction on Doppler ultrasound (based on velocity and flow direction of intrahepatic vessels), perform portal pressure gradient measurements

Abbreviations: TIPS, transjugular intrahepatic portal systemic shunt.

As mentioned, sequential combination therapy starting with antibiotics and a safe vasoactive drug at the time of (or even before) admission followed by EVL (ideally within 12 hours of admission) at the time of diagnostic endoscopy is the current standard management for AVH.

Bands in the Prevention of Recurrent Variceal Hemorrhage

As mentioned, EVL is superior to sclerotherapy in the secondary prophylaxis of variceal hemorrhage.[60] In fact, the use of sclerotherapy in this setting has been essentially abandoned. Meta-analysis of trials comparing EVL versus NSBB plus ISMN (optimal pharmacologic therapy) show that both therapies are equally effective regarding the prevention of overall rebleeding, with a tendency for a lower mortality with pharmacotherapy.[69]

According to a recent meta-analysis[41] and a summary of trials,[36] the combination of EVL plus pharmacologic therapy (NSBB alone or in combination with ISMN) has lower rebleeding rates than either therapy alone (**Fig. 1**). Because triple therapy is associated with more adverse events, the recommended therapy for prevention of recurrent variceal hemorrhage is EVL plus NSBB at the doses and schedules specified in **Tables 1** and **2**. In patients who are not candidates for EVL, the strategy would be to maximize portal pressure reduction by combining NSBB plus ISMN.[20]

SHUNTS

Portosystemic shunts, either surgical or placed via the jugular vein by an interventional radiologist (TIPS), divert blood from the portal vein to a systemic vein, circumventing mechanical resistance resulting from cirrhosis. This leads to a marked reduction and even to a normalization of portal pressure. Therefore, both types of shunts are very effective in preventing variceal hemorrhage with the lowest rates of recurrent variceal hemorrhage (**Fig. 1**).

However, shunts can lead to portosystemic encephalopathy and liver failure. In general, they do not seem to have a survival advantage over other treatments and may actually worsen survival in patients with varices without a history of variceal hemorrhage.[70] Because of this, shunts are generally recommended as second-line therapy for those who fail pharmacologic and endoscopic treatment. Moreover, a careful selection process is required to exclude patients that are at a high risk of death after shunt, namely those patients with the most advanced cirrhosis.

Surgical Shunts

Of the surgical shunts, the small-diameter (8–10 mm) portocaval H-graft shunt or the distal splenorenal shunt (DSRS) are probably the favored surgical options because the portal vein would still be available should liver transplantation be required.

The DSRS was designed to reduce the incidence of hepatic encephalopathy and liver failure after total portacaval shunt by partially maintaining portal liver perfusion while decreasing portal blood flow to varices. A meta-analysis of published trials comparing DSRS versus portacaval shunt show a trend toward less hepatic encephalopathy and a better survival with DSRS; however, the differences were not significant.[70]

In a small trial, the small-diameter portocaval H-graft shunt was shown to be effective in the control of variceal hemorrhage and was associated with a lower rate of hepatic encephalopathy when compared with total portacaval shunt.[71]

The performance of surgical shunts in the management of patients with portal hypertension has decreased dramatically in the last decade. This has occurred because of significant improvement in overall management of patients with portal hypertension, but mainly because of the introduction of the TIPS procedure, a less invasive way of decompressing the portal system. Presently, surgical shunts are reserved for patients in whom TIPS cannot be placed for technical reasons or for patients who live far from suitable medical services.

TIPS

TIPS is usually performed by an interventional radiologist and involves puncture of the jugular vein, from which a catheter is advanced though the right atrium and the inferior vena cava into a hepatic vein. A branch of the portal vein within the liver is then catheterized (the most challenging step) with placement of an expandable stent from the hepatic vein into the branch of the portal vein. The portosystemic pressure gradient should be decreased by 50% of its initial value or below the threshold of 12 mmHg. In most TIPS studies mentioned in this review, the type of stent placed was uncoated, the type with a high obstruction rate (20%–80% in 1 year) mostly owing to pseudointimal proliferation within the shunt. With the relatively new polytetrafluoroethylene-coated stents, pseudointimal proliferation is prevented, obstruction is minimal, and outcomes seem to be better.[72] After TIPS placement, surveillance is required and should ideally involve direct portography with portosystemic gradient measurement. However, Doppler ultrasound is principally used because it not invasive and does not expose the patient to additional radiation.[73]

Shunts in the Prevention of First Variceal Hemorrhage

Meta-analysis of early RCTs of shunt surgery in primary prophylaxis have shown conclusively that, although very effective in preventing first variceal hemorrhage, shunting blood away from the liver is accompanied by more frequent encephalopathy and a higher mortality.[70] These results can be extrapolated to TIPS because its physiology is the same as that of surgical shunts (ie, diversion of blood away from the liver).[73] Therefore, shunt therapy (surgery or TIPS) should not be used in the primary prevention of variceal hemorrhage.

Shunts in the Treatment of AVH

As discussed, the standard management for AVH is pharmacologic therapy and endoscopic banding (**Table 3**). However, failures to standard therapy (either bleeding that cannot be controlled or early recurrence of hemorrhage) occur in about 10%–20% of patients. There is no role for surgical shunt to manage these patients. TIPS is of proven clinical efficacy as salvage therapy for patients who fail standard therapy with immediate bleeding control in over 90% of the cases; however, mortality is very high (>35% during admission),[73] probably because by the time the patients have a TIPS placed, their liver disease has further deteriorated.

The identification of patients at a high risk of failing standard therapy is important so that more aggressive therapies can be attempted early on in these patients. The most important predictor of failure is an HVPG (measured within 24 hours of admission) above 20 mmHg[74,75]; however, these measurements are not feasible in most centers. It has been shown that Child–Pugh class correlates with the likelihood of having an HVPG above 20 mmHg, so that about 85% of Child C patients have this high pressure.[75] This finding led to 2 trials of early (preemptive) TIPS in patients with AVH at a high risk of failing standard therapy. In the first—a single-center trial—52 patients with an HVPG above 20 mmHg were randomized to (uncoated) TIPS within 24 hours of admission versus continuing standard therapy.[76] In the second trial, a multicenter European study, 63 Child class C patients (excluding those with the highest scores of 14 and 15) or Child class B patients with active hemorrhage were randomized to (polytetrafluoroethylene-coated) TIPS within 24 to 72 hours of admission versus continued standard therapy.[77] Both trials showed a significant advantage of TIPS with a reduction in composite outcomes (failure to control bleeding or early rebleeding) and, importantly, a significantly higher survival. This led to the recommendation that in the patients with variceal hemorrhage who are Child class C (<14 points) or are Child class B with active bleeding an early (preemptive) TIPS (<72 hours) should be considered.[21]

Importantly, the subpopulation of patients with variceal hemorrhage who would be candidates for early TIPS represent less than 20% of the patients admitted with this complication. In the rest of the patients, the majority, TIPS is considered second-line therapy and is reserved for patients who fail standard therapy.

Shunts in the Prevention of Recurrent Variceal Hemorrhage

Meta-analyses of RCTs that compare-TIPS versus endoscopic therapy (sclerotherapy or EVL) with or without propranolol show that TIPS placement is associated with a significantly lower incidence of rebleeding (**Fig. 1**), but with a significantly increased risk of encephalopathy and without any differences in survival.[78,79] One RCT compared TIPS with drug therapy (propranolol + ISMN) and found lower rates of bleeding with TIPS. However, drug therapy was associated with less encephalopathy, identical survival, and lower costs.[80] Based on these results, TIPS is recommended as

Table 4
Use of drugs, bands, and shunts in the different clinical settings of portal hypertension

	Drugs	Bands	Shunts	
			TIPS	Surgical Shunt
Prevention of varices	Not indicated	Not applicable	Not indicated	Not indicated
Prevention of first variceal hemorrhage				
Large varices	NSBB (or EVL)	EVL (or NSBB)	Not indicated	Not indicated
High-risk small varices[a]	NSBB	Not applicable?	Not indicated	Not indicated
Low risk small varices[b]	NSBB optional	Not indicated	Not indicated	Not indicated
Control of AVH				
Child A and B (without active hemorrhage at EGD)	Antibiotics + IV vasoconstrictor[c] + EVL (or sclerotherapy)	Antibiotics + IV vasoconstrictor[c] + EVL	2nd line (if 1st line fails)	Not indicated
Child C (<14 points) and B (with active hemorrhage at EGD)	Antibiotics + IV vasoconstrictor[c] + EVL (or sclerotherapy)	Antibiotics + IV vasoconstrictor[c] + EVL	Performed within 24-48 hours (preemptive)	Not indicated
Prevention of recurrent variceal hemorrhage	NSBB ± ISMN + Bands		2nd line (if 1st line fails)	2nd line in specific cases[d]

[a] Small varices with red wale marks or occurring in a Child C patient.
[b] Small varices without red wale marks and occurring in a Child A or B patient.
[c] Octreotide, somatostatin, or terlipressin.
[d] In noncandidates to TIPS and where TIPS is unavailable but surgical expertise is available.

second line therapy in patients who have failed secondary prophylaxis with EVL plus pharmacologic therapy.[20,42]

Regarding the selection of TIPS versus surgical shunt in patients who have failed first-line therapy, a recent multicenter RCT of TIPS versus DSRS in Child class A/B patients who rebled despite treatment with EVL plus pharmacologic therapy showed no significant differences in rebleeding, first encephalopathy, or survival.[81] Thrombosis, stenosis, and reintervention rates were significantly higher in the TIPS group. However, this trial was performed using uncoated TIPS stents and it is probable that with the use of polytetrafluoroethylene-coated stents, the number of reinterventions would not have been different. Coated stents are the stent of choice to be used in TIPS and have essentially replaced the use of uncoated stents. As mentioned, surgical shunts currently play a limited role in the management of portal hypertension and are restricted to patients who are not TIPS candidates or in places where the interventional radiology expertise is not available and surgical expertise is available.

SUMMARY

Drugs, bands, and shunts have all been used in the treatment of varices and variceal hemorrhage and have resulted in improved outcomes. However, the specific use of each of these therapies depends on the setting (primary or secondary prophylaxis, treatment of AVH) and on patient characteristics. The indications for each are summarized in **Table 4**.

REFERENCES

1. Pagliaro L, D'Amico G, Pasta L, et al. Portal hypertension in cirrhosis: natural history. In: Bosch J, Groszmann RJ, editors. Portal hypertension. Pathophysiology and treatment. Oxford (UK): Blackwell Scientific; 1994. p. 72–92.
2. Kovalak M, Lake J, Mattek N, et al. Endoscopic screening for varices in cirrhotic patients: data from a national endoscopic database. Gastrointest Endosc 2007;65: 82–8.
3. Garcia-Tsao G, Groszmann RJ, Fisher RL, et al. Portal pressure, presence of gastroesophageal varices and variceal bleeding. Hepatology 1985;5:419–24.
4. Groszmann RJ, Garcia-Tsao G, Bosch J, et al. Beta-blockers to prevent gastroesophageal varices in patients with cirrhosis. N Engl J Med 2005;353:2254–61.
5. Merli M, Nicolini G, Angeloni S, et al. Incidence and natural history of small esophageal varices in cirrhotic patients. J Hepatol 2003;38:266–72.
6. North Italian Endoscopic Club for the Study and Treatment of Esophageal Varices. Prediction of the first variceal hemorrhage in patients with cirrhosis of the liver and esophageal varices. A prospective multicenter study. N Engl J Med 1988;319:983–9.
7. Graham DY, Smith JL. The course of patients after variceal hemorrhage. Gastroenterology 1981;80:800–9.
8. Blei AT, Garcia-Tsao G, Groszmann RJ, et al. Hemodynamic evaluation of isosorbide dinitrate in alcoholic cirrhosis: pharmacokinetic-hemodynamic interactions. Gastroenterology 1987;93:576–83.
9. Garcia-Pagan JC, Villanueva C, Vila MC, et al. Isosorbide mononitrate in the prevention of first variceal bleed in patients who cannot receive beta-blockers. Gastroenterology 2001;121:908–14.
10. Gluud LL, Langholz E, Krag A. Meta-analysis: isosorbide-mononitrate alone or with either beta-blockers or endoscopic therapy for the management of oesophageal varices. Aliment Pharmacol Ther 2010;32:859–71.
11. Garcia-Tsao G, Grace N, Groszmann RJ, et al. Short term effects of propranolol on portal venous pressure. Hepatology 1986;6:101–6.

12. Fernandez M, Mejias M, Garcia-Pras E, et al. Reversal of portal hypertension and hyperdynamic splanchnic circulation by combined vascular endothelial growth factor and platelet-derived growth factor blockade in rats. Hepatology 2007;46:1208–17.
13. Mejias M, Garcia-Pras E, Tiani C, et al. Beneficial effects of sorafenib on splanchnic, intrahepatic, and portocollateral circulations in portal hypertensive and cirrhotic rats. Hepatology 2009;49:1245–56.
14. Storch CH, Hoeger PH. Propranolol for infantile haemangiomas: insights into the molecular mechanisms of action. Br J Dermatol 2010;163:269–74.
15. Lamy S, Lachambre MP, Lord-Dufour S, et al. Propranolol suppresses angiogenesis in vitro: inhibition of proliferation, migration, and differentiation of endothelial cells. Vascul Pharmacol 2010;53:200–8.
16. Garcia-Tsao G. Current management of the complications of cirrhosis and portal hypertension: varices and variceal hemorrhage, ascites and spontaneous bacterial peritonitis. Gastroenterology 2001;120:726–48.
17. Minano C, Garcia-Tsao G. Clinical pharmacology of portal hypertension. Gastroenterol Clin North Am 2010;39:681–95.
18. D'Amico G, Garcia-Pagan JC, Luca A, et al. HVPG reduction and prevention of variceal bleeding in cirrhosis. A systematic review. Gastroenterology 2006;131: 1611–24.
19. Albillos A, Banares R, Gonzalez M, et al. Value of the hepatic venous pressure gradient to monitor drug therapy for portal hypertension: a meta-analysis. Am J Gastroenterol 2007;102:1116–26.
20. Garcia-Tsao G, Bosch J. Management of varices and variceal hemorrhage in cirrhosis. N Engl J Med 2010;362:823–32.
21. de Franchis R. Revising consensus in portal hypertension: report of the Baveno V consensus workshop on methodology of diagnosis and therapy in portal hypertension. J Hepatol 2010;53:762–8.
22. Tandon P, Saez R, Berzigotti A, et al. A specialized, nurse-run titration clinic: a feasible option for optimizing beta-blockade in non-clinical trial patients. Am J Gastroenterol 2010;105:1917–21.
23. Longacre AV, Imaeda A, Garcia-Tsao G, et al. A pilot project examining the predicted preferences of patients and physicians in the primary prophylaxis of variceal hemorrhage. Hepatology 2008;47:169–76.
24. Serste T, Melot C, Francoz C, et al. Deleterious effects of beta-blockers on survival in patients with cirrhosis and refractory ascites. Hepatology 2010;52:1017–22.
25. Bernard B, Lebrec D, Mathurin P, et al. Beta-adrenergic antagonists in the prevention of gastrointestinal rebleeding in patients with cirrhosis: a meta-analysis. Hepatology 1997;25:63–70.
26. Senzolo M, Nadal E, Cholongitas E, et al. Is hydrophobia necessary for the hepatologist prescribing nonselective beta-blockers in cirrhosis? Hepatology 2011;56:2149–50.
27. D'Amico G, Pagliaro L, Bosch J. Pharmacological treatment of portal hypertension: an evidence-based approach. Semin Liver Dis 1999;19:475–505.
28. Bosch J, Abraldes JG, Berzigotti A, et al. Portal hypertension and gastrointestinal bleeding. Semin Liver Dis 2008;28:3–25.
29. Gluud LL, Klingenberg S, Nikolova D, et al. Banding ligation versus beta-blockers as primary prophylaxis in esophageal varices: systematic review of randomized trials. Am J Gastroenterol 2007;102:2842–8.
30. Bosch J, Berzigotti A, Garcia-Pagan JC, et al. The management of portal hypertension: rational basis, available treatments and future options. J Hepatol 2008;48(Suppl 1):S68–92.

31. Turnes J, Garcia-Pagan JC, Abraldes JG, et al. Pharmacological reduction of portal pressure and long-term risk of first variceal bleeding in patients with cirrhosis. Am J Gastroenterol 2006;101:506–12.

32. Villanueva C, Aracil C, Colomo A, et al. Acute hemodynamic response to beta-blockers and prediction of long-term outcome in primary prophylaxis of variceal bleeding. Gastroenterology 2009;137:119–28.

33. Merkel C, Marin R, Angeli P, et al. A placebo-controlled clinical trial of nadolol in the prophylaxis of growth of small esophageal varices in cirrhosis. Gastroenterology 2004;127:476–84.

34. Bosch J, Garcia-Pagan JC. Prevention of variceal rebleeding. Lancet 2003;361: 952–4.

35. Ripoll C, Tandon P, Garcia-Tsao G. Should the hepatic venous pressure gradient be sequentially measured to monitor beta-blocker therapy in the prophylaxis of variceal hemorrhage? In: Jensen DM, editor. Controversies in hepatology. Thorofare (NJ): Slack Incorporated; 2011. p. 123–31.

36. Garcia-Tsao G, Bosch J. Management of varices in cirrhosis. N Engl J Med 2010; 362:2331–2.

37. Albillos A, Garcia-Pagan JC, Iborra J, et al. Propranolol plus prazosin compared with propranolol plus isosorbide-5-mononitrate in the treatment of portal hypertension. Gastroenterology 1998;115:116–23.

38. Garcia-Pagan JC, Morillas R, Banares R, et al. Propranolol plus placebo versus propranolol plus isosorbide-5-mononitrate in the prevention of a first variceal bleed: a double-blind RCT. Hepatology 2003;37:1260–6.

39. Gournay J, Masliah C, Martin T, et al. Isosorbide mononitrate and propranolol compared with propranolol alone for the prevention of variceal rebleeding. Hepatology 2000;31:1239–45.

40. Lo GH, Chen WC, Lin CK, et al. Improved survival in patients receiving medical therapy as compared with banding ligation for the prevention of esophageal variceal rebleeding. Hepatology 2008;48:580–7.

41. Gonzalez R, Zamora J, Gomez-Camarero J, et al. Meta-analysis: combination endoscopic and drug therapy to prevent variceal rebleeding in cirrhosis. Ann Intern Med 2008;149:109–22.

42. Garcia-Tsao G, Sanyal AJ, Grace ND, et al. Prevention and management of gastroesophageal varices and variceal hemorrhage in cirrhosis. Hepatology 2007; 46:922–38.

43. Levacher S, Letoumelin P, Pateron D, et al. Early administration of terlipressin plus glyceryl trinitrate to control active upper gastrointestinal bleeding in cirrhotic patients. Lancet 1995;346:865–8.

44. Escorsell A, Bandi JC, Andreu V, et al. Desensitization to the effects of intravenous octreotide in cirrhotic patients with portal hypertension. Gastroenterology 2001;120: 161–9.

45. Buonamico P, Sabba C, Garcia-Tsao G, et al. Octreotide blunts post-prandial splanchnic hyperemia in cirrhotic patients: a double-blind randomized echo-Doppler study. Hepatology 1995;21:134–9.

46. Chen L and Groszmann RJ. Blood in the gastric lumen increases splanchnic blood flow and portal pressure in portal-hypertensive rats. Gastroenterology 1996;111: 1103–10.

47. D'Amico G, Pietrosi G, Tarantino I, et al. Emergency sclerotherapy versus medical interventions for bleeding oesophageal varices in cirrhotic patients. Cochrane Database Syst Rev 2002;1:CD002233.

48. Banares R, Albillos A, Rincon D, et al. Endoscopic treatment versus endoscopic plus pharmacologic treatment for acute variceal bleeding: a meta-analysis. Hepatology 2002;35:609–15.

49. Banares R, Moitinho E, Matilla A, et al. Randomized comparison of long-term carvedilol and propranolol administration in the treatment of portal hypertension in cirrhosis. Hepatology 2002;36:1367–73.

50. Tripathi D, Ferguson JW, Kochar N, et al. Randomized controlled trial of carvedilol versus variceal band ligation for the prevention of the first variceal bleed. Hepatology 2009;50:825–33.

51. Bosch J, Garcia-Tsao G, Pharmacological versus endoscopic therapy in the prevention of variceal hemorrhage: and the winner is. . . Hepatology 2009;50:674–7.

52. Abraldes JG, Rodriguez-Vilarrupla A, Graupera M, et al. Simvastatin treatment improves liver sinusoidal endothelial dysfunction in CCl4 cirrhotic rats. J Hepatol 2007;46:1040–6.

53. Abraldes JG, Albillos A, Banares R, et al. Simvastatin lowers portal pressure in patients with cirrhosis and portal hypertension: a randomized controlled trial. Gastroenterology 2009;136:1651–8.

54. Schepke M, Werner E, Biecker E, et al. Hemodynamic effects of the angiotensin II receptor antagonist irbesartan in patients with cirrhosis and portal hypertension. Gastroenterology 2001;121:389–95.

55. Tandon P, Abraldes JG, Berzigotti A, et al. Renin-angiotensin-aldosterone inhibitors in the reduction of portal pressure: a systematic review and meta-analysis. J Hepatol 2010;53:273–82.

56. Tandon P, Inayat I, Tal M, et al. Sildenafil has no effect on portal pressure but lowers arterial pressure in patients with compensated cirrhosis. Clin Gastroenterol Hepatol 2010;8:546–9.

57. Berzigotti A, Bellot P, De Gottardi A, et al. NCX-1000, a nitric oxide-releasing derivative of UDCA, does not decrease portal pressure in patients with cirrhosis: results of a randomized, double-blind, dose-escalating study. Am J Gastroenterol 2010;105:1094–101.

58. Bernard B, Grange JD, Khac EN, et al. Antibiotic prophylaxis for the prevention of bacterial infections in cirrhotic patients with gastrointestinal bleeding: a meta-analysis. Hepatology 1999;29:1655–61.

59. Hou MC, Lin HC, Liu TT, et al. Antibiotic prophylaxis after endoscopic therapy prevents rebleeding in acute variceal hemorrhage: a randomized trial. Hepatology 2004;39:746–53.

60. Laine L, Cook D. Endoscopic ligation compared with sclerotherapy for treatment of esophageal variceal bleeding. A meta-analysis. Ann Intern Med 1995;123:280–7.

61. de Franchis R, Primignani M. Endoscopic treatment for portal hypertension. Semin Liver Dis 1999;19:439–55.

62. Singh P, Pooran N, Indaram A, et al. Combined ligation and sclerotherapy versus ligation alone for secondary prophylaxis of esophageal variceal bleeding: a meta-analysis. Am J Gastroenterol 2002;97:623–9.

63. Khuroo MS, Khuroo NS, Farahat KL, et al. Meta-analysis: endoscopic variceal ligation for primary prophylaxis of oesophageal variceal bleeding. Aliment Pharmacol Ther 2005;21:347–61.

64. Garcia-Pagan JC, Bosch J. Endoscopic band ligation in the treatment of portal hypertension. Nat Clin Pract Gastroenterol Hepatol 2005;2:526–35.

65. Garcia-Tsao G, Bosch J, Groszmann RJ. Portal hypertension and variceal bleeding— unresolved issues. Summary of an American Association for the Study of Liver

Diseases and European Association for the Study of the Liver Single-Topic Conference. Hepatology 2008;47:1764–72.

66. Lo GH, Chen WC, Wang HM, et al. Controlled trial of ligation plus nadolol versus nadolol alone for the prevention of first variceal bleeding. Hepatology 2010;52:230–7.

67. Villanueva C, Piqueras M, Aracil C, et al. A randomized controlled trial comparing ligation and sclerotherapy as emergency endoscopic treatment added to somatostatin in acute variceal bleeding. J Hepatol 2006;45:560–7.

68. de Franchis R. Evolving consensus in portal hypertension: Report of the Baveno IV Consensus Workshop on methodology of diagnosis and therapy in portal hypertension. J Hepatol 2005;43:167–76.

69. Cheung J, Zeman M, van Zanten SV, et al. Systematic review: secondary prevention with band ligation, pharmacotherapy or combination therapy after bleeding from oesophageal varices. Aliment Pharmacol Ther 2009;30:577–88.

70. D'Amico G, Pagliaro L, Bosch J. The treatment of portal hypertension: a meta-analytic review. Hepatology 1995;22:332–54.

71. Fernandez-Aguilar JL, Bondia Navarro JA, Santoyo SJ, et al. Calibrated portacaval H-graft shunt in variceal hemorrhage. Long-term results. Hepatogastroenterology 2003;50:2000–4.

72. Bureau C, Garcia-Pagan JC, Otal P, et al. Improved clinical outcome using polytetrafluoroethylene-coated stents for TIPS: results of a randomized study. Gastroenterology 2004;126:469–75.

73. Boyer TD, Haskal ZJ. The role of transjugular intrahepatic portosystemic shunt in the management of portal hypertension. Hepatology 2005;41:386–400.

74. Moitinho E, Escorsell A, Bandi JC, et al. Prognostic value of early measurements of portal pressure in acute variceal bleeding. Gastroenterology 1999;117:626–31.

75. Abraldes JG, Villanueva C, Banares R, et al. Hepatic venous pressure gradient and prognosis in patients with acute variceal bleeding treated with pharmacologic and endoscopic therapy. J Hepatol 2008;48:229–36.

76. Monescillo A, Martinez-Lagares F, Ruiz-del-Arbol L, et al. Influence of portal hypertension and its early decompression by TIPS placement on the outcome of variceal bleeding. Hepatology 2004;40:793–801.

77. Garcia-Pagan JC, Caca K, Bureau C, et al. Early use of TIPS in patients with cirrhosis and variceal bleeding. N Engl J Med 2010;362:2370–9.

78. Luca A, D'Amico G, LaGalla R, et al. TIPS for prevention of recurrent bleeding in patients with cirrhosis: meta-analysis of randomized clinical trials. Radiology 1999; 212:411–21.

79. Khan S, Tudur SC, Williamson P, et al. Portosystemic shunts versus endoscopic therapy for variceal rebleeding in patients with cirrhosis. Cochrane Database Syst Rev 2006;4:CD000553.

80. Escorsell A, Banares R, Garcia-Pagan JC, et al. TIPS versus drug therapy in preventing variceal rebleeding in advanced cirrhosis: a randomized controlled trial. Hepatology 2002;35:385–92.

81. Henderson JM, Boyer TD, Kutner MH, et al. Distal splenorenal shunt versus transjugular intrahepatic portal systematic shunt for variceal bleeding: a randomized trial. Gastroenterology 2006;130:1643–51.

Hepatorenal Syndrome: Do the Vasoconstrictors Work?

Wesley Leung, MD, FRCPC, Florence Wong, MBBS, MD, FRACP, FRCPC*

KEYWORDS
- Hepatorenal syndrome • Liver transplantation
- Renal impairment • Terlipressin
- Transjugular intrahepatic portosystemic shunt
- Vasoconstrictors

Hepatorenal syndrome (HRS) is a potentially reversible clinical syndrome that occurs in patients with cirrhosis, ascites and liver failure, as well as in patients with acute liver failure or alcoholic hepatitis. It is characterized by impaired renal function, marked alterations in cardiovascular function and overactivity of the sympathetic nervous (SNS) and renin–angiotensin–aldosterone systems.[1]

The incidence of functional renal failure including HRS in nonazotemic patients with cirrhosis after the onset of ascites is estimated to be 23.6% at 1 year and 42% by 5 years.[2] Older age, higher Child–Pugh score, and higher baseline creatinine are strong predictors for the development functional renal failure including HRS,[2] reflecting that a longer duration of disease, and more severe liver and renal dysfunction are strong risk factors for the development of HRS.

The diagnosis of HRS must be based on excluding other causes of acute kidney injury, because there are no specific tests for the syndrome. The HRS is diagnosed by a serum creatinine higher than 1.5 mg/dL (133 μmol/L) after the exclusion of reversible functional renal failure with volume expansion using albumin at a dose of 1 g/kg body weight (maximum 100 g/d), and withdrawal of diuretic therapy for at least 2 days. The diagnostic criteria of HRS were updated by the International Ascites Club in 2007 (**Box 1**).[1]

Clinically, there are 2 types of HRS, each with different clinical presentation and different prognostic implications. Type 1 HRS (HRS-1) is a rapidly progressive acute renal failure that occurs in cirrhosis and ascites either spontaneously or in the context of various precipitating factors (**Box 2**). HRS-1 is diagnosed when the serum creatinine doubles from baseline to a level higher than 2.5 mg/dL (221 μmol/L) in less than 2 weeks. The patient is usually very ill with jaundice and marked coagulopathy. If untreated, median survival is several days.[3] In contrast, type 2 HRS (HRS-2) occurs in patients with cirrhosis and refractory ascites, and the renal function slowly deteriorates over the course of weeks to months as reflected by a chronic, slowly

Division of Gastroenterology, Department of Medicine, 9N/983, Toronto General Hospital, University of Toronto, 200 Elizabeth Street, Toronto, Ontario M5G2C4, Canada
* Corresponding author.
E-mail address: florence.wong@utoronto.ca

Gastroenterol Clin N Am 40 (2011) 581–598
doi:10.1016/j.gtc.2011.06.011
0889-8553/11/$ – see front matter © 2011 Elsevier Inc. All rights reserved.

Box 1
Criteria for diagnosis of HRS in cirrhosis

Cirrhosis with ascites.

Serum creatinine >133 μmol/L (1.5 mg/dL).

No improvement of serum creatinine (decrease to a level of ≤133 μmol/L) after ≥2 days with diuretic withdrawal and volume expansion with albumin. The recommended dose of albumin is 1 g/kg of body weight per day up to a maximum of 100 g/d.

Absence of shock.

No current or recent treatment with nephrotoxic drugs.

Absence of parenchymal kidney disease as indicated by proteinuria >500 mg/d, microhematuria (>50 red blood cells per high power field), and/or abnormal renal ultrasonography.

Data from Salerno F, Gerbes A, Ginès P, et al. Diagnosis, prevention and treatment of hepatorenal syndrome in cirrhosis. Gut 2007;56:1310–8.

---

progressive rise in serum creatinine eventually reaching 1.5 mg/dL (133 μmol/L). Because the major clinical problem in patients with HRS-2 is refractory ascites, they are usually less ill with lesser degrees of liver dysfunction. Their prognosis is therefore slightly better than patients with HRS-1 with median survival of several weeks to months.[3]

Recent recognition that serum creatinine may underestimate the severity of renal dysfunction has led to the proposal to diagnose renal dysfunction in cirrhosis with lower levels of serum creatinine than traditionally recognized (**Table 1**).[4] This is because even smaller rises of serum creatinine have been associated with poorer prognosis both in patients with cirrhosis and ascites[5] and in those without underlying liver disease.[6] If accepted, this will allow patients with cirrhosis and renal dysfunction to be treated at an earlier stage of renal impairment, potentially improving their overall prognosis.

PATHOGENESIS

The pathogenesis of HRS is complex, with several factors contributing to the gradual deterioration in renal function as cirrhosis advances, leading to the development of HRS-2 (**Fig. 1**). Any acute event that perturbs the systemic and renal hemodynamics can lead to a rapid decline in renal function, precipitating HRS-1. This can occur either

---

Box 2
Common precipitants for type I HRS

Spontaneous bacterial peritonitis.

Other bacterial infections.

Intravascular volume depletion: Overly rapid diuresis, excess vomiting, gastrointestinal bleeding.

Large volume paracentesis without adequate intravascular volume replacement.

Nephrotoxic drugs including radiocontrast dye.

Surgical jaundice.

Table 1	
Proposed diagnostic criteria of kidney dysfunction in cirrhosis	
Diagnosis	**Definition**
Acute kidney injury	A rise in serum creatinine of ≥50% from baseline, or a rise of serum creatinine by ≥0.3 mg/dL (≥26.4 μmol/L) in <48 hours. HRS type I is a specific form of acute kidney injury.
Chronic kidney disease	Glomerular filtration rate of <60 mL/min for >3 mos calculated using the MDRD6 formula. HRS type II is a specific form of chronic kidney disease.
Acute-on-chronic kidney disease	Rise in serum creatinine of ≥50% from baseline or a rise of serum creatinine by ≥0.3 mg/dL (≥26.4 μmol/L) in <48 hours in a patient with cirrhosis whose glomerular filtration rate is <60 mL/min for >3 mos calculated using the MDRD6 formula.

Note: Both the acute deterioration in renal function and the background chronic renal dysfunction can be functional or structural in nature.

Abbreviation: MDRD6, modification of diet in renal disease formula calculated using 6 variables of serum creatinine, age, gender, albumin, blood urea nitrogen and whether the patient is African-American or not.

Data from Wong F, Nadim M, Kellum J, et al. Working Party proposal for a revised classification system of renal dysfunction in patients with cirrhosis. Gut 2011;60:702–9.

in a patient with normal baseline renal function, or superimposed on preexisting HRS-2. The following is a summary of the major contributing factors to the development of HRS in cirrhosis.

Splanchnic and Systemic Arterial Vasodilatation

The development of cirrhosis is accompanied by the distortion of liver architecture, leading to obstruction to portal flow. As a result, increased shear stress on splanchnic vessel walls lead to increased production of various vasodilators; the most potent is nitric oxide.[7] This, together with development of mesenteric angiogenesis and decreased responsiveness to vasoconstrictors, leads to the development of splanchnic vasodilatation, with a consequent increase in portal venous blood flow. Splanchnic vasodilatation also means that there is pooling of blood volume in the splanchnic circulation. Both the increased portal blood flow and the obstruction to portal flow contribute to the development of portal hypertension.[8] The opening of portosystemic shunts as a result of the portal hypertension means that some vasodilators are channeled from the splanchnic to the systemic circulation, causing systemic vasodilatation. The physiologic response is one of increased cardiac output, together with an increase in total blood volume through renal sodium retention to maintain hemodynamic stability, and a hyperdynamic circulation develops.[9] However, the maldistribution of part of the total blood volume to the splanchnic circulation means that there is effectively a subtraction of volume from the systemic circulation, despite no actual loss of total blood volume, akin to a splanchnic steal syndrome. This is known as a reduction of the effective arterial blood volume (EABV).

Hemodynamic Response to a Reduction in EABV

A reduced EABV results in the compensatory activation of various vasoconstrictor systems, including the SNS, renin–angiotensin–aldosterone system, and arginine vasopressin. In addition, reduced EABV results in decreased renal perfusion pressure,

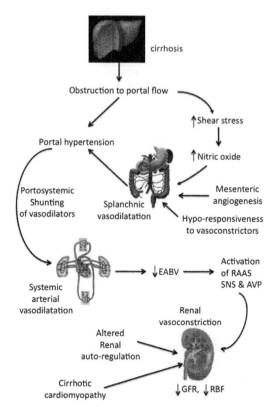

Fig. 1. Pathogenesis of HRS. AVP, arginine vasopressin; EABV, effective arterial blood volume; GFR, glomerular filtration rate; RBF, renal blood flow; SNS, sympathetic nervous system.

leading to reduced blood flow with consequent reduction in the glomerular filtration rate (GFR).[10] Initially, there is increased production of renal vasodilators such as prostaglandins and kallikrein; however, these soon become exhausted, resulting in an imbalance favoring renal vasoconstriction.[10] This renal hypoperfusion further increases the production of various intrarenal vasoconstrictors, including angiotensin II and endothelin, causing further deterioration of renal hemodynamics and renal function. Endothelin can cause mesangial constriction, further compromising the GFR.[11]

Altered Renal Autoregulation

Renal autoregulation is the process whereby regulatory mechanisms ensure that the kidneys receive a relatively constant blood supply regardless of fluctuations in blood pressure. Below a critical threshold of 65 mmHg, renal blood flow decreases in proportion to renal perfusion pressure that, in turn, depends on mean arterial pressure. When a patient progresses from pre-ascitic cirrhosis to the stages of diuretic-responsive, then diuretic-refractory ascites and eventually HRS, there is a progressive rightward shift of the renal autoregulation curve related to increasing SNS activity.[12] That is, for every given renal perfusion pressure, there is a gradual reduction of renal blood flow as liver disease advances. Therefore, the patient with cirrhosis is poised to develop renal failure simply because of the presence of advanced cirrhosis.

Cardiac Dysfunction in Cirrhosis

The hyperdynamic, high cardiac output state in decompensated cirrhosis means that these patients are encroaching on their cardiac reserve, and further reductions in systemic vascular resistance may not be met with further increases in cardiac output, with consequent fall in blood pressure. Failure to maintain blood pressure further compromises renal perfusion. In advanced cirrhosis, a relative inability to increase cardiac output during stress or systolic incompetence, part of a syndrome known as cirrhotic cardiomyopathy,[13] may be a risk factor for the development of the HRS. For example, cirrhotic patients who develop bacterial infections such as spontaneous bacterial peritonitis have further worsening of their arterial vasodilatation as a result of increased cytokine production from the bacteria. Those who went on to develop the HRS had significantly lower cardiac output at infection resolution when compared with baseline, when compared with those who did not develop the HRS at the time of infection resolution.[14] Recently, cardiac systolic dysfunction in cirrhotics has been found to be associated with increased risk of developing renal dysfunction and poorer survival.[15] This has been confirmed in a further study indicating a correlation between low cardiac output, low mean arterial pressure, and low renal blood flow.[16]

A PATHOPHYSIOLOGIC BASIS FOR USING VASOCONSTRICTORS IN HRS

The rationale for using vasoconstrictors in HRS is to reduce the extent of arterial vasodilatation in cirrhosis, thereby reducing the mismatch between circulatory capacitance and intravascular volume within it, with an overall improved EABV. This attenuates the activation of the various vasoconstrictor systems, leading to an improved renal perfusion pressure, and hence an improved GFR. Currently, there are 3 classes of vasoconstrictors that have been used in the management of HRS.

- *Vasopressin analogs:* Compounds such as ornipressin and vasopressin bind to the V1 receptors of the vascular smooth muscle cells to cause vasoconstriction in both the systemic and in the splanchnic circulations. The latter gives the added beneficial effects of reducing portal inflow, as well as reducing the extent of portal systemic shunting[17]; terlipressin, another vasopressin analog, has also been shown to dilate intrahepatic vessels, thereby reducing intrahepatic resistance to portal inflow.[18] The overall result is a reduction in portal pressure, which may have a direct effect on improving renal function.[17,19]
- *α-Adrenergic receptor agonists:* These include norepinephrine (NE) and midodrine. These act by binding to the α-1-adrenergic receptors on the vascular smooth muscle cells, which in turn leads to an increase in the intracellular calcium, thereby causing smooth muscle cell contraction and vasoconstriction.
- *Octreotide:* This is a somatostatin analog. It mediates its vasoconstrictive effects by inhibiting the release of glucagon and other vasodilatory peptides. It has been shown to have a vasoconstrictive effect in both the splanchnic[20] and systemic circulations.[21] Its portal hypotensive effects, however, are very short lived.[22]

To date, most of the studies using vasoconstrictor therapy have concentrated on patients with HRS-1, because they have the most disturbed hemodynamics that can derive the most benefits from vasoconstrictor therapy.

THE VASOCONSTRICTORS
Vasopressin Analogs

The proof-of-concept studies using a vasopressin analog in the management of HRS-1 employed ornipressin.[23,24] Complete response defined as either serum creatinine falling to less than 1.5 mg/dL or doubling of creatinine clearance to greater than 40 mL/min was observed in 57% to 75% patients with HRS-1. Median survival was prolonged to several months. However, because of the development of severe adverse events of an ischemic nature, ornipressin is not generally recommended for patients with HRS.

One of the most studied vasopressin analogs in HRS is terlipressin. Because terlipressin is a pro-drug, the active metabolite, lysine-vasopressin, is gradually released over several hours, thereby avoiding many of the ischemic side effects without any compromise of its potency. Its longer half-life also allows for more convenient intermittent intravenous dosing. There is no standardized dosing schedule for terlipressin administration because of the lack of dose-finding studies. Terlipressin is generally started at a dose of 1 mg every 4 to 6 hours and increased to a maximum of 2 mg every 4 to 6 hours if there is no reduction in serum creatinine of at least 25% compared with the baseline value on day 3 of therapy. Treatment is maintained until the serum creatinine has decreased below 1.5 mg/dL (133 μmol/L).[1] Response to therapy is characterized by a slowly progressive reduction in serum creatinine to below 1.5 mg/dL (133 μmol/L), and an increase in mean arterial pressure, urine volume, and serum sodium concentration. Median time to response is 14 days and the response time is usually dependent on the pretreatment serum creatinine level, being shorter in patients with lower baseline serum creatinine levels.[25] Recurrence after withdrawal of therapy is uncommon and retreatment with terlipressin is generally effective. It is important to emphasize that most studies excluded patients with known severe cardiovascular or ischemic conditions or patients with ongoing sepsis. In most studies, terlipressin was given in combination with albumin (1 g/kg of body weight on day 1 followed by 40 g/d) to improve the efficacy of treatment on circulatory function.[26]

Several small studies involving a total of 46 patients[27–30] with HRS examined the effects of terlipressin, with or without albumin, on systemic hemodynamics and renal function. Terlipressin, given at an initial dose of 0.5 to 1.0 mg every 4 to 6 hours, and titrating upward to 2.0 every 4 to 6 hours significantly improved mean arterial pressure by 13% to 28%. Serum creatinine reduced by at least 50% and the GFR doubled. In the 2 studies that measured plasma renin activity, the levels were reduced by at least 80%, suggesting that terlipressin improved the EABV and reduced the activation of the systemic vasoconstrictor systems. Ischemic side effects were significantly less with terlipressin than with ornipressin.

Two larger, randomized, controlled trials were subsequently published on the use of terlipressin for the treatment of HRS-1. In the first, Sanyal and the Terlipressin Study Group[31] evaluated the safety and efficacy of terlipressin plus albumin versus albumin alone in 112 patients with HRS-1 in a multinational study. Patients in the terlipressin group achieved significant improvement in serum creatinine (P<.009; **Fig. 2A**), mean day-14 Model of End-stage Liver Disease score (−4.1 vs −1.7; P<.008) and HRS reversal (44% vs 9%; P<.008) compared with the placebo group. However, there was no difference in 6-month overall survival or transplant-free survival. More patients in the terlipressin group experienced serious adverse cardiac events such as nonfatal myocardial infarction, nonsustained supraventricular tachycardia, and arrhythmias (10 vs 4 patients). In the second study, Martín-Llahí and The Terlipressin and Albumin for Hepatorenal Syndrome Investigators[32] compared terlipressin at 1 to 2 mg every 4 hours plus albumin to albumin alone in both HRS-1 and HRS-2 patients (n = 46). Similarly, in this trial, the terlipressin group experienced a significantly higher rate of improved renal function (by 0.7 mg/dL vs no change with placebo; **Fig. 2B**). Survival at 3 months, however, was not different. Once again, there was an increased

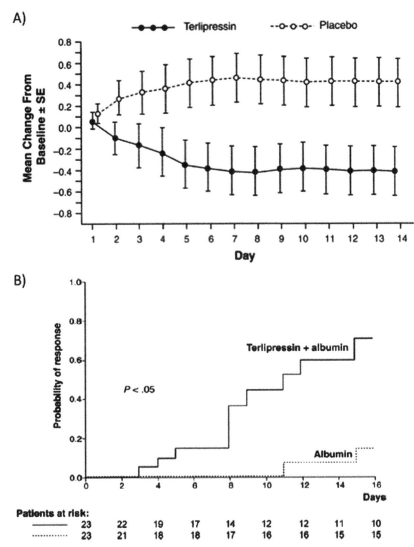

Fig. 2. (*A*) Mean change in serum creatinine from baseline to end of treatment in patients receiving terlipressin 1 mg every 6 hours plus albumin versus placebo plus albumin. (*From* Salerno F, Gerbes A, Ginès P, et al. Diagnosis, prevention and treatment of hepatorenal syndrome in cirrhosis. Gut 2007;56:1310–8; with permission.) (*B*) Inverse Kaplan–Meier curves estimating the cumulative incidence of improvement of renal function for patients with HRS on terlipressin 1 to 2 mg every 4 hours plus albumin versus albumin alone. (*From* Montoliu S, Ballesté B, Planas R, et al. Incidence and prognosis of different types of functional renal failure in cirrhotic patients with ascites. Clin Gastroenterol Hepatol 2010;8:616–22; with permission.)

rate of cardiovascular complications in the terlipressin group including myocardial ischemia, intestinal ischemia, arrhythmias, and volume overload (5 vs 1 patient).

The improvement in renal function after the administration of terlipressin in HRS-1 can be explained by its physiologic actions. Its vasoconstrictive effects on the systemic circulation can lead to an improvement in systemic hemodynamics, associated with an amelioration of the hyperdynamic circulation in cirrhosis.[33] The EABV becomes better filled, as reflected by a significant reduction in activities of the renin–angiotensin–aldosterone system and SNS. This in turn, leads to an improvement in GFR, and renal sodium excretion.[34]

There is preliminary evidence that when terlipressin is given as a continuous infusion rather than as boluses in the treatment of HRS-1, the same efficacy can be achieved with a lower total daily dose and with fewer side effects.[35,36] Pharmacodynamic studies have shown that continuous infusion of terlipressin provides a more sustained portal pressure-lowering effect than bolus injections,[37] thereby explaining the beneficial effects of a terlipressin infusion over bolus injections.

Although these studies have included a few patients with HRS-2, the data are difficult to abstract to determine the effects of terlipressin on renal function in patients with HRS-2. Studies specifically designed for HRS-2 patients are scant. However, given the fact that the pathophysiology of HRS-2 is similar to that of HRS-1, especially in terms of the splanchnic and systemic hemodynamic changes, there is every reason to believe that terlipressin should also work in patients with HRS-2. In a small study that included 11 patients with HRS-2, terlipressin given at a dose of 1 mg every 4 hours for at least 7 days resulted in a reduction in serum creatinine in 73% of patients, with 88% of the responders achieving a serum creatinine of less than 1.5 mg/dL (133 μmol/L).[38] Seven of the responders then went on to receive a transjugular intrahepatic portosystemic shunt (TIPS), making it difficult to assess whether HRS-2 recurred after completion of terlipressin therapy or not.

α-Adrenergic Receptor Agonists

Midodrine

The most widely used α-adrenergic receptor agonist is midodrine, a systemic vasoconstrictor that has been approved for the treatment of postural hypotension. The acute effects of midodrine on renal function was first assessed in 25 cirrhotic patients with ascites (17 patients without HRS and 8 with HRS-2).[39] In patients without HRS, midodrine was able to improve systemic and renal hemodynamics, increase urinary sodium excretion, associated with a decrease in plasma renin activity, and arginine vasopressin, as well as serum nitrite and nitrate levels. However, in the 8 patients with HRS, midodrine did not have any significant effects on renal function, or urinary sodium excretion.

However, the combination of midodrine and octreotide in patients with HRS-1 seems to have the same beneficial effects on renal function as midodrine alone in patients without HRS. Three studies, totaling 79 patients[40–42] reported HRS reversal as defined by a serum creatinine of less than 1.5 mg/dL (133 μmol/L) in 49% of patients when the combination was given for a median period of 17 days. Midodrine has been administered orally at an initial dose of 5 to 10 mg 3 times per day, and octreotide either subcutaneously at an initial dose of 100 μg 3 times daily, or as an intravenous infusion at an hourly dose of 25 μg/h after an initial bolus of 25 μg. If there is no increase in MAP of at least 15 mmHg, the dose of midodrine can be increased up to 15 mg 3 times daily and that of subcutaneous octreotide up to 200 μg 3 times daily. Another retrospective study evaluated the use of 7.5 to 15 mg midodrine combined with subcutaneous octreotide 100 to 200 μg 3 times per day and intravenous albumin 50 to 100 g/d for a mean of 8.4 $\pm$ 9.6 days in 75 patients with either HRS-1 (n = 49) or HRS-2 (n = 26).[43] The treatment group was compared with a pre-2001 historical control group of 87 patients with either HRS-1 (n = 53) or HRS-2 (n = 34) who did not receive the drug regimen. During a mean follow-up of almost 4 months, there was a significant improvement of GFR in the treatment group compared with the historical controls (48 vs 34 mL/min; P = .03). Median survival was significantly improved in patients who received the combination therapy for both HRS-1 (40 vs 17 days; P = .007) and HRS-2 patients (>12 months vs 22 days; P = .0004). The percentage of patients who underwent transplantation was increased only for patients with HRS-2 (58% vs 25%; P = .04).

One study found that the dose of midodrine was an important determinant in HRS-1 reversal. When midodrine was given at 15 mg 3 times daily, 88% patients had HRS-1 reversal compared with 33% in those receiving <12.5 mg 3 times daily.[42] Adverse events associated with midodrine use are generally mild and self-limiting and these include diarrhea and tingling without cardiovascular complications. Therefore, the combination of midodrine and octreotide is a alternative in the management of HRS, particularly in countries where terlipressin in unavailable.

NE

NE (at 0.5–3 mg/h) is another α-adrenergic receptor agonist that has been administered to patients with HRS because of its potent vasoconstrictive effects on both the venous and arterial vasculature. However, the number of patients treated with NE is small and no randomized, comparative studies with a control group of patients receiving no vasoconstrictor therapy have been performed to evaluate its efficacy.

The initial uncontrolled pilot study using NE showed a 83% reversal of HRS-1 in 12 patients after a median duration of treatment of 7 days.[44] NE also effectively improved serum sodium concentration, creatinine clearance, urine output, and renal sodium excretion. Systemic hemodynamics as indicated by mean arterial pressure, and fullness of the EABV, as indicated by plasma renin activity, and aldosterone levels also improved.

Two recent studies that were part of small, prospective, open-label, randomized studies of NE versus terlipressin found both vasoconstrictors to be equally effective in the treatment of HRS-1 with similar rates of side effects. One study compared the efficacy of NE versus terlipressin for treating HRS in 22 patients (9 with HRS-1 and 13 with HRS-2).[45] Patients received norepinephrine 0.1 to 0.7 μg/kg per minute plus albumin (n = 10) or terlipressin 1 to 2 mg every 4 hours plus albumin (n = 12) for up to 2 weeks. Reversal of HRS occurred in 70% of patients receiving NE versus 83% of patients receiving terlipressin (P = NS), indicating NE was not inferior to terlipressin in the management of HRS, although it was a small trial. Relapse after treatment discontinuation occurred in 29% of NE responders versus 60% of terlipressin responders (P = NS). The cost of NE therapy was significantly lower than that of terlipressin (107 vs 1536 Euros; P<.0001). To evaluate the efficacy of NE for treating patients with HRS-1, a randomized pilot study was conducted using NE infusion starting at 0.5 mg/h with stepwise increases of 0.5 mg/h every 4 hours titrated to the mean arterial pressure plus albumin (20 patients) versus intravenous terlipressin 0.5 to 2 mg every 6 hours plus albumin (20 patients).[46] NE significantly increased MAP (mean, 78.3–93.3 mmHg; P<.01), increased urine output (mean, 479–1278 mL/d; P<.01), and decreased serum creatinine from baseline (mean, 3.3–1.0 mg/dL; P<.01; **Fig. 3**). The renal function improvement between patients treated with NE and those treated with terlipressin was similar. The percentage of patients who responded to therapy was not different between the NE and terlipressin groups (50% vs 40%; P = .741), and no difference was noted in cumulative survival between groups (11.6 vs 12.6 days; P = .452).

At doses of 1.5 mg/h, NE has been associated with ventricular arrhythmias (7%) and myocardial hypokinesia (5%), both reversed with dose reduction. Given the much

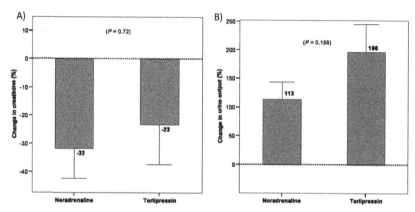

Fig. 3. (*A*) Percentage change in serum creatinine and (*B*) percentage change in urine output following the administration of either NE or terlipressin in patients with HRS-1. (*From* Lassnigg A, Schmidlin D, Mouhieddine M, et al. Minimal changes of serum creatinine predict prognosis in patients after cardiothoracic surgery: a prospective cohort study. J Am Soc Nephrol 2004;15:1597–605; with permission.)

lower cost and wider availability of NE, it can be considered a safe and effective alternative to terlipressin for HRS-1, especially in countries where terlipressin is not available or cost is a major concern. However, patients being given NE should be transferred to an intensive care unit where it can infused in a monitored environment.

Octreotide

Octreotide is a long-acting somatostatin analog that reduces portal hypertension and splanchnic hyperemia,[47] and it may also cause splanchnic vasoconstriction; however, these effects may be blunted in patients with cirrhosis.[48] Octreotide was evaluated in a randomized, double-blind, placebo-controlled, crossover study of 19 patients with either HRS-1 or HRS-2.[49] Patients received intravenous octreotide 50 μg/h or placebo with daily albumin of 50 g over two 4-day study periods. Of the 14 patients who completed both crossover periods of the study, no significant differences were noted in the number of patients who had a 20% decrease in serum creatinine from baseline or reductions in plasma renin activity, aldosterone levels, or glucagon levels. No adverse effects related to octreotide therapy were observed. A retrospective review of 43 patients with HRS also found no clear benefit with octreotide monotherapy or any additional benefit when added to vasopressin.[50] Based on the currently available literature, octreotide monotherapy does not seem to be any more effective than placebo for treating HRS. Octreotide is well-tolerated and may be useful when given as an adjunct therapy in patients with esophageal variceal hemorrhage or as a combination therapy with midodrine.

Albumin

Traditionally, albumin is seen as an effective intravascular volume expander, but recent evidence have shown that it also has ligand-binding, anti-oxidant, anti-inflammatory, and metabolic properties with beneficial effects beyond simple fluid resuscitation.[51] Albumin has not been established as a stand alone treatment for HRS, but is often used in conjunction with other vasoconstrictors for additional benefits. In recent studies comparing albumin alone versus albumin and vasoconstrictors in patients with HRS, albumin has not been shown to reverse HRS, or improve survival.[31,32,52]

Albumin followed by the administration of furosemide has been used in patients with cirrhosis.[53,54] The use of diuretics in patients with HRS has generally not been recommended because of the already reduced EABV. A pilot study evaluating albumin plus furosemide was conducted in 20 patients with HRS-1 or HRS-2.[55] Albumin 40 to 600 g was administered to increase and/or maintain central venous pressure above 3 cmH$_2$O. Patients were then administered furosemide 250 to 1500 mg/d if required to maintain a diuresis of more than 50 mL/h. Eleven patients (55%) had reversal of HRS with a mean of 275 $\pm$ 177 g of albumin over a mean period of 6.8 $\pm$ 4.9 days without the use of furosemide. Patients with higher baseline creatinine clearance and HRS-2 were more likely to respond to albumin infusion. If albumin is used, the admixture should provide a high percentage of albumin (eg, 20%–25% albumin) and the typical dosage is 1 g/kg of body weight (up to 100 g) on day 1, then 20 to 60 g/d thereafter. Given that albumin alone has not been proven to be efficacious in randomized, controlled trials of vasoconstrictors, the use of albumin alone as a treatment of HRS-1 cannot be recommended.

DO THE VASOCONSTRICTORS REALLY WORK FOR THE HRS?

To date, there are no meta-analyses combining all studies using various vasoconstrictors to answer the question as to whether vasoconstrictors can reverse HRS; the number of randomized, controlled trials is small, and many of the studies only included small number of patients. However, there are 2 recent meta-analyses assessing the efficacy of terlipressin in the treatment of HRS. The first meta-analysis[56] assessing 4 randomized, control trials[30–32,52] demonstrated that the use of terlipressin plus albumin was superior than albumin with or without placebo in improving renal function in patients with cirrhosis, ascites, and HRS-1. Reversal of HRS-1 defined as a reduction of serum creatinine to <1.5 mg/dL (133 μmol/L) was observed in 46.0% of patients who received terlipressin plus albumin versus 11.6% in the control group. The improvement was sustained in most patients during the follow-up of 90 to 180 days, and recurrence only occurred in 8% of patients. There was also a trend toward improved transplant-free survival. Prolongation of treatment beyond 7 days and up to 20 days seems to improve the likelihood of response. Overall, terlipressin seemed to be safe and well-tolerated.

A second systematic review of randomized studies using all vasoconstrictors performed a subanalysis on the efficacy of terlipressin as a treatment for HRS, and found that terlipressin plus albumin was more efficacious than albumin alone in terms of improving renal function or reversal of HRS[57] (**Fig. 4A**). The same study also reported that, when all randomized trials on vasoconstrictors alone or with albumin versus no intervention or albumin for HRS were assessed in a meta-analysis, there was a reduction in all-cause mortality favoring the vasoconstrictors (**Fig. 4B**).[57] Currently, a multicenter trial is being conducted to confirm whether terlipressin increases survival in HRS-1 patients. Finally, treatment with vasoconstrictors in patients with HRS-2 is also associated with an improvement in renal function,[43,58] but the recurrence rate is high. Nevertheless, the published information is still limited for vasoconstrictors to be routinely recommended as a treatment for HRS-2.

Despite the fact that the meta-analyses found that vasoconstrictor therapy was beneficial for patients with HRS, not every patient treated with vasoconstrictor therapy responded with an improvement in renal function. The identification of those patients who will not respond to vasoconstrictor therapy is critical when planning for other treatment options, especially for those patients awaiting liver transplantation.

less than 1.5 mg/dL (133 μmol/L), included a baseline serum bilirubin level of less than 10 mg/dL (170 μmol/L) and an increase in mean arterial pressure of more than 5 mmHg on day 3 of treatment. Another multicenter, randomized, double-blind, placebo-controlled trial of terlipressin for HRS-1 showed that only patients with baseline serum creatinine below 5.6 mg/dL (493 μmol/L) and receiving more than 3 days of terlipressin therapy achieved HRS reversal.[60] The corollary from these observations is that patients with severe liver and renal dysfunction should not receive terlipressin, because they are less likely to respond, especially if they do not have a hemodynamic response in the first 3 days of treatment.

COMBINED VASOCONSTRICTOR THERAPY AND TIPS

Because the use of vasoconstrictor therapy does not correct the renal dysfunction in every case of HRS, the addition of a treatment option that corrects another aspect of the pathophysiology of HRS would be a feasible alternative. The combination of vasoconstrictor therapy followed by a TIPS is one such alternative. The combination eliminates portal hypertension and reduces the extent of systemic arterial vasodilatation, and potentially could have an additive effect in improving renal function in patients with HRS. Midodrine, octreotide, and albumin were administered to 14 patients with HRS-1, and this improved but not normalized the renal function.[61] Among those patients who were deemed suitable to receive a TIPS, the insertion of TIPS eventually normalized renal function over the course of 12 months and allowed eventual elimination of ascites. The overall survival rate was 50%, with the longest patient surviving 30 months. In another study, 11 patients with HRS-2 received terlipressin together with albumin, which maintained the central venous pressure to 10 cmH$_2$O.[38] The placement of TIPS in 9 of the 11 patients eventually brought the serum creatinine down to 1.36 $\pm$ 0.3 mg/dL (120 μmol/L) at 1 month post-TIPS. As expected, TIPS improved 24-hour urinary volume in all patients, leading to a lower postprocedure diuretic requirement. Ascites also significantly decreased in all patients and eventually disappeared from the second week onward after TIPS.

LIVER TRANSPLANTATION

Liver transplantation is the definitive treatment for patients with HRS, because it eliminates liver dysfunction, portal hypertension, and the hemodynamic abnormalities in decompensated cirrhosis, which are central to the pathogenesis of HRS. Indeed, renal function improves in many patients with HRS after liver transplantation, associated with reductions in systemic vasoconstrictor levels.[62] However, renal recovery after liver transplant is not guaranteed; up to 40% of patients remain dependent on renal dialysis after liver transplantation.[63] Patients with renal failure at the time of liver transplantation tend to have more complications and longer stays in intensive care units compared with patients who receive liver transplantation without HRS.[63,64] In addition, these patients have poorer graft and patient survival compared with patients without pretransplant renal failure.[64,65] Therefore, treating the HRS preoperatively may improve long-term survival postoperatively, comparable with transplant recipients with previously normal renal function.[66] Indeed, pretransplant renal failure has been identified as an independent predictor for 30-day and 2-year mortality post liver transplantation.[67]

In those patients with prolonged renal dysfunction before liver transplantation, a combined liver-kidney transplant (CLKT) may be necessary.[68] Often, there is a further worsening of renal function in the immediate perioperative period.[69] The issue of whether to perform CLKT is difficult. HRS itself is not an indication for CLKT. CLKT is reserved for those patients with irreversible kidney injury, requiring hemodialysis for longer than 6 to 8 weeks, or progressive primary kidney disease.[70] Recent data suggested that patients with renal failure without undergoing dialysis pretransplantation did not benefit from CLKT.[71] Only patients who required dialysis pretransplantation showed an improved survival with CLKT when compared with patients who underwent liver transplantation alone.[71] Therefore, it has been proposed that patients who have had more than 8 to 12 weeks of dialysis should be considered for CLKT. Because the outcome after CLKT is inferior to that of liver transplant alone,[72] there is now a trend to perform a liver transplantation, alone even in the presence of pretransplant renal failure requiring dialysis, and then only to consider kidney transplant if there is no renal recovery after liver transplantation.

PROGNOSIS

The patient with advanced cirrhosis and HRS has a poor prognosis. If untreated, the median survival is approximately 10 days.[3] The advent of vasoconstrictor therapy has improved the prognosis of these patients significantly. Many patients can now survive sufficiently long to await a liver transplant after vasoconstrictor therapy. Correction of renal dysfunction before liver transplant also improves graft and patient survival. Conversely, failure to respond to treatment is a predictor of poor patient outcome.[73] In these patients, liver transplantation offers the best chance for survival. Currently, there are some parameters that predict response to vasoconstrictor therapy. However, the best strategy in the management of patients with advanced cirrhosis is to prevent the development of HRS, rather than treating HRS once it has occurred. Given that vasoconstrictors correct some of the pathophysiology of advanced cirrhosis, future studies may well include vasoconstrictors as part of this preventive approach to improve the overall outcome of these patients.

REFERENCES

1. Salerno F, Gerbes A, Ginès P, et al. Diagnosis, prevention and treatment of hepatorenal syndrome in cirrhosis. Gut 2007;56:1310–8.
2. Montoliu S, Ballesté B, Planas R, et al. Incidence and prognosis of different types of functional renal failure in cirrhotic patients with ascites. Clin Gastroenterol Hepatol 2010;8:616–22.
3. Ginès P, Guevara M, Arroyo V, et al. Hepatorenal syndrome. Lancet 2003;362:1819–27.
4. Wong F, Nadim M, Kellum J, et al. Working Party proposal for a revised classification system of renal dysfunction in patients with cirrhosis. Gut 2011;60:702–9.
5. Tsien C, Rabie R, Wong F. Are repeated episodes of acute renal dysfunction clinically significant in cirrhosis with ascites? [Abstract] Hepatology 2010;52(Suppl 1):891A.
6. Lassnigg A, Schmidlin D, Mouhieddine M, et al. Minimal changes of serum creatinine predict prognosis in patients after cardiothoracic surgery: a prospective cohort study. J Am Soc Nephrol 2004;15:1597–605.
7. Martin PY, Ginès P, Schrier RW. Nitric oxide as a mediator of hemodynamic abnormalities and sodium and water retention in cirrhosis. N Engl J Med 1998; 339:533–41.
8. Sanyal AJ, Bosch J, Blei A, et al. Portal hypertension and its complications. Gastroenterology 2008;134:1715–28.
9. Blendis L, Wong F. The hyperdynamic circulation in cirrhosis: an overview. Pharmacol Ther 2001;89:221–31.
10. Gines P, Schrier RW. Renal failure and cirrhosis. N Engl J Med 2009;361:1279–90.
11. Oliver JA, Verna EC. Afferent mechanisms of sodium retention in cirrhosis and hepatorenal syndrome. Kidney Int 2010;77:669–80.

12. Stadlbauer V, Wright GA, Banaji M, et al. Relationship between activation of the sympathetic nervous system and renal blood flow autoregulation in cirrhosis. Gastro-enterology 2008;134:111–9.
13. Wong F. Cirrhotic cardiomyopathy. Hepatol Int 2009;3:294–304.
14. Ruiz-del-Arbol L, Urman J, Fernandez J, et al. Systemic, renal, and hepatic hemody-namic derangement in cirrhotic patients with spontaneous bacterial peritonitis. Hepa-tology 2003;38:1210–8.
15. Ruiz-del-Arbol L, Monescillo A, Arocena C, et al. Circulatory function and hepatorenal syndrome in cirrhosis. Hepatology 2005;42:439–47.
16. Krag A, Bendtsen F, Henriksen JH, et al. Low cardiac output predicts development of hepatorenal syndrome and survival in patients with cirrhosis and ascites. Gut 2010; 59:105–10.
17. Narahara Y, Kanazawa H, Taki Y, et al. Effects of terlipressin on systemic, hepatic and renal hemodynamics in patients with cirrhosis. J Gastroenterol Hepatol 2009;24: 1791–7.
18. Kiszka-Kanewitz M, Henricksen JH, Hansen EF, et al. Effect of terlipressin on blood volume distribution in patients with cirrhosis. Scand J Gastroenterol 2004; 39:486–92.
19. Jalan R, Forrest EH, Redhead DN, et al. Reduction in renal blood flow following acute increase in the portal pressure: evidence for the existence of a hepatorenal reflex in man? Gut 1997;40:664–70.
20. Wiest R, Tsai MH, Groszmann RJ. Octreotide potentiates PKC-dependent vasocon-strictors in portal-hypertensive and control rats. Gastroenterology 2001;120:975–83.
21. Chatila R, Ferayorni L, Gupta T, et al. Local arterial vasoconstriction induced by octreotide in patients with cirrhosis. Hepatology 2000;31:572–6.
22. Baik SK, Jeong PH, Ji SW, et al. Acute hemodynamic effects of octreotide and terlipressin in patients with cirrhosis: a randomized comparison. Am J Gastroenterol 2005;100:631–5.
23. Guevara M, Ginès P, Fernández-Esparrach G, et al. Reversibility of hepatorenal syndrome by prolonged administration of ornipressin and plasma volume expansion. Hepatology 1998;27:35–41.
24. Gülberg V, Bilzer M, Gerbes AL. Long-term therapy and retreatment of hepatorenal syndrome type 1 with ornipressin and dopamine. Hepatology 1999;30:870–5.
25. Nazar A, Pereira GH, Guevara M, et al. Predictors of response to therapy to terlipressin and albumin in patients with cirrhosis and type 1 hepatorenal syndrome. Hepatology 2010;51:219–26.
26. Ortega R, Ginès P, Uriz J, et al. Terlipressin therapy with and without albumin for patients with hepatorenal syndrome: results of a prospective, nonrandomized study. Hepatology 2002;36:941–8.
27. Uriz J, Ginès P, Cárdenas A, et al. Terlipressin plus albumin infusion: an effective and safe therapy of hepatorenal syndrome. J Hepatol 2000;33:43–8.
28. Mulkay JP, Louis H, Donckier V, et al. Long-term terlipressin administration improves renal function in cirrhotic patients with type 1 hepatorenal syndrome: a pilot study. Acta Gastroenterol Belg 2001;64:15–9.
29. Ortega R, Ginès P, Uriz J, et al. Terlipressin therapy with and without albumin for patients with hepatorenal syndrome: results of a prospective, nonrandomized study. Hepatology 2002;36:941–8.
30. Solanki P, Chawla A, Garg R, et al. Beneficial effects of terlipressin in hepatorenal syndrome: a prospective, randomized placebo-controlled clinical trial. J Gastroen-terol Hepatol 2003;18:152–6.

31. Sanyal AJ, Boyer T, Garcia-Tsao G, et al. A randomized, prospective, double-blind, placebo-controlled trial of terlipressin for type 1 hepatorenal syndrome. Gastroenterology 2008;134:1360–8.
32. Martín-Llahí M, Pépin MN, Guevara M, et al. Terlipressin and albumin vs albumin in patients with cirrhosis and hepatorenal syndrome: a randomized study. Gastroenterology 2008;134:1352–9.
33. Krag A, Bendtsen F, Mortensen C, et al. Effects of a single Terlipressin administration on cardiac function and perfusion in cirrhosis. Eur J Gastroenterol Hepatol 2010;22: 1085–92.
34. Krag A, Moller S, Henriksen JH, et al. Terlipressin improves renal function in patients with cirrhosis and ascites without hepatorenal syndrome. Hepatology 2007;46:1863–71.
35. Angeli P, Fasolato S, Cavallin M, et al. Terlipressin given as continuous intravenous infusion is the more suitable schedule for the treatment of type 1 hepatorenal syndrome (HRS) in patients with cirrhosis: results of a controlled clinical trial [abstract]. Hepatology 2008;48(Suppl):378A.
36. Gerbes AL, Huber E, Gülberg V. Terlipressin for hepatorenal syndrome: continuous infusion as an alternative to i.v. bolus administration. Gastroenterology 2009;137: 1179.
37. Escorsell A, Bandi JC, Moitinho E, et al. Time profile of the haemodynamic effects of terlipressin in portal hypertension. J Hepatol 1997;26:621–7.
38. Alessandria C, Venon WD, Marzano A, et al. Renal failure in cirrhotic patients: role of terlipressin in clinical approach to hepatorenal syndrome type 2. Eur J Gastroenterol Hepatol 2002;14:1363–8.
39. Angeli P, Volpin R, Piovan D, et al. Acute effects of the oral administration of midodrine, an α-adrenergic agonist, on renal hemodynamics and renal function in cirrhotic patients with ascites. Hepatology 1998;28:937–43.
40. Angeli P, Volpin R, Gerunda G, et al. Reversal of type 1 hepatorenal syndrome with the administration of midodrine and octreotide. Hepatology 1999;29:1690–7.
41. Wong F, Pantea L, Sniderman K. The use of midodrine, octreotide and transjugular intrahepatic portosystemic stent shunt in the treatment of cirrhotic patients with ascites and renal dysfunction including hepatorenal syndrome. Hepatology 2004;40: 55–64.
42. Esrailian E, Pantangco ER, Kyulo NL, et al. Octreotide/Midodrine therapy significantly improves renal function and 30-day survival in patients with type 1 hepatorenal syndrome. Dig Dis Sci 2007;52:742–8.
43. Skagen C, Einstein M, Lucey MR, et al. Combination treatment with octreotide, midodrine, and albumin improves survival in patients with type 1 and type 2 hepatorenal syndrome. J Clin Gastroenterol 2009;43:680–5.
44. Duvoux C, Zanditenas D, Hezode C, et al. Effects of noradrenalin and albumin in patients with type I hepatorenal syndrome: a pilot study. Hepatology 2002;36: 374–80.
45. Alessandria C, Ottobrelli A, Debernardi-Venon W, et al. Noradrenalin vs terlipressin in patients with hepatorenal syndrome: a prospective, randomized, unblinded, pilot study. J Hepatol 2007;47:499–505.
46. Sharma P, Kumar A, Shrama BC et al. An open label, pilot, randomized controlled trial of noradrenaline versus terlipressin in the treatment of type 1 hepatorenal syndrome and predictors of response. Am J Gastroenterol 2008;103:1689–97.
47. Vorobioff JD, Ferretti SE, Zangroniz P, et al. Octreotide enhances portal pressure reduction induced by propranolol in cirrhosis: a randomized, controlled trial. Am J Gastroenterol 2007;102:2206–13.

48. Moller S, Brinch K, Henriksen JH, et al. Effect of octreotide on systemic, central, and splanchnic haemodynamics in cirrhosis. J Hepatol 1997;26:1026–33.
49. Pomier-Layrargues G, Paquin SC, Hassoun Z, et al. Octreotide in hepatorenal syndrome: a randomized, double-blind, placebo-controlled, crossover study. Hepatology 2003;38:238–43.
50. Kiser TH, Fish DN, Obritsch MD, et al. Vasopressin, not octreotide, may be beneficial in the treatment of hepatorenal syndrome: a retrospective study. Nephrol Dial Transplant 2005;20:1813–20.
51. Wong F. Drug insight: the role of albumin in the management of chronic liver disease. Nat Clin Pract Gastroenterol Hepatol 2007;4:43–51.
52. Neri S, Pulvirenti D, Malaguarnera M, et al. Terlipressin and albumin in patients with cirrhosis and type I hepatorenal syndrome. Dig Dis Sci 2008;53:830–5.
53. Gentilini P, Casini-Raggi V, Di Fiore G, et al. Albumin improves the response to diuretics in patients with cirrhosis and ascites: results of a randomized, controlled trial. J Hepatol 1999;30:639–45.
54. Romanelli RG, La Villa G, Barletta G, et al. Long-term albumin infusion improves survival in patients with cirrhosis and ascites: an unblinded randomized trial. World J Gastroenterol 2006;12:1403–7.
55. Peron JM, Bureau C, Gonzalez L, et al. Treatment o f hepatorenal syndrome as defined by the International Ascites Club by albumin and furosemide infusion according to the central venous pressure: a prospective pilot study. Am J Gastroenterol 2005;100:2702–7.
56. Sagi SV, Mittal S, Kasturi KS, et al. Terlipressin therapy for reversal of type 1 hepatorenal syndrome: a meta-analysis of randomized controlled trials. J Gastroenterol Hepatol 2010;25:880–5.
57. Gluud LL, Christensen K, Christensen E, et al. Systematic review of randomized trials on vasoconstrictor drugs for hepatorenal syndrome. Hepatology 2010;51:576–84.
58. Alessandria C, Debernardi-Venon W, Carello M, et al. Midodrine in the prevention of hepatorenal syndrome type 2 recurrence: a case-control study. Dig Liver Dis 2009; 41:298–302.
59. Nazar A, Pereira GH, Guevara M, et al. Predictors of response to therapy with terlipressin and albumin in patients with cirrhosis and type 1 hepatorenal syndrome. Hepatology 2010;51:219–26.
60. Boyer TD, Sanyal AJ, Garcia-Tsao G, et al. Predictors of response to terlipressin plus albumin in hepatorenal syndrome (HRS) type 1: relationship of serum creatinine to hemodynamics. J Hepatol 2010. [Epub ahead of print].
61. Wong F, Pantea L, Sniderman K. Midodrine, octreotide, albumin, and TIPS in selected patients with cirrhosis and type 1 hepatorenal syndrome. Hepatology 2004;40:55–64.
62. Cassinello C, Moreno E, Gozalo A, et al. Effects of orthotopic liver transplantation on vasoactive systems and renal function in patients with advanced liver cirrhosis. Dig Dis Sci 2003;48:179–86.
63. Marik PE, Wood K, Starzl TE. The course of type 1 hepatorenal syndrome post liver transplantation. Nephro Dial Transplant 2006;21:478–82.
64. Nair S, Verma S, Thuluvath PJ. Pre-transplant renal function predicts survival in patients undergoing orthotopic liver transplantation. Hepatology 2002;35:1179–85.
65. Gonwa TA, Klintmalm GB, Levy M, et al. Impact of pre-transplant renal function on survival after liver transplantation. Transplantation 1995;59:361–5.
66. Restuccia T, Ortega R, Guevara M, et al. Effects of treatment of hepatorenal syndrome before transplantation on post-transplantation outcome. A case-control study. J Hepatol 2004;40:140–6.

67. Weismuller TJ, Prokein J, Becker T, et al. Prediction of survival after liver transplantation by pre-transplant parameters. Scand J Gastroenterol 2008;43:736–46.
68. Papafragkakis H, Martin P, Akalin E. Combined liver and kidney transplantation. Curr Opin Organ Transplant 2010;15:263–8.
69. Wong LP, Blackley MP, Andreoni KA, et al. Survival of liver transplant candidates with acute renal failure receiving renal replacement therapy. Kidney Int 2005;68:362–70.
70. Davis CL, Feng S, Sung R, et al. Simultaneous liver-kidney transplantation: evaluation to decision making. Am J Transplant. 2007;7:1702–9.
71. Schmitt TM, Kumer SC, Al-Osaimi A, et al. Combined liver-kidney and liver transplantation in patients with renal failure outcomes in the MELD era. Transpl Int 2009;22: 876–83.
72. Locke JE, Warren DS, Singer AL, et al. Declining outcomes in simultaneous liver-kidney transplantation in the MELD era: ineffective usage of renal allografts. Transplantation 2008;85:935–42.
73. Schepke M, Appenrodt B, Heller J, et al. Prognostic factors for patients with cirrhosis and kidney dysfunction in the era of MELD: results of a prospective study. Liver Int 2006;26:834–9.

Hepatocellular Carcinoma: Locoregional and Targeted Therapies

Robert Wong, MD[a], Catherine Frenette, MD[b], Robert Gish, MD[c],*

KEYWORDS
- Radiofrequency ablation • Chemoembolization • Yttrium-90
- Sorafenib • Molecular targeted therapies

Hepatocellular carcinoma (HCC) is the sixth most common cancer and is the third leading cause of cancer-related deaths worldwide.[1–3] The continued rise in HCC incidence and mortality emphasizes the need for novel therapeutic approaches. The ability to significantly impact disease epidemiology hinges on 2 important factors: cancer screening and surveillance programs and the existence of effective therapeutic tools. The success of any cancer screening program relies on principles of early detection of cancer among at-risk populations affording greater therapeutic options and more effective treatment potential. Many factors can influence HCC risk, chief among them HCC etiology, and recent updates by the American Association for the Study of Liver Diseases attempt to better define at risk groups for which routine HCC screening is recommended, including those with cirrhosis from any cause, and certain populations of patients with hepatitis B without cirrhosis.[1]

The clinical evaluation and management of HCC encompasses a multidisciplinary assessment combining comprehensive therapeutic approaches along with cancer surveillance implementation.[4–8] Therapeutic options available to patients with HCC span a spectrum that includes less invasive locoregional therapies that utilize localized thermal ablation or intra-arterial infusion and embolization therapies, potentially curative operative resection or transplantation, and more novel molecular-based targeted therapies and external beam radiotherapy. The challenging aspect of HCC management revolves around optimizing available therapy for each individual patient,

Dr Frenette is a speaker for Onyx and Gilead. Dr Gish is a consultant for Astellas OSI and is a consultant and speaker for Bayer and Onyx.

[a] Stanford University School of Medicine, Division of Gastroenterology and Hepatology, Alway Building, Room M211, 300 Pasteur Drive, MC: 5187, Stanford, CA 94305-5187, USA
[b] The Methodist Hospital, Methodist Transplant Center, Department of Liver Transplantation, 6550 Fannin, SM1001, Houston, TX 77030, USA
[c] Division of Gastroenterology and Hepatology, University of California, 200 West Arbor Drive, MC8413, San Diego, CA 92103-8413, USA
* Corresponding author.
E-mail address: rgish@ucsd.edu

an often difficult task that involves selecting appropriate candidates for appropriate therapies in an effort to maximize benefits and minimize harms in an era of limited resources.

Updates in the management of HCC continue to push the limits of conventional therapies, attempting to expand qualifying criteria for potentially curative surgical resection and liver transplantation. The role of locoregional approaches such as radiofrequency ablation (RFA)/microwave ablation (MWA) and transarterial chemo-embolization (TACE), bead embolization, and radioembolization continue to play important roles either as primary treatment modalities for patients not appropriate for surgery or as neoadjuvant therapy in potential transplant candidates. The advent of molecular targeted therapies, namely inhibitors of angiogenesis and other molecular pathways in HCC [eg, sorafenib (Nexavar)], may provide patients and practitioners with another viable option in their treatment armamentarium. Although currently approved for primary treatment among advanced HCC, the greatest potential benefits of these molecular agents lie in their possible roles as adjuvant or neoadjuvant therapy in conjunction with other locoregional therapies or surgical modalities. In this article, we review recent updates in HCC treatment with a focus on well-established locoregional and molecular targeted therapies.

SURGICAL APPROACHES

Early detection of HCC with cancer screening and surveillance programs allows implementation of the most appropriately aggressive therapy. The surgical approach, whether via potentially curative resection or transplantation, offers the greatest benefit among patients with small, localized tumors. Postresection 5-year survival rates for solitary tumors in noncirrhotic patients exceed 70% in some studies.[9–13] Although the presence of cirrhosis or multiple foci of tumor is not an absolute contraindication for operative resection, postresection outcomes are less ideal owing to higher rates of hepatic decompensation and/or tumor recurrence. Selection of the most appropriate candidates for resection involves an accurate assessment of multiple factors including tumor characteristics, comorbidities, liver functional status, presence of portal hypertension, and evidence of decompensated disease. The most ideal candidates for surgical resection are patients with small, solitary tumors with good liver functional status. Among patients with advanced disease or significant cirrhosis and impaired liver functional status, the role of surgical resection is less beneficial and may in fact contribute to the development of liver failure. Although large tumor size is not an absolute contraindication to resection, larger tumors harbor greater risks of underlying vascular invasion and dissemination, resulting in higher rates of postresection recurrence.[14,15] When it does occur, the approach to postresection tumor recurrence is not well-studied, and repeat resection is complex; patients often demonstrate multifocal presentations reflective of disseminated disease. These patients may be more suitable to undergo salvage liver transplantation, or other locoregional therapies with or without oral multikinase inhibitors.

Liver transplantation remains a viable option for patients with disease or tumor characteristics that are not appropriate for primary surgical resection. Often in conjunction with less invasive neoadjuvant locoregional therapies, outcomes among appropriate candidates are promising, with posttransplant 5-year survival rates exceeding 70%.[15–18] However, liver transplantation is not appropriate for all individuals and a comprehensive evaluation and selection process are necessary to best allocate the scarce resources available.

The Milan criteria, defined by the presence of a solitary tumor less than 5 cm or up to 3 tumors, each no more than 3 cm, has emerged as the international standard by which potential transplant candidates are evaluated.[15] When these guidelines are utilized, the posttransplant 5-year survival rates reach 70% to 80% and tumor recurrence rates are approximately 10%.[15–19] Whereas several studies have investigated the potential expansion of these criteria, those proposed by the University of California, San Francisco (UCSF) group have demonstrated the most promising results.[20–24] Using the UCSF criteria (solitary lesion ≤6.5 cm, ≤3 lesions, each ≤4.5 cm with the total combined tumor diameter not exceeding 8 cm) the initial report by Yao and colleagues demonstrated acceptable survival rates (90% 1-year survival and 75% 5-year survival), similar to those achieved with the Milan criteria.[23,24] Further challenging the limits of current transplantation criteria, recent studies have focused on preoperative "downstaging" approaches whereby patients with HCC beyond transplant criteria are treated with locoregional therapies to decrease tumor burden and downgrade lesions to fall within transplantation guidelines.[25–27] One recent prospective intention-to-treat analysis by Yao and colleagues[27] implemented a downstaging protocol using TACE and/or RFA in HCC patients exceeding the UCSF criteria.[27] Early results from this 61-patient cohort are promising, with 96.2% 1-year and 92.1% 4-year posttransplant survival rates. The success of these recent studies continue to raise debate about the need for reevaluation of transplantation criteria and the potential expansion of selection guidelines for patients who currently are not eligible based on Milan criteria. Whereas advances in both surgical and adjuvant medical therapy lead to more significant improvements in posttransplant outcomes, the complexity of the selection process for liver transplantation will continue to evolve along with the novel ideas that bring forth such challenges.

LOCOREGIONAL ABLATION THERAPIES

When a patient's disease burden or comorbidities are significant enough to make the prospect of surgical intervention inappropriate, nonsurgical invasive therapies play an important role in managing HCC. Either as a primary mode of therapy or adjuvant to transplantation, locoregional treatments include a spectrum of therapeutic tools that include both localized ablative techniques and chemoembolization.[8] Percutaneous ablation therapies involve localized destruction of tumor cells through direct exposure to toxic substances (eg, ethanol) or modifying the temperature (eg, radiofrequency, microwave). The most common ablation modalities include percutaneous ethanol injection (PEI) and RFA. Among patients with tumors less than 2 cm in size, PEI and RFA have similar efficacies, achieving tumor necrosis in 90% to 100%.[28–31] The performance of PEI among larger tumors is less consistent, and generally requires a greater number of treatment sessions compared with RFA. Given the fewer number of treatment sessions needed, greater tolerability, and better survival outcomes in recent studies, RFA is often preferred over PEI even in patients with smaller tumors.[30–34] Regardless of modality, the overall efficacy of any ablation technique declines with increasing tumor size, and tumors larger than 3 cm generally do not have consistently successful outcomes.

Although RFA remains the most utilized locoregional ablative therapy, newer techniques that incorporate novel ideas and alternative methods of tumor destruction continue to be developed. MWA is an emerging form of thermal ablation for the treatment of HCC that utilizes electromagnetic waves with frequencies greater than 900 kHz to irradiate and ablate tumor foci.[35–37] Unlike RFA, which relies primarily on passive heating, MWA utilizes active heating, which by virtue of its form of heat distribution, enables continuous and uniform ablation. This method is able to generate higher temperatures and larger zones of ablation, leading to higher rates of tumor necrosis compared with more conventional ablative techniques. MWA therapy also overcomes the "heat sink" effect, a common limitation of RFA that involves the cooling of blood flow in the immediate proximity of tumors, which can lead to incomplete ablation and necrosis. This ability to overcome the "heat sink" is related to the ability of MWA to heat the tumor faster and hotter, but may also result in increased risk of damage to nearby structures, including blood vessels. The clinical advantages of MWA over RFA, and its potential to demonstrate a greater rate of tumor necrosis with fewer treatment sessions owing to more rapid and thorough tumor heating, needs to be investigated further in large clinical trials.

LOCOREGIONAL CHEMOEMBOLIZATION

In addition to ablation-based therapies, the treatment approach to the nonsurgical management of HCC includes utilizing methods of chemoembolization. The underlying mechanism by which chemoembolization achieves its therapeutic potential hinges on principles of cytotoxicity and induced ischemia. The concept of TACE involves localized intra-arterial injection of chemotherapy agents followed by angiographically induced ischemia via selective embolization of the tumor's vascular supply. The success of conventional TACE, which utilizes a lipiodol-suspended emulsion of chemotherapy for drug delivery was demonstrated by one of the early systematic reviews by Llovet and Bruix, reporting improved 2-year survival among advanced HCC treated with chemoembolization when compared with more conservative therapies.[38] As is the case with surgical approaches, the success of TACE depends on appropriate patient selection. Subsequent subset analyses demonstrated that, although TACE was generally associated with improved outcomes when compared with conservative symptom-directed therapy among nonsurgical candidates, the improved survival was most significant among patients without evidence of decompensated cirrhosis, vascular invasion, or extrahepatic spread of tumor.[8,38–42]

Although there has been greater experience with conventional forms of lipiodol-based TACE, the recent advent of embolic, drug-eluting microspheres offers a promising alternative. The success of drug-eluting spheres has resulted in replacement of conventional TACE at many institutions with this new therapy. The major advantages of embolic microspheres loaded with doxorubicin include the ability to deliver therapy in a controlled, sustained fashion to tumor foci. This method not only improves drug delivery, but also helps to minimize the effects of systemic chemotherapy exposure.[43–45] Several recent studies have compared the performance of doxorubicin (Adriamycin)-eluting beads (DEB) with conventional methods of TACE. The PRECISION V study—a multicenter, phase II, randomized, controlled trial—demonstrated a trend toward greater treatment response rate and tumor necrosis among patients treated with DEB when compared with conventional TACE.[43] A subset analysis of patients with more advanced tumor stages demonstrated significantly greater treatment responses. However, patients randomized to the conventional TACE group achieved higher than expected treatment response rates (44% compared with an expected 35%), resulting in criticisms that this trial was underpowered to detect a significant difference between the DEB and conventional TACE groups. Furthermore, the lack of evaluating differences in progression-free and overall survival raises questions about the impact of greater treatment responses on actual patient outcomes.

One of the major theoretical advantages of a targeted drug delivery system is the ability to minimize toxicities that arise from undesired systemic distribution of the drug. Although some of the early studies comparing DEB and conventional TACE have raised questions about the clinical significance of study outcomes on patient survival, DEB–TACE therapies have demonstrated better tolerability and safety.

DEB–TACE is associated with significantly lower rates of serious liver toxicity and lower rates of chemotherapy related side effects, the major limitations of conventional TACE.[43–47] A recent study by Malagari and colleagues[47] further investigated the safety profiles of DEB–TACE therapies, focusing primarily on complications associated with microsphere bead diameters, the extent of embolization, and quantity of loaded beads, reflecting amount of doxorubicin delivered. This large, descriptional study reported no increased risk of complications associated with smaller bead diameters, and emphasized the safety profiles of DEB therapies, even among patients treated with higher doses of doxorubicin.[47] The advent of chemotherapy-eluting microspheres has created a new treatment regimen for patients with intermediate and advanced stages of HCC. The improved safety and tolerability profile offers an advantage to conventional therapies, and the greater treatment response rates indicate promise for this form of therapy. The potential impact of DEB–TACE alone on patient survival outcomes is unclear, but large, randomized, controlled trials combining DEB–TACE with sorafenib that are currently enrolling patients may revitalize interest in DEB–TACE as an adjuvant form of therapy.

LOCOREGIONAL RADIOEMBOLIZATION

The role of radiation therapy in the treatment of HCC has traditionally been avoided secondary to the exacerbation of liver disease by the radiation treatment itself. Radiation-induced liver disease, which had previously been noted as radiation-induced hepatitis, results from accumulated parenchymal damage, especially in cirrhotic livers that have low tolerances to radiation-induced injuries. The advent of microsphere-based technology for chemoembolization therapies raised the clinical idea of potentially utilizing this method for delivery of radiation treatments. The underlying treatment regimen relies on similar concepts that form the basis for TACE. Utilizing the hypervascularity of tumors, microspheres can be preferentially delivered to tumor foci, allowing targeted treatment and limiting systemic toxicities. The development of yttrium-90 (Y90)-coated microspheres hinges on these concepts in an attempt to offer novel treatment alternatives to patients with intermediate and advanced HCC.[48–55] In addition, the safety profile of Y90-based treatments, especially its minimally embolic effects, allows it to be utilized in patients with portal vein thrombosis. However, Y90 is absolutely contraindicated in patients with significant hepatopulmonary shunting, which could result in very high levels of pulmonary radiation exposure.

Several recent studies have demonstrated efficacy for Y90 therapies.[48–55] In 1 study by Riaz and colleagues,[55] an analysis of patients who underwent Y90 radioembolization before transplantation demonstrated complete pathologic necrosis in 61% of the cohort.[55] Although no randomized, controlled trials have compared Y90 head to head with other locoregional therapies, several nonrandomized trials report promising results that demonstrate a trend toward improved outcomes among those treated with Y90. One recent large study by Salem and colleagues[54] evaluated 245 patients with unresectable HCC that had received locoregional therapies (122 received chemoembolization and 123 received radioembolization). Over 80% of patients were Barcelona Clinic Liver Cancer stage A or B, and the majority of patients had hepatitis C. Overall, patients treated with radioembolization demonstrated a trend toward higher treatment response rates (49% vs 36%; $P = .104$), significantly longer time to progression (13.3 vs 8.4 months; $P = .046$), but no difference in median survival times (20.5 vs 17.4 months; $P = .232$) when compared with those treated with chemoembolization. Although no randomized, controlled trials have been published demonstrating clinical benefit of Y90 compared with more established treatment modalities, many studies have reported on the efficacy of Y90-based therapies and the potential trend toward improved outcomes for patients with intermediate and advanced HCC. Future studies evaluating Y90 treatment in randomized, controlled trials are needed and further investigation of Y90 in combination with other locoregional or systemic therapies in treating intermediate and advanced staged HCC may hold promise for novel approaches to the management of HCC.

MOLECULAR TARGETED THERAPIES

The field of systemic therapies for the treatment of HCC has been limited. Traditional cytotoxic chemotherapy regimens have failed to demonstrate significant improvements in HCC survival, and their extensive toxicity profile further contributed to their lack of efficacy. However, research in the area of angiogenesis inhibition in the management of cancer has contributed to a novel approach for the treatment of HCC. The rationale for targeting angiogenesis as a treatment approach is supported by its integral role in tumor growth and progression.[56-60] Angiogenesis promotes development of vascular networks, and thereby enables tumor growth via enhanced delivery of nutrients and oxygen to tumor foci. Furthermore, tumor invasion and metastasis are enabled as the vascular supply links tumor foci with more distant sites. HCC is a hypervascularized malignancy, whose growth and progression relies heavily on angiogenesis; thus, the use of anti-angiogenic agents is a reasonable approach to systemic treatment of HCC.

One of the earlier models of success in targeting angiogenesis as a treatment approach for HCC, sorafenib, a multitargeted tyrosine kinase inhibitor, was the first molecular targeted therapy to be approved by the US Food and Drug Administration for the treatment of unresectable HCC. The SHARP trial demonstrated a 2.8-month survival advantage among patients with advanced HCC treated with sorafenib compared with best supportive care (10.7 vs 7.9 months; hazard ratio, 0.69; $P <$ .001).[61] Furthermore, the time to radiologic progression of tumor was also significantly extended among the sorafenib group (5.5 vs 2.8 months; $P<.001$). Although subsequent studies continued to demonstrate significantly improved survival among patients treated with sorafenib, the early trials had limited data for Asian subpopulations, a cohort that often harbored concomitant hepatitis B infection and impaired liver functional status.[62-70] A subsequent randomized, phase III trial that evaluated sorafenib among Asians with advanced HCC demonstrated results similar to the SHARP trial, with significant improvements in both survival and time to progression.[64] Mounting evidence clearly supports the efficacy of sorafenib in treatment of advanced HCC among a more diverse patient cohort and current guidelines by the American Association for the Study of Liver Diseases recommend sorafenib as first-line therapy among patients with unresectable HCC who are not appropriate candidates for percutaneous ablation or TACE, but maintain preserved liver function.[1]

Given the success of sorafenib, several additional anti-angiogenic agents currently under investigation demonstrate great promise. Brivanib is an anti-angiogenesis agent that inhibits both fibroblast growth factor and vascular endothelial growth factor pathways. The major theoretical advantage of this dual inhibitory mechanism of action is its potential to overcome development of compensatory signaling and subsequent loss of drug efficacy. Early phase II trials with brivanib in patients with advanced HCC demonstrated significantly improved survival outcomes, with a mean overall survival of 10 months.[71,72] In addition, this early phase II evaluation reported low incidences of adverse events, and current phase III trials are underway to further elucidate the efficacy of this emerging therapeutic agent. Other agents such as sunitinib (Sutent) and bevacizumab (Avastin) have been less successful in the management of HCC owing to treatment-related toxicities and lack of survival efficacy.

Erlotinib (Tarceva) is an epidermal growth factor receptor (EGFR) tyrosine kinase inhibitor that has played a major role in the treatment of patients with advanced non-small cell lung cancer. Recent studies have investigated the role of EGFR in the tumorigenesis of HCC.[73–76] Prior studies have indicated that EGFR is expressed frequently in HCC cells and have postulated that an EGFR-mediated mechanism may be involved in promoting tumor growth and metastasis. Early studies on human HCC cells demonstrated the efficacy of erlotinib to induce growth inhibition, apoptosis, and cell-cycle arrest.[74] A recent phase II study of erlotinib in patients with advanced unresectable HCC yielded promising results with improved progression-free survival and overall survival among treated patients.[75,76] Whereas the majority of prior research evaluated the efficacy of erlotinib as monotherapy, the inhibition of EGFR-mediated pathways has been postulated to enhance the therapeutic potential of other therapies. The combination of erlotinib and sorafenib in the treatment of advanced colorectal and non–small-cell lung cancers have shown promising results in early reports.[77,78] Further studies evaluating the role of erlotinib in the treatment of HCC are needed. Although early reports demonstrate great promise for erlotinib as mono-therapy in HCC patients, the potential for treatment synergy in combination with other targeted therapies will likely yield the greatest potential.

Another emerging class of molecular targeted therapies are the mammalian targets of rapamycin (mTOR) inhibitors. The antineoplastic potential of mTOR inhibitors hinges on its multilevel modulation of tumor proliferation and metabolism. Although not traditionally considered an angiogenesis inhibitor, mTOR also modulates angiogenesis through indirect regulation of vascular endothelial growth factor expression.[79] One of the early mTOR inhibitors demonstrating promise as an antineoplastic therapy is everolimus (Zortress; Afinitor). Early studies demonstrated efficacy in treatment of patients with advanced renal cell cancer, and recently the US Food and Drug Administration approved everolimus for treatment of renal cell cancer in patients who have disease progression on sunitinib (Sutent), sorafenib, or both,[80,81] Given the similar tumorigenic pathways involved in HCC and the previously reported efficacy of anti-angiogenic therapies on advanced HCC, recent studies have investigated the antineoplastic potential of everolimus among HCC patients.[82,83] In a phase I/II study evaluating 28 patients with advanced HCC, everolimus demonstrated promising results, producing a mean progression-free survival of 3.9 months and a disease control rate of 44%.[84] Currently, a large, multicenter, phase III, randomized, double-blind, placebo-controlled trial (EVOLVE-1) is underway to compare everolimus with best supportive care in patients with advanced HCC who failed sorafenib therapy. As with the spectrum of targeted therapies currently available and under investigation, the role of everolimus as monotherapy and/or combination therapy continue to offer patients and practitioners greater tools to treat and manage HCC.

Many additional targeted therapies are currently under investigation.[85–88] The success of sorafenib in particular has set a precedent for the emergence of molecular targeted therapies for the management of HCC. As newer agents continue to push the limits of improving morbidity and mortality among patients with HCC, the role of these novel agents in conjunction with operative resection, liver transplantation, ablation therapies, and/or concurrent oral systemic therapies that target different components of malignancy progression in an adjuvant or neoadjuvant fashion will likely offer the most potential and is under active investigation.[88] The application of advancing locoregional approaches to the management of HCC in earlier staged disease may offer not only benefits in prolonged survival, but perhaps a potential cure.

SUMMARY

HCC is a leading cause of morbidity and mortality worldwide. Advances in cancer screening and surveillance have allowed for earlier detection of tumors, affording greater treatment potential. The advent of locoregional therapies has generated greater treatment options for patients with HCC. Either alone or in combination as an adjuvant or neoadjuvant therapy, these novel approaches continue to hold promise for improving morbidity and/or mortality of patients with HCC. The emergence of systemic molecular targeted therapies increases the role of translational science. Whereas surgical resection and transplantation conventionally form the cornerstone of curative approaches, the advancement of locoregional therapies holds great promise in adding to the curative armamentarium.

REFERENCES

1. Bruix J, Sherman M. Management of hepatocellular carcinoma: an update. Hepatology 2011;53:1020–2.
2. El-Serag HB, Marrero JA, Rudolph L, et al. Diagnosis and treatment of hepatocellular carcinoma. Gastroenterology 2008;134:1752–63.
3. Jemal A, Siegel R, Xu J, Ward E. Cancer statistics, 2010. CA Cancer J Clin 2010;60:277–300.
4. Gish RG, Marrero JA, Benson AB. A multidisciplinary approach to the management of hepatocellular carcinoma. Gastroenterol Hepatol 2010;6(Suppl 7):1–14.
5. Schwartz M, Roayaie S, Konstadoulakis M. Strategies for the management of hepatocellular carcinoma. Nat Clin Pract Oncol 2007;4:424–32.
6. Asmis T, Balaa F, Scully L, et al. Diagnosis and management of hepatocellular carcinoma: results of a consensus meeting of The Ottawa Hospital Cancer Centre. Curr Oncol 2010;17:6–12.
7. Lopez PM, Villanueva A, Llovet JM. Systematic review: evidence-based management of hepatocellular carcinoma: an updated analysis of randomized controlled trials. Aliment Pharmacol Ther 2006;23:1535–47.
8. Lencioni R. Loco-regional treatment of hepatocellular carcinoma. 2010;52:762-73.
9. Arii S, Yamaoka Y, Futagawa S, et al. Results of surgical and nonsurgical treatment for small-sized hepatocellular carcinomas: a retrospective and nationwide survey in Japan. The Liver Cancer Study Group of Japan. Hepatology 2000;32:1224–9
10. Takayama T, Makuuchi M, Hirohashi S, et al. Early hepatocellular carcinoma as an entity with a high rate of surgical cure. Hepatology 1998;28:1241–6.
11. Llovet JM, Fuster J, Bruix J. Intention-to-treat analysis of surgical treatment for early hepatocellular carcinoma: resection versus transplantation. Hepatology 1999;30:1434–40.
12. Nathan H, Schulick RD, Choti MA, et al. Predictors of survival after resection of early hepatocellular carcinoma. Ann Surg 2009;249:799–805.
13. Poon RT, Fan ST, Ng IO, et al. Significance of resection margin in hepatectomy for hepatocellular carcinoma: a critical reappraisal. Ann Surg 2000;231:544–51.
14. Llovet JM, Schwartz M, Mazzaferro V. Resection and liver transplantation for hepatocellular carcinoma. Semin Liver Dis 2005;25:181–200.
15. Mazzaferro V, Regalia E, Doci R, et al. Liver transplantation for the treatment of small hepatocellular carcinomas in patients with cirrhosis. N Engl J Med 1996;334:693–9.
16. Bismuth H, Majno PE, Adam R. Liver transplantation for hepatocellular carcinoma. Semin Liver Dis 1999;19:311–22.
17. Bismuth H, Chiche L, Adam R, et al. Surgical treatment of hepatocellular carcinoma in cirrhosis: liver resection or transplantation? Transplant Proc 1993;25:1066–7.

18. Llovet JM, Bruix J, Fuster J, et al. Liver transplantation for small hepatocellular carcinoma: the tumor-node-metastasis classification does not have prognostic power. Hepatology 1998;27:1572–7.

19. Jonas S, Bechstein WO, Steinmuller T, et al. Vascular invasion and histopathologic grading determine outcome after liver transplantation for hepatocellular carcinoma in cirrhosis. Hepatology 2001;33:1080–6.

20. Mazzaferro V, Llovet JM, Miceli R, et al. Predicting survival after liver transplantation in patients with hepatocellular carcinoma beyond the Milan criteria: a retrospective, exploratory analysis. Lancet Oncol 2009;10:35–43.

21. Toso C, Trotter J, Wei A, et al. Total tumor volume predicts risk of recurrence following liver transplantation in patients with hepatocellular carcinoma. Liver Transpl 2008;14:1107–15.

22. Yao FY, Ferrell L, Bass NM, et al. Liver transplantation for hepatocellular carcinoma: comparison of the proposed UCSF criteria with the Milan criteria and the Pittsburgh modified TNM criteria. Liver Transpl 2002;8:765–74.

23. Yao FY, Xiao L, Bass NM, et al. Liver transplantation for hepatocellular carcinoma: validation of the UCSF-expanded criteria based on preoperative imaging. Am J Transplant 2007;7:2587–96.

24. Yao FY, Ferrell L, Bass NM, et al. Liver transplantation for hepatocellular carcinoma: expansion of the tumor size limits does not adversely impact survival. Hepatology 2001;33:1394–403.

25. Yao FY. Expanding criteria for hepatocellular carcinoma: down-staging with a view to liver transplantation—yes. Semin Liver Dis 2006;26:239–47.

26. Yao FY, Hirose R, LaBerge J, et al. A prospective study on down-staging of hepatocellular carcinoma prior to liver transplantation. Liver Transpl 2005;11:1505–14.

27. Yao FY, Kerlan RK Jr, Hirose R, et al. Excellent outcome following down-staging of hepatocellular carcinoma prior to liver transplantation: an intention-to-treat analysis. Hepatology 2008;48:819–27.

28. Okada S. Local ablation therapy for hepatocellular carcinoma. Semin Liver Dis 1999;19:323–8.

29. Ishii H, Okada S, Nose H, et al. Local recurrence of hepatocellular carcinoma after percutaneous ethanol injection. Cancer 1996;77:1792–6.

30. Lencioni RA, Allgaier HP, Cioni D, et al. Small hepatocellular carcinoma in cirrhosis: randomized comparison of radio-frequency thermal ablation versus percutaneous ethanol injection. Radiology 2003;228:235–40.

31. Livraghi T, Goldberg SN, Lazzaroni S, et al. Small hepatocellular carcinoma: treatment with radio-frequency ablation versus ethanol injection. Radiology 1999;210:655–61.

32. Cho YK, Kim JK, Kim MY, et al. Systematic review of randomized trials for hepatocellular carcinoma treated with percutaneous ablation therapies. Hepatology 2009;49:453–9.

33. Lin SM, Lin CJ, Lin CC, et al. Radiofrequency ablation improves prognosis compared with ethanol injection for hepatocellular carcinoma < or =4 cm. Gastroenterology 2004;127:1714–23.

34. Shiina S, Teratani T, Obi S, et al. A randomized controlled trial of radiofrequency ablation with ethanol injection for small hepatocellular carcinoma. Gastroenterology 2005;129:122–30.

35. Shibata T, Iimuro Y, Yamamoto Y, et al. Small hepatocellular carcinoma: comparison of radio-frequency ablation and percutaneous microwave coagulation therapy. Radiology 2002;223:331–7.

36. Yu NC, Lu DS, Raman SS, et al. Hepatocellular carcinoma: microwave ablation with multiple straight and loop antenna clusters—pilot comparison with pathologic findings. Radiology 2006;239:269–75.
37. Martin RC, Scoggins CR, McMasters KM. Safety and efficacy of microwave ablation of hepatic tumors: a prospective review of a 5-year experience. Ann Surg Oncol 2010;17:171–8.
38. Llovet JM, Real MI, Montaña X, et al. Barcelona Liver Cancer Group. Arterial embolisation or chemoembolisation versus symptomatic treatment in patients with unresectable hepatocellular carcinoma: a randomized controlled trial. Lancet 2002;359: 1734–9.
39. Cammà C, Schepis F, Orlando A, et al. Transarterial chemoembolization for unresectable hepatocellular carcinoma: meta-analysis of randomized controlled trials. Radiology 2002;224:47–54.
40. Llovet JM, Bruix J. Systematic review of randomized trials for unresectable hepatocellular carcinoma: chemoembolization improves survival. Hepatology 2003;37:429–42.
41. Lewandowski RJ, Kulik LM, Riaz A, et al. A comparative analysis of transarterial downstaging for hepatocellular carcinoma: chemoembolization versus radioembolization. Am J Transplant 2009;9:1920–8.
42. Bruix J, Castells A, Montanya X, et al. Phase II study of transarterial embolization in European patients with hepatocellular carcinoma: need for controlled trials. Hepatology 1994;20:643–50.
43. Lammer J, Malagari K, Vogl T, et al; PRECISION V Investigators. Prospective randomized study of doxorubicin-eluting-bead embolization in the treatment of hepatocellular carcinoma: results of the PRECISION V study. Cardiovasc Intervent Radiol 2010;33:41–52.
44. Dhanasekaran R, Kooby DA, Staley CA, et al. Comparison of conventional transarterial chemoembolization (TACE) and chemoembolization with doxorubicin drug eluting beads (DEB) for unresectable hepatocellular carcinoma (HCC). J Surg Oncol 2010; 101:476–80.
45. Nicolini A, Martinetti L, Crespi S, et al. Transarterial chemoembolization with epirubicin-eluting beads versus transarterial embolization before liver transplantation for hepatocellular carcinoma. J Vasc Interv Radiol 2010;21:327–32.
46. Reyes DK, Vossen JA, Kamel IR, et al. Single-center phase II trial of transarterial chemoembolization wit drug-eluting beads for patients with unresectable hepatocellular carcinoma: initial experience in the United States. Cancer J 2009;15:526–32.
47. Malagari K, Pomoni M, Spyridopoulos TN, et al. Safety profile of sequential transcatheter chemoembolization with DC Bead: results of 237 hepatocellular carcinoma (HCC) patients. Cardiovasc Intervent Radiol 2010 Dec 24. [Epub ahead of print].
48. Salem R, Lewandowski RJ, Kulik L, et al. Radioembolization results in longer time-to-progression and reduced toxicity compared with chemoembolization in patients with hepatocellular carcinoma. Gastroenterology 2010;140:497–507.
49. Geschwind JF, Salem R, Carr BI, et al. Yttrium-90 microspheres for the treatment of hepatocellular carcinoma. Gastroenterology 2004;127:S194–S205.
50. Salem R, Lewandowski RJ, Atassi B, et al. Treatment of unresectable hepatocellular carcinoma with use of 90Y microspheres (TheraSphere): safety, tumor response, and survival. J Vasc Interv Radiol 2005;16:1627–39.
51. Sangro B, Bilbao JI, Boan J, et al. Radioembolization using 90Y-resin microspheres for patients with advanced hepatocellular carcinoma. Int J Radiat Oncol Biol Phys 2006;66:792–800.

52. Kooby DA, Egnatashvili V, Srinivasan S, et al. Comparison of yttrium-90 radioembolization and transcatheter arterial chemoembolization for the treatment of unresectable hepatocellular carcinoma. J Vasc Interv Radiol 2010;21:224–30.

53. Kulik LM, Carr BI, Mulcahy MF, et al. Safety and efficacy of 90Y radiotherapy for hepatocellular carcinoma with and without portal vein thrombosis. Hepatology 2008; 47:71–81.

54. Salem R, Lewandowski RJ, Mulcahy MF, et al. Radioembolization for hepatocellular carcinoma using yttrium-90 microspheres: a comprehensive report of long-term outcomes. Gastroenterology 2010;138:52–64.

55. Riaz A, Kulik L, Lewandowski RJ, et al. Radiologic-pathologic correlation of hepatocellular carcinoma treated with internal radiation using yttrium-90 microspheres. Hepatology 2009;49:1185–93.

56. Carmeliet P, Jain RK. Angiogenesis in cancer and other diseases. Nature 2000;407: 249–57.

57. Ribatti D, Vacca A, Dammacco F. The role of the vascular phase in solid tumor growth: a historical review. Neoplasia 1999;1:293–302.

58. Mignatti P, Rifkin DB. Biology and biochemistry of proteinases in tumor invasion. Physiol Rev 1993;73:161–95.

59. Aznavoorian S, Murphy AN, Stetler-Stevenson WG, et al. Molecular aspects of tumor cell invasion and metastasis. Cancer 1993;71:1368–83.

60. Birchmeier C, Birchmeier W, Gherardi E, et al. Met, metastasis, motility and more. Nat Rev Mol Cell Biol 2003;4:915–25.

61. Llovet JM, Ricci S, Mazzaferro V, et al. Sorafenib in advanced hepatocellular carcinoma. N Engl J Med 2008;359:378–90.

62. Kane RC, Farrell AT, Madabushi R, et al. Sorafenib for the treatment of unresectable hepatocellular carcinoma. Oncologist 2009;14:95–100.

63. Okita K, Imanaka K, Chida N, et al. Phase III study of sorafenib in patients in Japan and Korea with advanced hepatocellular carcinoma (HCC) treated after transarterial chemoembolization (TACE). 2010 Gastrointestinal Cancers Symposium. Abstract LBA128.

64. Cheng AL, Kang YK, Chen Z, et al. Efficacy and safety of sorafenib in patients in the Asia-Pacific region with advanced hepatocellular carcinoma: a phase III randomized, double-blind, placebo-controlled trial. Lancet Oncol 2009;10:25–34.

65. Yau T, Chan P, Ng KK, et al. Phase 2 open-label study of single-agent sorafenib in treating advanced hepatocellular carcinoma in a hepatitis B-endemic Asian population: presence of lung metastasis predicts poor response. Cancer 2009;115:428–36.

66. Pinter M, Sieghart W, Graziadei I, et al. Sorafenib in unresectable hepatocellular carcinoma from mild to advanced stage liver cirrhosis. Oncologist 2009;14:70–76.

67. Abou-Alfa GK, Amadori D, Santoro A, et al. Is sorafenib (S) safe and effective in patients (pts) with hepatocellular carcinoma (HCC) and Child-Pugh B (CPB) cirrhosis? J Clin Oncol 2008;26(Suppl):abstr 4518.

68. Schwartz M, Roayaie S, Uva P. Treatment of HCC in patients awaiting liver transplantation. Am J Transplant 2007;7:1875–81.

69. Kim R, Menon N, Aucejo F. Safe use of sorafenib in a patient undergoing salvage liver transplantation for recurrent hepatocellular carcinoma after hepatic resection. Med Oncol 2010 Jul 16. [Epub ahead of print].

70. Vitale A, Volk ML, Pastorelli D, et al. Use of sorafenib in patients with hepatocellular carcinoma before liver transplantation: a cost-benefit analysis while awaiting data on sorafenib safety. Hepatology 2010;51:165–73.

71. Finn RS, Park J-W, Kang Y-K, et al. Time-to-progression sub-analysis of second-line treatment with brivanib after failure of prior anti-angiogenic therapy in patients with

unresectable, locally advanced, or metastatic hepatocellular carcinoma. Presented at the 60th Annual Meeting of the American Association for the Study of Liver Disease. Boston (MA), October 30 to November 3, 2009.

72. Park J-W, Finn RS, Kim JS, et al. Phase II, open-label study of brivanib as first-line therapy in patients with advanced hepatocellular carcinoma. Clin Cancer Res 2011; 17:1973–83.

73. Huether A, Hopfner M, Sutter AP, et al. Erlotinib induces cell cycle arrest and apoptosis in hepatocellular cancer cells and enhances chemosensitivity towards cytostatics. J Hepatol 2005;43:661–9.

74. Pore N, Jiang Z, Gupta A, et al. EGFR tyrosine kinase inhibitors decrease VEGF expression by both hypoxia-inducible factor (HIF)-1-independent and HIF-1-dependent mechanisms. Cancer Res 2006;66:3197–204.

75. Thomas MB, Chadha R, Glover K, et al. Phase 2 study of erlotinib in patients with unresectable hepatocellular carcinoma. Cancer 2007;110:1059–67.

76. Philip PA, Mahoney MR, Allmer C, et al. Phase II study of erlotinib (OSI-774) in patients with advanced hepatocellular cancer. J Clin Oncol 2005;23:6657–63.

77. Martinelli E, Troiani T, Morgillo F, et al. Synergistic antitumor activity of sorafenib in combination with epidermal growth factor receptor inhibitors in colorectal and lung cancer cells. Clin Cancer Res 2010;16:4990–5001.

78. Lind JS, Dingemans AM, Groen HJ, et al. A multicenter, phase 2 study of erlotinib and sorafenib in chemotherapy-naive patients with advanced non-small cell lung cancer. Clin Cancer Res 2010;16:3078–87.

79. Yuan R, Kay A, Berg WJ, et al. Targeting tumorigenesis: development and use of mTOR inhibitors in cancer therapy. J Hematol Oncol 2009;27:2–45.

80. Chan HY, Grossman AB, Bukowski RM. Everolimus in the treatment of renal cell carcinoma and neuroendocrine tumors. Adv Ther 2010;27:495–511.

81. Motzer RJ, Escudier B, Oudard S, et al. Efficacy of everolimus in advanced renal cell carcinoma: a double-blind, randomised, placebo-controlled phase III trial. Lancet 2008;372:449–56.

82. Treiber G. mTOR inhibitors for hepatocellular cancer: a forward-moving target. Expert Rev Anticancer Ther 2009;9:247–61.

83. Villanueva A, Chiang DY, Newell P, et al. Pivotal role of mTOR signaling in hepatocellular carcinoma. Gastroenterology 2008;135:1972–83.

84. Blaszkowsky LS, Abrams TA, Miksad RA, et al. Phase I/II study of everolimus in patients with advanced hepatocellular carcinoma (HCC). J Clin Oncol 2010;28(Suppl):abstr e14542.

85. Spratlin JL, Cohen RB, Eadens M, et al. Phase I pharmacologic and biologic study of ramucirumab (IMC-1121B), a fully human immunoglobulin G1 monoclonal antibody targeting the vascular endothelial growth factor receptor-2. J Clin Oncol 2010;28: 780–7.

86. Albert DH, Tapang P, Magoc TJ, et al. Preclinical activity of ABT-869, a multitargeted receptor tyrosine kinase inhibitor. Mol Cancer Ther 2006;5:995–1006.

87. Toh H, Chen P, Carr BI, et al. A phase II study of ABT-869 in hepatocellular carcinoma (HCC): interim analysis. J Clin Oncol 2009;27:15(Suppl):abstr 4581.

88. Yau T, Chan P, Epstein R, et al. Management of advanced hepatocellular carcinoma in the era of targeted therapy. Liver Int 2009;29:1–7.

Alcoholic Hepatitis: Prognostic Models and Treatment

Ashwani K. Singal, MD[a], Vijay H. Shah, MD[b],*

KEYWORDS
- Alcoholic hepatitis • Corticosteroids • Pentoxifylline
- Tumor necrosis factor-α • Liver transplantation

SEVERITY SCORES FOR ALCOHOLIC HEPATITIS

Alcoholic hepatitis (AH) is a distinct subset of patients with alcoholic liver disease and has a potential for high mortality within 3 to 6 months after clinical presentation.[1] Mild forms of AH usually improve with conservative management. However, patients with severe AH have been reported to have 30-day mortality of up to 50%.[2] Therefore, assessment of the disease severity becomes an important and practical issue for clinicians involved in the management of patients with AH. Many scoring systems have been developed for use in clinical practice.

Discriminant Function Index

The discriminant function index (DFI) was initially described by Maddrey and colleagues[3] in a placebo-controlled study to assess the benefit of corticosteroid (CS) therapy in 55 patients with AH. Using the formula: 4.6 × prothrombin time (PT) in seconds + serum bilirubin (mg/dL), patients with a DFI above 93 and treated with placebo had a 28-day survival of 25%, whereas those with a score of 93 or lower had 100% survival.[3] In 1989, this score was modified (modified discriminant function or mDF) using prolongation of PT in seconds (over control) instead of absolute value of PT (**Table 1**).[4] Patients without treatment and mDF score of 32 or higher and/or the presence of encephalopathy had a 28-day survival of about 65%. A recent analysis confirmed this observation with untreated patients having 28-day survival of 68% among patients with mDF of 32 or higher.[5] The American College of Gastroenterology recommends that AH patients with mDF score of 32 or higher should be considered for CS therapy.[6]

[a] Division of Gastroenterology and Hepatology, Mayo Clinic, 200 First Street SW, Rochester, MN 55905-0001, USA
[b] Division of Gastroenterology and Hepatology, Mayo Clinic College of Medicine, 200 First Street SW, Rochester, MN 55905-0001, USA
* Corresponding author.
E-mail address: shah.vijay@mayo.edu

Gastroenterol Clin N Am 40 (2011) 611–639
doi:10.1016/j.gtc.2011.06.008
0889-8553/11/$ – see front matter © 2011 Elsevier Inc. All rights reserved.
gastro.theclinics.com

Table 1
Scoring systems for assessment of severity of acute AH

Scoring System	Parameters	Formula				Severe Disease
DFI	SB and PT	4.6 × (patient's PT – control PT in seconds) + SB				≥32
CPT	SB, PT, serum albumin, ascites, and PSE		1	2	3	≥7
		SB	<2	2–3	>3	
		PT ↑	<4	4–6	>6	
		Albumin	>3.5	2.8–3.5	<2.8	
		Ascites	Absent	Slight	Tense	
		PSE	None	Grade I–II	Grade III–IV	
MELD score	Age, SB, INR, and SC	$9.57 \log_e (SC) + 3.78 \log_e (SB) + 11.2 \log_e (INR) + 6.43$ Available at: www.mayoclinic.org/meld/ mayomodel7.html				≥21
GAHS	Age, BUN, WBC, SB, and INR		1	2	3	≥9
		Age	<50	≥50	—	
		WBC	<15	≥15	—	
		BUN	<14	≥14	—	
		SB	<7.3	7.3–14.6	>14.6	
		Tc>INR	<1.5	1.5–2.0	>2.0	
Lille score	Age, labs at day 0 (SB, albumin, and PT), and change in SB at day 7	3.19–0.101 × age in yrs + 0.147 × albumin (g/L) on day 0 +0.0165 × change in SB (μmol/L) – 0.206 × RI (0 if absent and 1 if present) −0.0065 × SB on day 0 (μmol/L) −0.0096 × PT (in seconds)				≥0.45
ABIC score	Age, bilirubin, INR, and creatinine	(age × 0.1) + (SB × 0.08) + (SC × 0.3) + (INR × 0.8)				≥9

Patients with a CTP score of 5–6 have CTP stage A; 7–9, stage B; and 10–15, stage C.
Abbreviations: ABIC, Age, bilirubin, INR, creatinine; CTP, Child–Turcotte–Pugh score; DFI, discriminant function index; GAHS, Glasgow alcoholic hepatitis score; INR, International Normalized Ratio; MELD, Model for End-Stage Liver Disease; RI, renal insufficiency; PT, prothrombin time in seconds; SB, serum bilirubin in mg/dL; SC, serum creatinine in mg/dL; WBC, white blood count in 10^9/L.

The advantages of the mDF are its simplicity of calculation and validation in many clinical trials. However, nonstandardization of the PT testing with laboratory to laboratory variation depending on the type of thromboplastin used by the laboratory is a limitation.[7] Because patients with a DFI greater than 32 and an absence of encephalopathy are not considered for specific treatment, the mDF should have an accuracy of close to 100% in predicting their survival. However, patients with an mDF of less than 32 may have a 28-day mortality rates of about 7% to 17%.[5,8] Overall sensitivity and specificity of predicting mortality in 1 study was 67% and 62%, respectively.[8] One of the ways to tackle this issue is to lower the threshold score for initiating treatment. However, the risk benefit ratio does not favor CS treatment of patients with mDF score of less than 32.

Child–Turcotte–Pugh Score

This scoring system is based on 3 objective (serum bilirubin, serum albumin, and PT) and 2 subjective (hepatic encephalopathy and ascites) variables and categorize into 3 stages (A–C) with a total score of 5 to 6, 7 to 9, and greater than 9, respectively.[9] The score is traditionally used for cirrhotic patients with mortality rates of about 10% to 15%, 25% to 30%, and 70% to 80% at 1 year for stages A, B, and C, respectively. Although not a traditional scoring system for AH patients, the Child–Turcot–Pugh (CTP) score was useful in predicting mortality at 3 to 6 months (see **Table 1**).[10–12] Presently, the CTP score is not widely used for assessing severity of AH.

Model for End-Stage Liver Disease Score

Model for End-Stage Disease (MELD) score is being widely used for prediction of mortality in end-stage liver disease and is universally used to prioritize patients for liver transplantation (LT).[13,14] Some studies have examined the use of MELD in assessing severity of AH.[11,15,16] In a study on 34 patients with AH, the area under receiver operating characteristic curve (AUROC) for the MELD score was 0.82 with sensitivity and specificity in predicting 30-day mortality for a MELD score above 11 being 86% and 81%, respectively.[16] In another study on 73 patients with AH, MELD score of 21 had highest sensitivity and specificity to predict mortality at 30 and 90 days.[15] In yet another study on 202 patients, a first week MELD score of 20 or greater and an increase of MELD score at 1 week of 2 or more points had the highest sensitivity and specificity in predicting mortality.[11] Recently, MELD-Na has been shown to be superior than MELD score among AH patients and ascites.[17]

The advantage of MELD score is the use of the International Normalized Ratio (INR) (instead of PT). This is more comparable across laboratories, because the calculation accounts for the sensitivity of the thromboplastin reagent used in the test.[18] However, the formula for calculating MELD is complex; however, this can be easily overcome using a computer program or calculating the MELD score online (see **Table 1**). Another problem with the use of MELD score is variation across studies in the best cutoff score in predicting mortality from 11,[16] 18,[11,19] to 21 to 22.[15,20] Much of the variability, though, is due to use of original versus newer iterations of the MELD score that assign points differently. American Association for Study of Liver Diseases guidelines on the management of acute liver disease suggest that a cutoff MELD score of 18 be taken to predict severe AH and be the criterion for initiating treatment.[21]

Glasgow Alcoholic Hepatitis Score

The Glasgow alcoholic hepatitis score (GAHS) was introduced in 2005 to assess AH severity (see **Table 1**).[22] The score ranges between 5 and 12; a GAHS of 9 or higher at days 1 and 7 was more accurate than the mDF in predicting survival at 28 days ($P = .0016$ and $P = .0038$, respectively) and at 84 days ($P = .0179$ and $P = .0477$, respectively). GAHS at day 7 but not at day 1 was better in predicting 28-day outcome than the MELD score ($P = .0339$ and $P = .069$). GAHS at days 1 and 7 was more accurate than the MELD score in predicting the 84-day outcome ($P = .0005$ for both scores).[22] GAHS was reliable in predicting mortality irrespective of the use of INR or PT for determination of coagulation status or use of liver biopsy for diagnosis of AH. GAHS was confirmed in a validation cohort of 195 patients in this study; however, the score has not been validated outside the United Kingdom.[22]

Recently, the GAHS has been shown to predict response to CS treatment.[23] In this retrospective study, 144 AH patients with an mDF of 32 or higher were included. Of this group, 73 (51%) with a GAHS of 9 or greater were treated with CS. Patients with a GAHS below 9 did not differ on 28- and 84-day survival whether or not treated with CS (84% vs 80% and 73% vs 68%, respectively). However, the survival of patients with a GAHS of 9 or greater was better with CS treatment at day 28 (78% vs 52%; P = .002) and at day 84 (59% vs 38%; P = .02).[23]

Age–Bilirubin–INR–Creatinine Score

A new score, the age–bilirubin–INR–creatinine (ABIC) score, has been suggested for prognostic stratification of patients with AH (see **Table 1**).[24] Using the cutoff values of 6.71 and 9.0, authors identified patients with low, intermediate, and high risk of death at 90 days (100%, 70%, and 25% of survival rate, respectively; $P<.0001$). Using the same cutoff values, the ABIC score also stratified patients according to their risk of death at 1 year. The AUROC for predicting mortality at 90 days using ABIC score was 0.82 (95% confidence interval [CI], 0.73–0.91; P = .0001). In comparison, AUROC values were lower for the mDF score, MELD score, and GAHS: 0.70 (95% CI, 0.56–0.84; P = .008), 0.76 (95% CI, 0.64–0.88; P = .0004), and 0.75 (95% CI, 0.63–0.86; P = .001), respectively. On multivariate analysis, ABIC score was the best independent predictor of 90-day mortality (hazard ratio, 2.78; 95% CI, 1.90–4.09; P = .0001).

Early Change in Bilirubin Level

In a retrospective study on 238 biopsy-proven AH patients, a decrease in serum bilirubin at 1 week or early change in bilirubin level (ECBL) was a predictor for survival. A total of 73% patients showed ECBL at 1 week (4.9–4.4) and 83% of them survived. In contrast, the remaining cases did not show ECBL, with only 23% survival.[25] In another study reported from France assessing role of N-acetylcysteine (NAC) in combination with CS, decrease in bilirubin at day 14 was a significant predictor of survival.[26]

Lille Model

About 40% of patients with severe AH fail to respond to treatment with steroids.[27] In a prospective study on 320 biopsy-proven severe AH, nonresponders to steroids (NRS) could be identified based on ECBL and other five variables. This led to the development of Lille score (see **Table 1**).[27]

Survival at 6 months was lower for patients with a Lille score of 0.45 or higher compared with patients with Lille score of less than 0.45 (25% vs 85%; $P<.0001$). The AUROC value for the Lille score cutoff of 0.45 was higher than the CTP score (0.89 vs 0.62; $P<.00001$) or mDF score (0.89 vs 0.66; $P<.00001$). The authors concluded that CS be discontinued for patients with a Lille score of 0.45 or greater at 1 week.[27] The Lille score maintains accuracy in predicting the survival when used across a range. In a retrospective study on 641 biopsy-proven AH, a linear correlation with survival was seen among groups with Lille score of less than 0.16, 0.16 to 0.56, or greater than 0.56 with survival rates of 87%, 70%, and 21%, respectively, at 6 months.[28] Although this score has not been validated outside France, the score has been validated prospectively in other studies from the same center.[29,30] Unfortunately, the score does not guide initiation of treatment because it cannot be calculated at admission.

Comparison of Scores

Many studies have compared available scoring systems assessing severity of AH. MELD and DFI have been compared among 6 studies.[11,12,15,16,19,20] The data have shown differences across studies (**Table 2**).

Table 2
Comparison of different scoring systems for assessing the severity of AH

Author (Year)	Country	Comparison of	Type of Study	n	Diagnosis of AH	Outcome	Score Cutoff	Findings
Sheth et al (2002)[16]	USA	MELD and DFI	Retrospective	34	Clinical	30-day mortality	MELD 11 DFI 32	MELD: Sensitivity 82%, specificity 82%, AUROC 0.82 DFI: Sensitivity 86%, specificity 48%, AUROC 0.86
Said et al (2004)[10]	USA	MELD and CTP	Retrospective	98[a]	Clinical	3- and 6-month mortality	MELD and CTP as continuous scores	3-month mortality: AUROC MELD vs CTP (0.85 vs 0.85; $P = .5$) 6-month mortality: AUROC MELD vs CTP (0.83 vs 0.81; $P = .33$)
Dunn et al (2005)[15]	USA	MELD and DFI	Retrospective	73	Clinical	30-day mortality 90-day mortality[b]	MELD 22 DFI 41 MELD 21 DFI 37	MELD: Sensitivity 75%, specificity 75% AUROC 0.83 DFI: Sensitivity 75% specificity 69%, AUROC 0.74 MELD: Sensitivity 75%, specificity 75%, AUROC 0.86 DFI: Sensitivity 88% specificity 65% AUROC 0.83
Forrest et al (2005)[22]	UK	GAHS and DFI	Retrospective[c]	241	Clinical	28-day mortality 84-day mortality	GAHS 9 DFI 32 Same	Sensitivity and specificity GAHS vs DFI at admission (54/89 vs 82/39; $P = .002$) and at day 6-9 (66/85 vs 92/41; $P = .04$) Sensitivity and specificity GAHS vs DFI at admission (43/90 vs 79/40; $P = .018$) and at days 6-9 (56/88 vs 88/44; $P = .048$)

(continued on next page)

Table 2
(continued)

Author (Year)	Country	Comparison of	Type of Study	n	Diagnosis of AH	Outcome	Score Cutoff	Findings
Srikureja (2005)[11]	USA	MELD, DFI, and CTP[d]	Retrospective[d]	202	Clinical	In-hospital mortality	DFI 32 MELD 18 CTP 12	Sensitivity/specificity/AUROC MELD vs DFI vs CTP at admission (85/84/0.89 vs 83/60/0.81 vs 76/80/0.87; P = NS) At 1 wk AUROC MELD vs DFI: 0.91 vs 0.85; P = .33 and MELD vs CTP 0.91 vs 0.85; P = .35 Change in score at 1 wk AUROC: MELD vs DFI 0.85 vs 0.71; 0.059 and MELD vs CTP 0.85 vs 0.57; P = .0004
Verma (2006)[19]	USA	MELD and DFI	Retrospective[e]	99	Clinical	Septic events, HRS, and short-term mortality	MELD 20 DFI 32	MELD score and not DFI was independent predictor for outcomes with OR [95% CI] for septic event, HRS, and short-term mortality: 2.8 [1–8; P = .04]; 4.0 [1–17; P = .05]; and 6.4 [1–38; P = .03], respectively
Forrest et al (2007)[23]	UK	GAHS and DFI	Retrospective[f]	144	Clinical	28- and 84-day survival on CS treatment	GAHS 9 DFI 32	GAHS < 9: No difference in survival among treated and untreated patients at 28 days (84% vs 80%) and 84 days (73% vs 68%) GAHS ≥ 9: Survival better with treatment at 28 days (78% vs 52%; P = .002) and 84 days (59% vs 38%; P = .02).

(continued on next page)

Table 2
(continued)

Author (Year)	Country	Comparison of	Type of Study	n	Diagnosis of AH	Outcome	Score Cutoff	Findings
Jeong et al (2007)[12]	Korea	DFI, CPT, and MELD	Retrospective	74	Clinical	90-day mortality	Not available	On multivariate regression analysis, CTP and DFI scores but not MELD could predict the outcome; overall mortality at 90 days was 16%
Zapata-Irrison et al (2008)[20]	Mexico	MELD and DFI	Retrospective	67	Clinical	Mortality	MELD 21 DFI 32	Sensitivity/specificity/AUROC of MELD: 96/10/0.73 and of DFI: 100/7/0.69 (P = NS)

Abbreviations: CI, confidence interval; HRS, hepatorenal syndrome; NS, not significant; OR, odds ratio.

[a] Study performed on 1016 patients with liver disease of various causes, including 98 AH patients.

[b] MELD and DFI similar in predicting mortality; however, on multivariate regression analysis, MELD independently predicted 90-day mortality.

[c] No patient was treated with CS or pentoxifylline, but antioxidants were allowed. Score validated on a prospective cohort of 195 biopsy-proven AH patients

[d] Patients with DFI of ≥32 were treated with pentoxifylline and none treated with CS. AUROC for MELD score at admission (cutoff 18), at 1 week (cutoff 20), and change in MELD at 1 week (cutoff 2) was similar.

[e] Patients with severe AH (DFI ≥ 32) were included. Treatment was with pentoxifylline (as per treating physician discretion) and none of the patients received CS.

[f] Patients with severe AH (DFI ≥ 32) were included and of this cohort 73% received CS.

Similarly, the MELD and CPT scores have been compared and were found to be similar in predicting survival.[10] Two studies compared MELD, DFI, and CPT scores. Admission scores were similar in predicting mortality; however, MELD was better than other scores when an increase in respective scores was analyzed at 1 week.[11] In contrast, another study found that DFI and CPT but not MELD scores independently predicted survival.[12]

Two studies from the same center compared GAHS and DFI scores. The first study showed that the GAHS is superior to DFI in predicting survival at 28 and 84 days.[22] In another study, the GAHS was shown to be superior to DFI for predicting the response to CS treatment.[23]

The retrospective design of these studies, small sample size, and heterogeneity of the sample population are some of the potential reasons for the conflicting observations among various studies. Some of the reasons for heterogeneous population are variations in (1) proportion of use of liver biopsy in diagnosis of AH, (2) proportion of patients having concomitant cirrhosis, (3) inclusion and exclusion criteria, (4) proportion of patients receiving specific treatment, and (5) time at which survival is estimated. A recent study overcoming some of these limitations has compared the ABIC, GAHS, DFI, MELD, and DFI scores in a prospective cohort of 332 biopsy-proven AH patients.[31] The Lille score was found to be superior to all other scores with an AUROC of 0.84. However, the MELD and ABIC scores were also useful with AUROC of 0.7 or higher.[31]

An ideal score should be simple, accurate, credible, objective, and validated in a prospective cohort both within and outside the country of origin. Furthermore, the score should be able to guide treatment initiation and response. However, we still do not have a single scoring system that passes all these criteria (**Table 3**). Until the search for an ideal scoring system is completed, the mDF score will continue to be used for initiating treatment and the Lille score for guiding treatment response. The MELD and GAHS scores are also currently useful for initiating treatment with cutoffs at 18 and 9, respectively. One novel area of investigation would be to examine whether a combination of existing scoring systems can meet the criteria for an ideal score for assessing AH patients.

TREATMENT OF AH
Abstinence From Alcohol

Abstinence is of paramount importance in the treatment of AH and has been shown to significantly improve long-term survival.[32,33] The success rate of achieving abstinence varies across different studies using different treatment approaches for achieving alcohol abstinence.[34] Factors associated with long-term abstinence are patient's awareness of the consequences of alcohol consumption, adequate social support, lack of illicit drug use, and absence of psychiatric comorbidities.[35] Incorporation of behavior modification and Alcoholics Anonymous increases the abstinence rates and is recommended for patients who have difficulty in abstaining.

Pharmacologic therapy such as naltrexone (an opioid receptor antagonist), acamprosate (GABA analog), and baclofen (GABA agonist) can be used to maintain abstinence.[36–38] However, only baclofen has been tried in patients with cirrhosis and liver failure.[38] In this study, patients with alcoholic decompensated cirrhosis were randomized to receive baclofen (n = 42) or placebo (n = 42). At 3 months, abstinence rates were better with use of baclofen compared with placebo-treated patients (71% vs 29%; P = .0001) with longer cumulative abstinence duration (63 vs 31 days; P = .001). No side effects were reported with the use of baclofen in these patients with advanced cirrhosis.[38]

Table 3
Characteristics of an ideal scoring system for assessing the severity of AH

	Simplicity	Accuracy	Credibility	Objectivity	Validity	International Validation	Direction for Treatment	Treatment Response
CTP score	++	+	+	+/−	++	++	−	−
mDF score	++	++	++	++	++	++	++	+/−
MELD score	+/−	++	++	++	++	++	+/−	+/−
GAHS	++	+	+	++	++	−−	+/−	+
Lille score	+/−	++	++	++	++	−−	−−	++
ABIC score	+/−	+	+	++	+	−	+/−	−−

Management of Alcohol Withdrawal

In patients with a history of alcohol abuse, it is crucial to recognize symptoms of alcohol withdrawal, including insomnia, irritability, nausea, vomiting, headache, anxiety, cardiac arrhythmia, hypoglycemia, and diaphoresis. Rarely, withdrawal tonic clonic seizures may occur which can proceed to delirium tremens (DT). DT defined by hallucinations, disorientation, cardiac arrhythmia, hypertension, fever, agitation, and diaphoresis, usually occurs 48 to 96 hours after the patient's last alcohol drink. Risk factors for the development of DT include chronic alcohol use, history of DT in the past, elevated serum alcohol levels, and presence of concomitant illness. Mortality rate of DT approaches 5% and is usually owing to arrhythmia and complicating illness (pancreatitis, hepatitis, or pneumonia). Benzodiazepines are used for prophylaxis and acute withdrawal with lorazepam and oxazepam being the preferred agents because of their relatively short half-lives. Refractory DT may be treated with the addition of phenobarbital to benzodiazepine therapy. Propofol has also been utilized to control symptoms. Patients who require phenobarbital or propofol will likely need endotracheal intubation and mechanical ventilation.

Treatment of Complications of Chronic Liver Disease

About 40% to 50% of patients with AH may have underlying cirrhosis.[1] Therefore, these patients may frequently have complications of cirrhosis such as ascites, infection particularly spontaneous bacterial peritonitis, variceal bleeding, altered mental status, and renal insufficiency with hepatorenal syndrome (HRS). The management of these complications is similar to any other patient with cirrhosis.[39] This will not be detailed here and only a brief outline is provided (**Table 4**).

Malnutrition

Patients with AH frequently present with protein caloric malnutrition due to a number of factors such as poor intake, decreased small intestinal absorption, and alcoholic diarrhea.[40] Maintaining an adequate nutritional status is crucial because the outcome is directly related to the nutritional status of these patients.[41,42] Physical examination and laboratory evaluation should be performed for mid-arm circumference, triceps skin-fold thickness, creatinine height index, total lymphocyte count, and prealbumin levels to provide a comprehensive nutritional status of the patient.[42] Patients who are found to be malnourished should specially be targeted for providing rigorous nutritional support.

Many studies have assessed the role of nutritional supplementation in the treatment of AH. A randomized controlled trial (RCT) compared CS therapy (40 mg/d) with enteral diet (2000 kcal/d). Overall mortality in both groups was similar. However, the enteral nutrition group had a lower incidence of infections.[43] In another RCT, 263 patients with moderate to severe AH were randomized to receive prednisolone, oxandrolone, or placebo. Patients receiving oxandrolone and nutritional supplementation had a better outcome as opposed to oxandrolone alone.[44]

It is important to achieve nutritional goals with positive nitrogen balance to improve survival, therefore an energy intake of 35 to 40 kcal/kg per day and protein intake of 1.2 to 1.5 g/kg per day is recommended. Proteins should not be restricted even in patients with encephalopathy, provided they can tolerate the protein load and encephalopathy does not worsen. The use of a daily caloric count and the help of a professional dietitian are crucial to identify patients who need additional supplementation.[45] Enteral supplementation is preferred and enteral tubes can be safely placed even in patients with unbanded esophageal varices.[46]

Table 4
Treatment of complications of cirrhosis

Complication	Initial Evaluation	Treatment Measures	Treatment if Refractory to Routine Measures
Variceal bleeding	CBC, LFTs, BMP	Octreotide infusion, antibiotics, EGD and EVL	TIPS; Shunt surgery for compensated cirrhosis
Ascites	LFTs, ascetic fluid analysis	Diuretics, IV albumin, paracentesis	TIPS
Spontaneous bacterial peritonitis	Ascitic fluid analysis with gram stain and C/S, blood C/S	Antibiotics, IV albumin	Change antibiotics based on C/S
Hepatic encephalopathy	Detailed history and evaluation to identify precipitant	Treat the precipitant factor, lactulose	Rifaximin
Hepatorenal syndrome	LFTs, BUN, SC, UA, infection work-up, fluid challenge and discontinue diuretics	Midodrine, octreotide, terlipressin	TIPS

Abbreviations: BMP, basic metabolic panel; BUN, blood urea nitrogen; CBC, complete blood count; C/S, culture and sensitivity; EGD, esophagogastroduodenoscopy; EVL, endoscopic variceal ligation; LFT, liver function tests; SC, serum creatinine; TIPS, transjugular intrahepatic portosystemic shunt; UA, urine analysis.

Specific Pharmacologic Agents for the Treatment of AH

Because patients with severe AH have a mortality rate of about 40% to 50% in first 6 months, they should be treated with specific pharmacologic agents.[1] Many agents have been tried (**Fig. 1**) and CS use is recommended by some as the initial drug of choice.[21]

Corticosteroids

Over the last about 3 decades, 12 placebo-controlled RCTs have been performed to assess benefit of CS in AH (**Table 5**).[3,4,47–56] Data are conflicting with only 5 studies showing a survival benefit (see **Table 5**). Variations in sample size, inclusion/exclusion criteria especially on the use of liver biopsy for diagnosis, disease severity, endpoints, type of CS used, and treatment duration could explain the differences among studies. Meta-analyses on the efficacy of steroids in AH have also shown conflicting data.[5,57–59] However, when the individual patient data on 132 patients with severe AH (mDF ≥32) from 3 RCTs were pooled, CS were found to be beneficial in improving survival at 28 days as compared with placebo (85% vs 65%; $P = .001$; **Fig. 2**).[5] The benefits of CS for patients with severe AH were also confirmed in a Cochrane analysis despite the heterogeneous data.[59]

CS act by reducing inflammatory cytokines such as tumor necrosis factor (TNF)-α, intercellular adhesion molecule-1, interleukin (IL)-6, and IL-8.[60,61] A decrease in the cytokines and other inflammatory markers was shown in a randomized study among

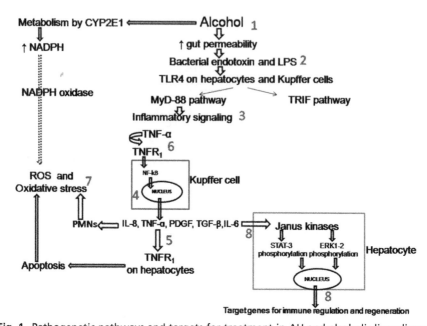

Fig. 1. Pathogenetic pathways and targets for treatment in AH and alcoholic liver disease. Alcohol increases the gut permeability allowing transmigration of gut derived bacteria to enter the portal circulation. Lipopolysaccharide (LPS) of the bacterial endotoxin is recognized by the Toll like receptors (TLRs), which are present on the hepatocytes, Kupffer cells, and vascular endothelial cells. Stimulation of TLRs leads to stimulation of inflammatory cascade and pathways via the myeloid differentiation factor (MyD88) pathway with release of TNF-α. Through its receptor TNFR1, TNF-α enters the Kupffer cells located within the sinusoids. This leads to increased expression of genes for nuclear factor-κB, which further translocates to the nucleus of the cell and causes increased expression of genes for various cytokines, such as interleukins (IL-6, IL-8, IL-10, IL-22), TNF-α, platelet-derived growth factor (PDGF), tumor growth factor (TGF)-β. IL-8 is a chemotactic agent for attracting polymorphonuclear cells (PMNs) at the site enhancing further the inflammation and liver injury. TNF-α activates caspases in the hepatocytes leading to apoptosis of these cells. Another major component of the pathogenesis of AH is generation of ROS via oxidative stress (OS). ROS are generated via (a) NADPH oxidase of the neutrophils, (b) apoptotic hepatocytes, and (c) metabolism of alcohol via CYP2E1 (cytochrome P 450, family 2, subfamily E, polypeptide 1) enzyme system. An important component is the effect of various cytokines on the hepatocytes prominent of which are IL-6 and IL-22. These cytokines enter the hepatocytes and stimulate janus-associated kinase (JAK). This stimulates phosphorylation of signal transducer and activator of transcription 3 (STAT-3) and extracellular signal regulated kinase (ERK) 1/2. Phosphorylated products then translocate to the nucleus to initiate increased expression of genes for proteins needed to regulate the immune system and for hepatic regeneration including growth factors. Treatment for AH can be targeted at various levels: (1) Alcohol being the primary mediator of the disease and hence most important being abstinence from alcohol; (2) antibiotics and probiotics killing or modulating the gut flora respectively; (3) TLR4 antagonists; (4) CS through their anti-inflammatory action decrease the inflammatory mediators, cytokines, and PMN recruitment; (5) pentoxifylline (PTX) neutralizing the effect of TNF-α on the hepatocytes and Kupffer cells; (6) anti-TNF agents, which block the release of TNF-α; (7) Antioxidants decreasing the OS and generation of ROS; and (8) newer agents: IL-6 or IL-22 helping hepatic regeneration and targeting other genes uniquely expressed in the liver in AH. TRIF, TIR-domain containing adaptor.

Table 5
Randomized studies to assess CS for treatment of acute AH

Author/Year	Sample Size	Mean Age (y)	Males (%)	Drug Schedule	Time to Survival	Survival (Treated vs Placebo)	Secondary Findings
Helman et al[47] (USA) 1971[e]	37 (20)	48	32	Prednisolone 40 mg/d × 4 wks	28 days	Benefit only for severe AH (93% vs 60%; P<.01).	No difference on histology at 4 wks and no effect on prevention to cirrhosis.
Porter et al[48] (USA) 1971	20 (11)	45	64	6-MP 40 mg/d × 10 d	In hospital	45% vs 22%; P = NS	No effect on biochemical parameters
Campra et al[49] (USA) 1973[c]	45 (20)	43	75	prednisone 0.5 mg/k/d × 3wks then 0.25 mg/k/d × 3 wks	6 weeks	36% vs 35%; P = NS	No effect on biochemical parameters and trend for improved survival with HE (P = .2)
Blitzer et al[50] (USA) 1973	28 (16)	48	NR	Prednisolone 40 mg × 14 days then tapering × 2 wks	In hospital	50% vs 69%; P = NS	No effect on biochemical parameters.
Shumaker et al[51] (USA) 1978	27 (12)	44	75	6-methyl prednisolone 80 mg/d × 4–7 d PO	In hospital	50% vs 53%; P = NS	Patients with CI to steroids had higher mortality. Causes of death in the 2 groups were similar with >50% dying from GIB
Maddrey et al[3] (USA) 1978	55	40	60	prednisolone 40 mg/d × 28–32 days	30 days	96% vs 80%; P = .1	SB > 20, PT > 8 sec prolonged and encephalopathy predicted mortality. No effect on development of portal hypertension.
Lesesne et al[52] (USA) 1978[a]	14 (7)	49	NR	Prednisolone 40 mg/d ×30 d then 2 wks of tapering	NR	71% vs 0%; P<.01	Infrequent complications from steroids could be cause of death.

(continued on next page)

Table 5
(continued)

Author/Year	Sample Size	Mean Age (y)	Males (%)	Drug Schedule	Time to Survival	Survival (Treated vs Placebo)	Secondary Findings
Depew et al[53] (USA) 1980[9]	28 (15)	49	66	Prednisolone 40 mg/d × 28 d then taper × 14 d	60 days	53% vs 54%; P = NS	No effect on biochemical parameters and complications higher with steroids.
Theodossi et al[54] (UK) 1982[c]	55 (27)	NR	70	Methylprednisolone 1 g/d × 3d	28 days	37% vs 43%; P = NS	Survival predicted by: HE, DF >93, bilirubin 20 mg/dL, creatinine 3 mg/dL, and histologic evidence of cirrhosis.
Mendenhall et al[55] (USA) 1984[b]	263 (90)	51	100	Prednisone tapered over 28 days	30 days	Survival similar	Overall mortality 13% for moderate and 29% for severe AH. Oxandrolone improved long-term survival.
Carithers et al[4] (USA) 1989[d]	66 (35)	43	62	Methylprednisolone 32 mg/d for 28 days then tapered over 2 weeks	28 days	94% vs 65%; P = .0006	Survival with HE: 93% vs 53%; P = .02
Ramond et al[56] (USA) 1992[d,e]	61 (32)	48	NR	Prednisolone 40 mg/d × 28 d [IV if unable to take PO]	66 days	84% vs 45%; P = .002 irrespective of HE (21/23 vs 10/19; P<.001).	Death in steroids group occurred early.

Abbreviations: CI, contraindication; DF, discriminant function; HE, hepatic encephalopathy; HRS, hepatorenal syndrome; IL, interleukin; NR, not reported; NS, not significant; SB, serum bilirubin; TNF, tumor necrosis factor.

[a] Includes patients with hepatic encephalopathy and compared prednisolone to caloric supplements with 1600 kcal/d.
[b] One hundred thirty-two patients had moderate and 131 severe AH; 85 received oxandrolone and 88 received placebo.
[c] Included severe AH patients defined based on clinical grounds or serum bilirubin > 5 mg/dL, or hepatic encephalopathy.
[d] Included severe AH patients defined by mDF ≥ 32 and/or hepatic encephalopathy.
[e] Included liver biopsy proven patients with AH.

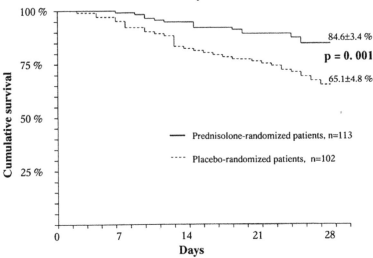

28-DAY SURVIVAL OF PATIENTS WITH DF ≥ 32:
Individual Data Analysis of the Three RCTs

Fig. 2. Kaplan–Meier curve showing 28-day survival of patients with severe AH (mDF ≥ 32 or hepatic encephalopathy): Comparison of 113 patients treated with CS and 102 patients receiving placebo. Pooled analysis of individual patient data from 3 RCTs. The results show that CS treatment is beneficial with improved survival (85% vs 65%; log-rank P = .001). (*From* Mathurin P, Abdelnour M, Ramond MJ, et al. Early change in bilirubin levels is an important prognostic factor in severe alcoholic hepatitis treated with prednisolone. Hepatology 2003; 38:1363–9; reproduced with permission).

patients given CS for 8 days as compared with patients receiving placebo.[62] Peripheral white blood cell count above 5500/mm³ and amount of polymorphonuclear leukocytic infiltration on the liver biopsy specimen have been shown to predict response and survival on CS treatment.[63] Recently, insensitivity of lymphocytes to steroids has been shown in patients with AH, which improves on recovery among those who respond to steroids.[64] In the same study, ex vivo use of theophylline reversed the lymphocyte insensitivity to CS, suggesting a possible adjunctive role of theophylline in the treatment of AH.[64]

Although many agents have been used across different studies, prednisolone is preferred (but not demonstrated to be better) over prednisone because prednisone requires conversion within the liver to its active form, prednisolone. The drug is given orally in a dose of 40 to 60 mg/d for a total duration of 4 weeks. The treatment is then tapered over next 2 to 3 weeks. If the patient is unable to take orally owing to nausea, vomiting, or altered sensorium, an intravenous preparation such as methylprednisolone may be used until the patient is capable to take medication by mouth.

It is prudent to screen patients for any contraindication before starting steroids. One of the most important contraindications is the presence of infection, which is fairly common among patients with severe AH. This used to be considered an absolute contraindication for steroids.[6] However, if patients are adequately treated for an established infection, CS can be safely administered and improve the outcome. In a prospective study on 246 severe AH patients, about 25% had infection requiring antibiotic treatment before starting CS. Survival at 2 months in this group was similar

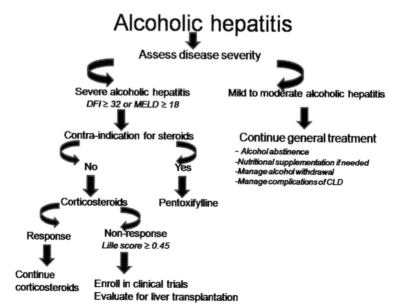

Fig. 3. Treatment algorithm for management of patients with AH.

to patients who were not infected (71% vs 72%; P = .99).[65] Other contraindications are an active gastrointestinal bleeding, renal failure, acute pancreatitis, active tuberculosis, uncontrolled diabetes, and psychosis.

Patients who achieve decrease in bilirubin at 1 week of starting CS have a better survival at 6 months compared with those whose bilirubin does not change or increases (83% vs 23%; P<.0001).[25] Patients with a Lille score of 0.45 or higher are defined as NRS and this is accurate in predicting 75% of deaths at 3 to 6 months.[27] Patients with NRS at 1 week do not benefit from continuing CS and are at risk for infection and sepsis.[65]

Pentoxifylline
Pentoxifylline (PTX), a TNF-α inhibitor and nonspecific phosphodiesterase inhibitor is an alternative option for patients with AH (**Fig. 3**).[66] Based on the pilot study on the efficacy of PTX in AH patients,[67] a pivotal double-blind, placebo-controlled RCT showed survival benefit at 1 month as compared with placebo (76% vs 54%; P = .037).[68] This benefit was mainly due to the prevention of the HRS among patients treated with PTX (50% vs 92%; P<.05).[68] Later, many studies (reported as abstracts) confirmed this observation of beneficial effect of PTX in the prevention of HRS (**Table 6**).[69–71] However, the latest Cochrane systematic review of 5 RCTs (4 reported as abstracts) concluded that there is not enough evidence for survival benefit of PTX in the treatment of AH.

A study published recently comparing steroids with PTX showed superiority of PTX in the treatment of AH patients with better survival rate at 3 months (85% vs 65%; P = .04).[72] This was again mainly owing to prevention of HRS by PTX (6 of 34 patients receiving steroids developed HRS compared with none of 34 receiving PTX).[72] The question of whether PTX can be a salvage option for patients with NRS was answered by a placebo controlled RCT on NRS at 1 week.[73] Steroids were continued and use

Table 6
Randomized studies to assess PTX for treatment of severe AH (mDF ≥ 32 and/or hepatic encephalopathy)

Author/Year	Sample Size	Mean Age (y)	Males (%)	Drug Schedule	Time to Survival	Survival (Treated vs Placebo)	Secondary Findings
McHutchison et al[67] (USA) 1991[a]	22 (12 PTX)	NR	NR	PTX 400 mg TID ×10 d	30 days	91% vs 70%; P = NS	Decreased renal dysfunction with PTX. Plasma TNF increased in controls only.
Akriviadis et al[68] (USA) 2000	101 (49 PTX)	42	71	PTX 400 mg TID ×28 d	In hospital	75% vs 54%; P = .037	Age, creatinine, and PTX treatment predicted survival. TNF levels were no different. However, among nonsurvivors TNF levels decreased more in PTX group.
Paladugu et al[69] (India) 2006[a]	30 (14)	50	100	PTX	28 days	71% vs 54%; P = .09.	Time to death 21 vs 18 days (0.041). TNF levels unchanged in both groups.
Sidhu et al[70] (India) 2006[a]	50	NR	NR	PTX 400 mg TID ×28 d	28 days	76% vs 60%; P = NS	PTX reduced creatinine, TNF, mDF, PT.
Lebrec et al[71] (France) 2007[a]	132	NR	NR	PTX	2 and 6 months	86% vs 84%; P = .77 and 73% vs 69%; P = .3 respectively	Subgroup with renal dysfunction also did not get benefit with PTX.

TID, 3 times a day; NS, not significant.
[a] Abstract publication.

of additional PTX failed to demonstrate survival advantage at 2 months (36% vs 31%; $P>.05$). Because patients with NRS are prone to develop infectious complications, this might have abrogated the benefit of PTX. Occurrence of infective complications and/or sepsis as cause of death was not reported in this study. Although the evidence for efficacy of PTX for severe AH is not so deep, this drug is an option in clinical practice.

PTX is given orally at a dose of 400 mg 3 times a day for a total duration of 28 days. Although an anti-TNF agent, TNF levels were not shown to be different among patients receiving PTX as compared with those receiving placebo.[68] The drug neutralizes the action of TNF-α with a consequent decrease in the inflammatory mediators. PTX is also known to decrease fibroblast proliferation and augment hepatic regeneration through increase in IL-6 levels.[74,75] Neutralization of TNF-α by PTX may explain the protective effect of this drug on HRS, although the exact mechanism is not clear.[76]

Agents that block TNF-α
Alcohol-induced stress leads to increased TNF-α production, which further mediates inflammatory signaling.[77] Further, use of anti-TNF agents in animal models resulted in beneficial effects. [78] Therefore, TNF-α was studied as a target for therapeutic intervention.

Infliximab An initial open study on 12 patients using single 5 mg/kg infliximab infusion showed efficacy with 10 of 12 patients being alive at 15 months. Two patients developed septicemia and died.[79] Similar beneficial results were shown in another open-label study.[80] These studies laid the foundation for assessing this molecule in randomized studies. A pilot placebo-controlled RCT on 20 patients with biopsy-proven severe AH showed the efficacy of a single infliximab (5 mg/kg) infusion as an adjuvant to CS in reducing the mDF score at day 28 (39 to 12; $P<.05$). However, patients receiving CS and placebo infusion did not show any improvement in mDF (44 to 22; $P>.05$). Infliximab infusions were well-tolerated.[81] However, another placebo controlled study did not show any benefit of infliximab. In fact, the study had to be stopped prematurely because 7 patients in the infliximab group and 3 in the placebo group died within 2 months. The frequency of severe infections was higher in the infliximab group. Three serial infusions of 10 mg/kg each were used in this study.[82] In contrast, a single infliximab infusion was used in other studies with dose of 5 mg/kg in two,[79,81] and 10 mg/kg in one.[80] Furthermore, patients with DFI were excluded in one study.[81]

Etanercept Another anti-TNF agent, its efficacy was examined in a pilot study (25 mg subcutaneously on days 4, 8, and 12) on 13 patients with moderate or severe AH. Although, 30-day survival was 92%, several adverse events were reported (infection, hepatorenal decompensation, gastrointestinal bleeding) requiring premature discontinuation of etanercept in 23% of patients.[83] A double-blind, placebo-controlled RCT of 48 patients with moderate to severe AH assessed 3-week course of etanercept (25 mg on days 1, 4, 8, 11, 15, and 18). Compared with placebo, the mortality rate with etanercept was similar at 1 month (36.4% and 22.7%; odds ratio, 1.8; 95% CI, 0.5–6.5) and higher at 6 months (58% vs 23%; $P = .017$). Higher rate of serious infections was reported in the etanercept group (34.6% vs 9.1%; $P = .04$).[84]In summary, TNF-α inhibitors are not effective agents for treating AH and pose a risk of serious infections. Studies have shown beneficial effects of TNF-α and other cytokines on the hepatic regenerative capacity and immune function (see **Fig. 1**).[85–87]

Blocking these important beneficial effects of TNF-α with the use of anti-TNF agents probably explain lack of benefit and increased risk of infections in AH patients.[88]

Antioxidants

Oxidative stress (OS) is an important component in the pathogenesis of AH (see **Fig. 1**) with frequent existence of OS markers in these patients.[89,90] Like other liver diseases, antioxidants have been studied for treatment of patients with severe AH.

Initial open-label studies and RCTs did not show a benefit to the use of antioxidant cocktails, NAC, and vitamin E.[91–94] Use of NAC improves survival of patients with acute liver failure due to acetaminophen overdose as well as non–acetaminophen-related causes.[95,96] Based on these, use of NAC (100 mg/kg daily infusion) was assessed in a multicenter placebo controlled RCT on 174 patients with severe AH and reported in abstract form. NAC was given for 5 days and both the groups received CS for 4 weeks. Mortality at 1 and 2 months was lower among the patients who received steroids and NAC (8% vs 24% and 15% vs 33%; $P = .007$). The complication rate at 6 months was lower in the group receiving NAC as compared with placebo (19% vs 42%; $P = .001$).[97] Until more data are available on the efficacy of NAC in the treatment of AH, it may be an attractive option as an adjunct for patients who do not benefit from CS.

Probiotics and antibiotics

Intestinal permeability to gut-derived micro-organisms is increased in patients with AH.[98] Toll-like receptors in the liver are pattern recognition receptors and recognize bacterial lipopolysaccharides leading to further inflammatory signaling (see **Fig. 1**).[99] Several studies have shown that patients with liver disease have abnormal bowel flora overgrowth and thus probiotics, which help to restore normal bowel flora, have been proposed as a possible treatment for alcoholic liver disease.[100–102] Probiotic use has also shown to reverse abnormal phagocytic activity of neutrophils and ex vivo endotoxin stimulated levels of TNF receptors and IL-10.[103] Rifaximin, a nonabsorbable antibiotic and a derivative of rifamycin, has broad activity against many gastrointestinal organisms and is being studied to assess its efficacy in improving liver function in alcoholic cirrhosis (AC).[104] A recent study showed that rifaximin use for 28 days significantly decreased plasma endotoxin levels compared with baseline levels in systemic (1.45 vs 0.7; $P<.0001$) and splanchnic circulation (1.8 vs 0.8; $P<.0001$). This was associated with decrease in hepatic venous pressure gradient (HVPG) from 18 mmHg on day 0 to 14.7 mmHg on day 29 ($P<.0001$).[105] Similarly, use of norfloxacin reduced serum endotoxin concentrations with partial reversal of hyperdynamic circulatory state in cirrhotics. However, there was no significant effect on the HVPG.[106,107]

Miscellaneous agents

Some of the treatment strategies that have been tried but have not shown any clear benefit are amlodipine, a calcium channel antagonist,[108] amino acids infusion,[109] colchicine,[110] insulin–glucagon infusion,[111] propylthiouracil,[112] and betaine.[113]

Based on the evidence for existence for qualitative functional defects of neutrophils in AH,[114] granulocytapheresis, a technique that removes up to 60% of activated granulocytes and monocytes from circulating blood, was used in AH patients. Although the procedure was tolerated well in a case series on 6 patients with severe AH (5 of them being NRS), no clinical benefit was seen.[115] In another RCT, the use of granulocyte colony stimulating factor for 7 days improved hepatic proliferative and regenerative capacity. However, there were no differences on histology or cytokine levels.[116]

The molecular adsorbent recirculating system used in an open study on 8 patients with severe AH (estimated survival of 20% at 3 months) showed 50% survival at 3 months.[117] Patients showed improved liver chemistry, renal function, hepatic encephalopathy, and systemic hemodynamics. In another study, molecular adsorbent recirculating system use in 7 patients and hemofiltration in 3 patients reduced HVPG to less than 12 mmHg within 6 hours and the effect was persistent for another 18 hours.[118]

Future Targets

Apart from mediating inflammation, cytokines also have beneficial effects on the liver, such as (1) induction of hepatic proliferative activity with hepatic regeneration and (2) immune modulation with prevention of infection. Therefore, use of cytokines as therapeutic agents in conjunction with CS is an attractive option (see **Fig. 1**). IL-6 use is limited by their potential side effects such as fever and inflammation.[119] IL-22 has minimal side effects with a potential for use in AH patients. The beneficial effect of IL-22 is mediated via STAT-3 activation.[120] Further, use of genome-wide association studies have identified multiple target genes and chemokines which are upregulated in AH patients.[121–123] These include IL-8; growth related gene product, NADPH oxidase, angiotensin-converting enzyme, and epithelial neutrophil activating protein-78 (ENA-78) genes.[122,123] Their levels are also correlated with survival and portal hypertension.[122] Growth regulated oncogene-alpha (GRO-α), a member of the IL-8, family binds to chemokine type X receptor-2 on the target cells. NADPH oxidase helps generation of reactive oxygen species (ROS) mediating OS. However, to avoid infections, it is crucial to selectively inhibit nonphagocytic NADPH oxidase.[123]

A recent genome-wide association studies study reported from Spain on 44 biopsy-proven AH patients showed a 58-fold upregulation of osteopontin (an extracellular matrix protein that attracts neutrophils) in AH livers.[124] In addition, TNG superfamily receptor, TNF-like weak inducer of apoptosis and its receptor, Fn 14, is upregulated exclusively in AH patients and is an important mediator of immune regulation, liver proliferation, and tissue remodeling.[125]

LT IN ACUTE AH: CURRENT STATUS AND FUTURE DEVELOPMENT

With a survival benefit of only about 50% with specific treatment of severe AH and about 75% mortality among NRS, there is a need for more definitive treatment option for these critically sick patients with severe AH.[5,27,126]

LT is an accepted treatment modality for patients with AC. The outcome after LT for AC is as good as for other causes of liver disease.[127] LT as a treatment option for patients with severe AH remains controversial despite the fact that it is an established treatment option for most etiologies of acute liver failure. Barriers precluding use of LT in AH include (1) ethical concerns of transplanting patients with active alcohol abuse, (2) the risk of recidivism to alcohol drinking after LT, and (3) the lack of applicability of 6-month abstinence rule with active drinking.

Ethical Concerns and Issues

One of the major ethical concerns is a shortage of organs for LT. The public opinion is that AH is self-inflicted by the patient and should be their own responsibility.[128] However, there are other liver diseases such as hepatitis B, hepatitis C, nonalcoholic fatty liver disease, and acetaminophen overdose where patient behavior is an important component either in the acquisition of these diseases or in management and yet transplant is liberally considered.

Recidivism After LT

The rate of alcohol relapse after LT varies from 3% to 49%, with graft dysfunction and death ranging from 0% to 27% and 0% to 6.5%, respectively.[129] Heavy drinking after LT in alcoholic liver disease as a whole is reported in fewer than 10% of patients.[130] However, the definition of harmful drinking varies from study to study.[131] Furthermore, documenting alcohol use by history is not always accurate because patients may not always be truthful.[132] In a retrospective study on long-term follow-up (median follow-up, 7.5 years) patients who relapsed to harmful drinking had poorer survival as compared with abstainers (45% vs 86%; $P<.05$).[133] In a systematic review on 22 studies, McCallum and colleagues[131] identified factors consistently associated with recidivism: younger age, associated polysubstance abuse, lack of social support, family history of alcohol abuse in a first-degree relative, poor response to previous rehabilitation programs, and noncompliance. Concomitant mental and psychiatric disorders and lack of insight did not predict recidivism.[131]

Six Months Abstinence Rule

Patients with AC qualify for LT if they are abstinent for 6 months or longer.[134] The same "6-month rule" is being applied currently in the United States for patients with AH.[135,136] Although the pre-LT abstinence duration was a predictor on the frequency as well as time to relapse to alcohol abuse after LT, only 40% of patients abstaining for 36 months before LT were sober after LT.[137] The lack of correlation of post-LT recidivism with 6 months abstinence before LT was also shown by McCallum and colleagues[131] in their systematic review of 11 studies, of which 9 studies did not show an association between 6 months pre-LT abstinence and post-LT recidivism.

Retrospective analyses of patients undergoing LT for AC have shown similar survival rates, irrespective of histologic changes of AH in the explants.[138–141] However, histologic changes of AH can persist for a long duration, even after response to treatment, and these data may not apply to a population with active clinical disease.[140] Prospective data on LT in patients with severe AH are scant. In a recently reported multicenter study from Europe, 20 patients with severe AH with NRS (Lille score ≥0.45) were studied prospectively to assess the role of LT.[30] Criteria for receiving the LT were very strict. Each case was matched with a control patient (who did not undergo LT) for age, gender, and Lille score. At the end of 1 year, patient survival in the transplanted group was higher compared with those not receiving LT (83% vs 44%; $P = .009$).[30] Among the nontransplanted patients, 50% to 90% of deaths occurred within first 2 months. None except one patient relapsed to social drinking about 2.5 years after LT.[30] Long-term follow-up data after LT are needed in the light of data showing that 5-year survival of patients with alcoholic liver disease who receive LT is offset by the occurrence of extrahepatic cancer.[142]

In summary, the approach to a patient with AH starts with assessment of the disease severity. Apart from instituting general measures, patients with severe AH are treated with CS with pentoxifylline reserved for those with contraindications to CS (see **Fig. 3**). At 1 week, CS should be discontinued among those with a Lille score of 0.45 or greater. With no effective treatment options currently for patients with NRS, these patients should be enrolled into clinical trials for development of more effective drugs or to evaluate role of LT. Before we routinely use LT as a definitive treatment for patients with NRS, we need to (1) derive long-term outcome of patients and graft in this setting, (2) determine criteria to identify candidates with the least risk of recidivism to harmful drinking, and (3) develop homogeneity in the definition of harmful drinking, drinking patterns, and alcohol abuse questionnaire. Then we will be able to implement guidelines that are fair and scientifically sound for the optimal utilization of available organs in the setting of AH. Although the destination is far, there seems to be light at the end of the tunnel, which will allow us to make the right decision to improve outcome of patients with severe AH.

REFERENCES

1. Lucey MR, Mathurin P, Morgan TR. Alcoholic hepatitis. N Engl J Med 2009;360: 2758–69.
2. Naveau S, Giraud V, Borotto E, et al. Excess weight risk factor for alcoholic liver disease. Hepatology 1997;25:108–11.
3. Maddrey WC, Boitnott JK, Bedine MS, et al. Corticosteroid therapy of alcoholic hepatitis. Gastroenterology 1978;75:193–9.
4. Carithers RL Jr, Herlong HF, Diehl AM, et al. Methylprednisolone therapy in patients with severe alcoholic hepatitis. A randomized multicenter trial. Ann Intern Med 1989;110:685–90.
5. Mathurin P, Mendenhall CL, Carithers RL Jr, et al. Corticosteroids improve short-term survival in patients with severe alcoholic hepatitis (AH): individual data analysis of the last three randomized placebo controlled double blind trials of corticosteroids in severe AH. J Hepatol 2002;36:480–7.
6. McCullough AJ, O'Connor JF. Alcoholic liver disease: proposed recommendations for the American College of Gastroenterology. Am J Gastroenterol 1998; 93:2022–36.
7. Tripodi A, Caldwell SH, Hoffman M, et al. Review article: the prothrombin time test as a measure of bleeding risk and prognosis in liver disease. Aliment Pharmacol Ther 2007;26:141–8.
8. Kulkarni K, Tran T, Medrano M, et al. The role of the discriminant factor in the assessment and treatment of alcoholic hepatitis. J Clin Gastroenterol 2004;38: 453–9.
9. Child CG, Turcotte JG. Surgery and portal hypertension. Philadelphia: WB Saunders; 1964.
10. Said A, Williams J, Holden J, et al. Model for end stage liver disease score predicts mortality across a broad spectrum of liver disease. J Hepatol 2004;40:897–903.
11. Srikureja W, Kyulo NL, Runyon BA, et al. MELD score is a better prognostic model than Child-Turcotte-Pugh score or Discriminant Function score in patients with alcoholic hepatitis. J Hepatol 2005;42:700–6.
12. Jeong JY, Sohn JH, Son BK, et al. [Comparison of model for end-stage liver disease score with discriminant function and child-Turcotte-Pugh scores for predicting short-term mortality in Korean patients with alcoholic hepatitis]. Korean J Gastroenterol 2007;49:93–9.
13. Kamath PS, Wiesner RH, Malinchoc M, et al. A model to predict survival in patients with end-stage liver disease. Hepatology 2001;33:464–70.
14. Kamath PS, Kim WR. The model for end-stage liver disease (MELD). Hepatology 2007;45:797–805.
15. Dunn W, Jamil LH, Brown LS, et al. MELD accurately predicts mortality in patients with alcoholic hepatitis. Hepatology 2005;41:353–8.
16. Sheth M, Riggs M, Patel T. Utility of the Mayo End-Stage Liver Disease (MELD) score in assessing prognosis of patients with alcoholic hepatitis. BMC Gastroenterol 2002;2:2.
17. Vaa BE, Asrani SK, Dunn W, et al. Influence of serum sodium on MELD-based survival prediction in alcoholic hepatitis. Mayo Clin Proc 2011;86:37–42.

18. Kamath PS, Kim WR. Is the change in MELD score a better indicator of mortality than baseline MELD score? Liver Transpl 2003;9:19–21.
19. Verma S, Ajudia K, Mendler M, et al. Prevalence of septic events, type 1 hepatorenal syndrome, and mortality in severe alcoholic hepatitis and utility of discriminant function and MELD score in predicting these adverse events. Dig Dis Sci 2006;51: 1637–43.
20. Zapata-Irrison L, Jurado-Nunez J, Altamirano-Gomez J. [do MELD or Maddrey? Comparison of 2 forecasting models in patients with hepatitis toxic alcohol. Rev Gastroenterol Mex 2008;73:57–62.
21. O'Shea RS, Dasarathy S, McCullough AJ. Alcoholic liver disease. Hepatology 2010;51:307–28.
22. Forrest EH, Evans CD, Stewart S, et al. Analysis of factors predictive of mortality in alcoholic hepatitis and derivation and validation of the Glasgow alcoholic hepatitis score. Gut 2005;54:1174–9.
23. Forrest EH, Morris AJ, Stewart S, et al. The Glasgow alcoholic hepatitis score identifies patients who may benefit from corticosteroids. Gut 2007;56:1743–6.
24. Dominguez M, Rincon D, Abraldes JG, et al. A new scoring system for prognostic stratification of patients with alcoholic hepatitis. Am J Gastroenterol 2008;103: 2747–56.
25. Mathurin P, Abdelnour M, Ramond MJ, et al. Early change in bilirubin levels is an important prognostic factor in severe alcoholic hepatitis treated with prednisolone. Hepatology 2003;38:1363–9.
26. Nguyen-Khac E TT, Piquet MA, Benferhat S, et al. Treatment of severe acute alcoholic hepatitis (AAH) with corticoids plus N-acetylcysteine (C+NAC) versus corticoids alone (C): a multicenter, randomized, controlled trial. J Hepatology 2010; 52(Suppl 1):S38.
27. Louvet A, Naveau S, Abdelnour M, et al. The Lille model: a new tool for therapeutic strategy in patients with severe alcoholic hepatitis treated with steroids. Hepatology 2007;45:1348–54.
28. Louvet AA, Wartel F, O'Grady JG, et al. A response guided therapy for a better management of patients with severe alcoholic hepatitis treated with corticosteroids. Hepatology 2010;52(4 Suppl):1109A.
29. Nguyen-Khac ETT, Piquet MA, Benferhat S, et al. Treatment of severe acute alcoholic hepatitis (AAH) with corticoids plus N-acetylcysteine (C+NAC) versus corticoids alone (C): a multicenter, randomized, controlled trial. Hepatology 2009; 50(4 Suppl):346A.
30. Castel H, Moreno C, Antonini TM, et al. Early transplantation improves survival of non-responders to steroids in severe alcoholic hepatitis: a challenge to the 6-month rule of abstinence. J Hepatology 2009;52(Suppl 1):S13.
31. Louvet AA, Diaz E, Wartel F, et al. Prognostic scores are efficient in patients with severe alcoholic hepatitis treated with corticosteroids: comparison of available models. Hepatology 2010;52(4 Suppl):1108A–9A.
32. Pessione F, Ramond MJ, Peters L, et al. Five-year survival predictive factors in patients with excessive alcohol intake and cirrhosis. Effect of alcoholic hepatitis, smoking and abstinence. Liver Int 2003;23:45–53.
33. Morgan MY. The prognosis and outcome of alcoholic liver disease. Alcohol Alcohol Suppl 1994;2:335–43.
34. Tripodi SJ, Bender K, Litschge C, et al. Interventions for reducing adolescent alcohol abuse: a meta-analytic review. Arch Pediatr Adolesc Med 2010;164:85–91.
35. Chung T, Martin CS, Winters KC. Diagnosis, course, and assessment of alcohol abuse and dependence in adolescents. Recent Dev Alcohol 2005;17:5–27.

36. Garbutt J, Kranzler H, O'Malley S, et al. Efficacy and tolerability of long-acting injectable naltrexone for alcohol dependence: a randomized controlled trial. JAMA 2005;293:1617–25.

37. Rosner S, Hackl-Herrwerth A, Leucht S, et al. Acamprosate for alcohol dependence. Cochrane Database Syst Rev 2010;9:CD004332.

38. Addolorato G, Leggio L, Ferrulli A, et al. Effectiveness and safety of baclofen for maintenance of alcohol abstinence in alcohol-dependent patients with liver cirrhosis: randomised, double-blind controlled study. Lancet 2007;370:1915–22.

39. Garcia-Tsao G, Lim JK. Management and treatment of patients with cirrhosis and portal hypertension: recommendations from the Department of Veterans Affairs Hepatitis C Resource Center Program and the National Hepatitis C Program. Am J Gastroenterol 2009;104:1802–29.

40. Mendenhall CL, Anderson S, Weesner RE, et al. Protein-calorie malnutrition associated with alcoholic hepatitis. Veterans Administration Cooperative Study Group on Alcoholic Hepatitis. Am J Med 1984;76:211–22.

41. Leevy C, Moroianu S. Nutritional aspects of alcoholic liver disease. Clin Liver Dis 2005;9:67–81.

42. Mendenhall CL, Moritz TE, Roselle GA, et al. Protein energy malnutrition in severe alcoholic hepatitis: diagnosis and response to treatment. The VA Cooperative Study Group #275. JPEN J Parenter Enteral Nutr 1995;19:258–65.

43. Cabré E, Rodríguez-Iglesias P, Caballería J, et al. Short- and long-term outcome of severe alcohol-induced hepatitis treated with steroids or enteral nutrition: a multi-center randomized trial. Hepatology 2000;32:36–42.

44. Mendenhall CL, Moritz TE, Roselle GA, et al. A study of oral nutritional support with oxandrolone in malnourished patients with alcoholic hepatitis: results of a Department of Veterans Affairs cooperative study. Hepatology 1993;17:564–76.

45. Morgan TR, Moritz TE, Mendenhall CL, et al. Protein consumption and hepatic encephalopathy in alcoholic hepatitis. VA Cooperative Study Group #275. J Am Coll Nutr 1995;14:152–8.

46. Plauth M, Cabre E, Riggio O, et al. ESPEN Guidelines on Enteral Nutrition: Liver disease. Clin Nutr 2006;25:285–94.

47. Helman RA, Temko MH, Nye SW, et al. Alcoholic hepatitis. Natural history and evaluation of prednisolone therapy. Ann Intern Med 1971;74:311–21.

48. Porter HP, Simon FR, Pope CE 2nd, et al. Corticosteroid therapy in severe alcoholic hepatitis. A double-blind drug trial. N Engl J Med 1971;284:1350–5.

49. Campra JL, Hamlin EM Jr, Kirshbaum RJ, et al. Prednisone therapy of acute alcoholic hepatitis. Report of a controlled trial. Ann Intern Med 1973;79:625–31.

50. Blitzer BL, Mutchnick MG, Joshi PH, et al. Adrenocorticosteroid therapy in alcoholic hepatitis. A prospective, double-blind randomized study. Am J Dig Dis 1977;22:477–84.

51. Shumaker JB, Resnick RH, Galambos JT, et al. A controlled trial of 6-methylprednisolone in acute alcoholic hepatitis. With a note on published results in encephalopathic patients. Am J Gastroenterol 1978;69:443–9.

52. Lesesne HR, Bozymski EM, Fallon HJ. Treatment of alcoholic hepatitis with encephalopathy. Comparison of prednisolone with caloric supplements. Gastroenterology 1978;74:169–73.

53. Depew W, Boyer T, Omata M, et al. Double-blind controlled trial of prednisolone therapy in patients with severe acute alcoholic hepatitis and spontaneous encephalopathy. Gastroenterology 1980;78:524–9.

54. Theodossi A, Eddleston AL, Williams R. Controlled trial of methylprednisolone therapy in severe acute alcoholic hepatitis. Gut 1982;23:75–9.

55. Mendenhall CL, Anderson S, Garcia-Pont P, et al. Short-term and long-term survival in patients with alcoholic hepatitis treated with oxandrolone and prednisolone. N Engl J Med 1984;311:1464–70.
56. Ramond MJ, Poynard T, Rueff B, et al. A randomized trial of prednisolone in patients with severe alcoholic hepatitis. N Engl J Med 20 1992;326:507–12.
57. Daures JP, Peray P, Bories P, et al. [Corticoid therapy in the treatment of acute alcoholic hepatitis. Results of a meta-analysis]. Gastroenterol Clin Biol 1991;15: 223–8.
58. Imperiale TF, McCullough AJ. Do corticosteroids reduce mortality from alcoholic hepatitis? A meta-analysis of the randomized trials. Ann Intern Med 1990;113: 299–307.
59. Rambaldi A, Saconato HH, Christensen E, et al. Systematic review: glucocortico-steroids for alcoholic hepatitis—a Cochrane Hepato-Biliary Group systematic review with meta-analyses and trial sequential analyses of randomized clinical trials. Aliment Pharmacol Ther 2008;27:1167–78.
60. Spahr L, Rubbia-Brandt L, Pugin J, et al. Rapid changes in alcoholic hepatitis histology under steroids: correlation with soluble intercellular adhesion molecule-1 in hepatic venous blood. J Hepatol 2001;35:582–9.
61. Taieb J, Mathurin P, Elbim C, et al. Blood neutrophil functions and cytokine release in severe alcoholic hepatitis: effect of corticosteroids. J Hepatol 2000;32:579–86.
62. Richardet JD, Mal F, Roulot D, et al. Influence of corticosteroids (CS) on plasma cytokines concentrations in patients with severe alcoholic hepatitis (HA): results of a randomized study. J Hepatol 1993;18:S75.
63. Mathurin P, Duchatelle V, Ramond MJ, et al. Survival and prognostic factors in patients with severe alcoholic hepatitis treated with prednisolone. Gastroenterology 1996;110:1847–53.
64. Kendrick SF, Henderson E, Palmer J, et al. Theophylline improves steroid sensitivity in acute alcoholic hepatitis. Hepatology;52:126–31.
65. Louvet A, Wartel F, Castel H, et al. Infection in patients with severe alcoholic hepatitis treated with steroids: early response to therapy is the key factor. Gastroenterology 2009;137:541–8.
66. Reuter BK, Wallace JL. Phosphodiesterase inhibitors prevent NSAID enteropathy independently of effects on TNF-alpha release. Am J Physiol 1999;277:G847–54.
67. McHutchison JR, Draduesku JO, et al. Pentoxifylline may prevent renal impairment (hepatorenal syndrome) in severe acute alcoholic hepatitis. Hepatology 1991;14:96A.
68. Akriviadis E, Botla R, Briggs W, et al. Pentoxifylline improves short-term survival in severe acute alcoholic hepatitis: a double-blind, placebo-controlled trial. Gastroenterology 2000;119:1637–48.
69. Paladugu H, Sawant, P, Dalvi, L, et al. Role of pentoxifylline in treatment of severe acute alcoholic hepatitis—a randomized controlled trial. J Gastrenterol Hepatol 2006;21:A459.
70. Sidhu S, Singla M, Bhatia KL. Pentoxifyline reduces disease severity and prevents renal impairment in severe acute alcoholic hepatitis: a double blind, placebo controlled trial. Hepatology 2006;44:A373–4.
71. Lebrec D, Dominique T, Oberti F, et al. Pentoxifylline for the treatment of patients with advanced cirrhosis. A randomized placebo controlled double blind trial. Hepatology 2007;46:A249–50.
72. De BK, Gangopadhyay S, Dutta D, et al. Pentoxifylline versus prednisolone for severe alcoholic hepatitis: a randomized controlled trial. World J Gastroenterol 2009;15: 1613–9.

73. Louvet A, Diaz E, Dharancy S, et al. Early switch to pentoxifylline in patients with severe alcoholic hepatitis is inefficient in non-responders to corticosteroids. J Hepatol 2008;48:465–70.

74. Morgan TR, McClain CJ. Pentoxifylline and alcoholic hepatitis. Gastroenterology 2000;119:1787–91.

75. Petrowsky H, Breitenstein S, Slankamenac K, et al. Effects of pentoxifylline on liver regeneration: a double-blinded, randomized, controlled trial in 101 patients undergoing major liver resection. Ann Surg 2010;252:813–22.

76. Lebrec D, Thabut D, Oberti F, et al. Pentoxifylline does not decrease short-term mortality but does reduce complications in patients with advanced cirrhosis. Gastroenterology;138:1755–62.

77. Strieter RM, Kunkel SL, Bone RC. Role of tumor necrosis factor-alpha in disease states and inflammation. Crit Care Med 1993;21(10 Suppl):S447–63.

78. Iimuro Y, Gallucci RM, Luster MI, et al. Antibodies to tumor necrosis factor alfa attenuate hepatic necrosis and inflammation caused by chronic exposure to ethanol in the rat. Hepatology 1997;26:1530–7.

79. Tilg H, Jalan R, Kaser A, et al. Anti-tumor necrosis factor-alpha monoclonal antibody therapy in severe alcoholic hepatitis. J Hepatol 2003;38:419–25.

80. Sharma P, Kumar A, Sharma BC, et al. Infliximab monotherapy for severe alcoholic hepatitis and predictors of survival: an open label trial. J Hepatol 2009;50:584–91.

81. Spahr L, Rubbia-Brandt L, Frossard JL, et al. Combination of steroids with infliximab or placebo in severe alcoholic hepatitis: a randomized controlled pilot study. J Hepatol 2002;37:448–55.

82. Naveau S, Chollet-Martin S, Dharancy S, et al. A double-blind randomized controlled trial of infliximab associated with prednisolone in acute alcoholic hepatitis. Hepatology 2004;39:1390–7.

83. Menon KV, Stadheim L, Kamath PS, et al. A pilot study of the safety and tolerability of etanercept in patients with alcoholic hepatitis. Am J Gastroenterol 2004;99:255–60.

84. Boetticher NC, Peine CJ, Kwo P, et al. A randomized, double-blinded, placebo-controlled multicenter trial of etanercept in the treatment of alcoholic hepatitis. Gastroenterology 2008;135:1953–60.

85. Yamada Y, Kirillova I, Peschon JJ, et al. Initiation of liver growth by tumor necrosis factor: deficient liver regeneration in mice lacking type I tumor necrosis factor receptor. Proc Natl Acad Sci U S A 18 1997;94:1441–6.

86. Hajeer AH, Hutchinson IV. TNF-alpha gene polymorphism: clinical and biological implications. Microsc Res Tech 2000;50:216–28.

87. Yamada Y, Fausto N. Deficient liver regeneration after carbon tetrachloride injury in mice lacking type 1 but not type 2 tumor necrosis factor receptor. Am J Pathol 1998;152:1577–89.

88. Akerman P, Cote P, Yang SQ, et al. Antibodies to tumor necrosis factor-alpha inhibit liver regeneration after partial hepatectomy. Am J Physiol 1992;263:G579–85.

89. Dey A, Cederbaum AI. Alcohol and oxidative liver injury. Hepatology 2006;43 (2 Suppl 1):S63–74.

90. Loguercio C, Federico A. Oxidative stress in viral and alcoholic hepatitis. Free Radic Biol Med 2003;34:1–10.

91. Phillips M, Curtis H, Portmann B, et al. Antioxidants versus corticosteroids in the treatment of severe alcoholic hepatitis—a randomised clinical trial. J Hepatol 2006; 44:784–90.

92. Stewart S, Prince M, Bassendine M, et al. A randomized trial of antioxidant therapy alone or with corticosteroids in acute alcoholic hepatitis. J Hepatol 2007;47:277–83.

93. Moreno C, Langlet P, Hittelet A, et al. Enteral nutrition with or without N-acetylcysteine in the treatment of severe acute alcoholic hepatitis: a randomized multicenter controlled trial. J Hepatol 2010;53:1117–22.

94. Mezey E, Potter JJ, Rennie-Tankersley L, et al. A randomized placebo controlled trial of vitamin E for alcoholic hepatitis. J Hepatol 2004;40:40–6.

95. Mazer M, Perrone J. Acetaminophen-induced nephrotoxicity: pathophysiology, clinical manifestations, and management. J Med Toxicol 2008;4:2–6.

96. Lee WM, Hynan LS, Rossaro L, et al. Intravenous N-acetylcysteine improves transplant-free survival in early stage non-acetaminophen acute liver failure. Gastroenterology 2009;137:856–64.

97. Ngyen-Khac ETT, Piquet MA, Benferhat S, et al. Treatment of severe acute alcoholic hepatitis (AAH) with corticoids plus N-acetylcysteine (C+NAC) versus corticoids alone (C): a multicenter randomized controlled trial [abstract]. Hepatology 2009; 50(Suppl):346A.

98. Bjarnason I, Peters TJ, Wise RJ. The leaky gut of alcoholism: possible route of entry for toxic compounds. Lancet 1984;1:179–82.

99. Mandrekar P, Szabo G. Signalling pathways in alcohol-induced liver inflammation. J Hepatol 2009;50:1258–66.

100. Liu Q, Duan ZP, Ha DK, et al. Symbiotic modulation of gut flora: effect on minimal hepatic encephalopathy in patients with cirrhosis. Hepatology 2004;39:1441–9.

101. Zhao HY, Wang HJ, Lu Z, et al. Intestinal microflora in patients with liver cirrhosis. Chin J Dig Dis 2004;5:64–7.

102. Kirpich IA, Solovieva NV, Leikhter SN, et al. Probiotics restore bowel flora and improve liver enzymes in human alcohol-induced liver injury: a pilot study. Alcohol 2008;42:675–82.

103. Stadlbauer V, Mookerjee RP, Hodges S, et al. Effect of probiotic treatment on deranged neutrophil function and cytokine responses in patients with compensated alcoholic cirrhosis. J Hepatol 2008;48:945–51.

104. Gillis JC, Brogden RN. Rifaximin. A review of its antibacterial activity, pharmacokinetic properties and therapeutic potential in conditions mediated by gastrointestinal bacteria. Drugs 1995;49:467–84.

105. Vlachogiannakos J, Saveriadis AS, Viazis N, et al. Intestinal decontamination improves liver haemodynamics in patients with alcohol-related decompensated cirrhosis. Aliment Pharmacol Ther 2009;29:992–9.

106. Albillos A, de la Hera A, Gonzalez M, et al. Increased lipopolysaccharide binding protein in cirrhotic patients with marked immune and hemodynamic derangement. Hepatology 2003;37:208–17.

107. Rasaratnam B, Kaye D, Jennings G, et al. The effect of selective intestinal decontamination on the hyperdynamic circulatory state in cirrhosis. A randomized trial. Ann Intern Med 2003;139:186–93.

108. Bird GL, Prach AT, McMahon AD, et al. Randomised controlled double-blind trial of the calcium channel antagonist amlodipine in the treatment of acute alcoholic hepatitis. J Hepatol 1998;28:194–8.

109. Mezey E, Caballeria J, Mitchell MC, et al. Effect of parenteral amino acid supplementation on short-term and long-term outcomes in severe alcoholic hepatitis: a randomized controlled trial. Hepatology 1991;14:1090–6.

110. Trinchet JC, Beaugrand M, Callard P, et al. Treatment of alcoholic hepatitis with colchicine. Results of a randomized double blind trial. Gastroenterol Clin Biol 1989;13:551–5.

111. Trinchet JC, Balkau B, Poupon RE, et al. Treatment of severe alcoholic hepatitis by infusion of insulin and glucagon: a multicenter sequential trial. Hepatology 1992;15: 76–81.
112. Rambaldi A, Gluud C. Propylthiouracil for alcoholic liver disease. Cochrane Database Syst Rev 2002;2:CD002800.
113. Samara K, Liu C, Soldevila-Pico C, et al. Betaine resolves severe alcohol-induced hepatitis and steatosis following liver transplantation. Dig Dis Sci 2006;51:1226–9.
114. Jaeschke H. Neutrophil-mediated tissue injury in alcoholic hepatitis. Alcohol 2002; 27:23–7.
115. Morris JM, Dickson S, Neilson M, et al. Granulocytapheresis in the treatment of severe alcoholic hepatitis: a case series. Eur J Gastroenterol Hepatol 2010;22: 457–60.
116. Spahr L, Lambert JF, Rubbia-Brandt L, et al. Granulocyte-colony stimulating factor induces proliferation of hepatic progenitors in alcoholic steatohepatitis: a randomized trial. Hepatology 2008;48:221–9.
117. Jalan R, Sen S, Steiner C, et al. Extracorporeal liver support with molecular adsorbents recirculating system in patients with severe acute alcoholic hepatitis. J Hepatol 2003;38:24–31.
118. Sen S, Mookerjee RP, Cheshire LM, et al. Albumin dialysis reduces portal pressure acutely in patients with severe alcoholic hepatitis. J Hepatol 2005;43:142–8.
119. Kammuller ME. Recombinant human interleukin-6: safety issues of a pleiotropic growth factor. Toxicology 1995;105:91–107.
120. Ki SH, Park O, Zheng M, et al. Interleukin-22 treatment ameliorates alcoholic liver injury in a murine model of chronic-binge ethanol feeding: role of signal transducer and activator of transcription 3. Hepatology Oct;52:1291–300.
121. Seth D, Gorrell MD, Cordoba S, et al. Intrahepatic gene expression in human alcoholic hepatitis. J Hepatol 2006;45:306–20.
122. Dominguez M, Miquel R, Colmenero J, et al. Hepatic expression of CXC chemokines predicts portal hypertension and survival in patients with alcoholic hepatitis. Gastroenterology 2009;136:1639–50.
123. Colmenero J, Bataller R, Sancho-Bru P, et al. Hepatic expression of candidate genes in patients with alcoholic hepatitis: correlation with disease severity. Gastroenterology 2007;132:687–97.
124. Morales OD, Juez E, Moreno M, et al. Osteopontin is a novel therapeutic target in patients with alcoholic hepatitis. J Hepatol 2010;52(Suppl 1):S23.
125. Tirnitz-Parker JE, Viebahn CS, Jakubowski A, et al. Tumor necrosis factor-like weak inducer of apoptosis is a mitogen for liver progenitor cells. Hepatology 2010;52:291–302.
126. Whitfield K, Rambaldi A, Wetterslev J, et al. Pentoxifylline for alcoholic hepatitis. Cochrane Database Syst Rev 2009;4:CD007339.
127. Neuberger J, Tang H. Relapse after transplantation: European studies. Liver Transpl Surg 1997;3:275–9.
128. Neuberger J, Adams D, MacMaster P, et al. Assessing priorities for allocation of donor liver grafts: survey of public and clinicians. BMJ 1998;317:172–5.
129. Anantharaju AVT. Liver transplantation for alcoholic liver disease. Bethesda (MD): National Institute of Alcohol Abuse and Alcoholism; 2004.
130. Mackie J, Groves K, Hoyle A, et al. Orthotopic liver transplantation for alcoholic liver disease: a retrospective analysis of survival, recidivism, and risk factors predisposing to recidivism. Liver Transpl 2001;7:418–27.
131. McCallum S, Masterton G. Liver transplantation for alcoholic liver disease: a systematic review of psychosocial selection criteria. Alcohol Alcohol 2006;41:358–63.

132. Weinrieb RM, Van Horn DH, McLellan AT, et al. Interpreting the significance of drinking by alcohol-dependent liver transplant patients: fostering candor is the key to recovery. Liver Transpl 2000;6:769–76.

133. Pfitzmann R, Schwenzer J, Rayes N, et al. Long-term survival and predictors of relapse after orthotopic liver transplantation for alcoholic liver disease. Liver Transpl 2007;13:197–205.

134. Lucey MR, Brown KA, Everson GT, et al. Minimal criteria for placement of adults on the liver transplant waiting list: a report of a national conference organized by the American Society of Transplant Physicians and the American Association for the Study of Liver Diseases. Liver Transpl Surg 1997;3:628–37.

135. Mathurin P. Is alcoholic hepatitis an indication for transplantation? Current management and outcomes. Liver Transpl 2005(11 Suppl 2):S21–4.

136. Dureja P, Lucey MR. The place of liver transplantation in the treatment of severe alcoholic hepatitis. J Hepatol 2010;52:759–64.

137. DiMartini A, Day N, Dew MA, et al. Alcohol consumption patterns and predictors of use following liver transplantation for alcoholic liver disease. Liver Transpl 2006;12:813–20.

138. Tome S, Martinez-Rey C, Gonzalez-Quintela A, et al. Influence of superimposed alcoholic hepatitis on the outcome of liver transplantation for end-stage alcoholic liver disease. J Hepatol 2002;36:793–8.

139. Wells JT, Said A, Agni R, et al. The impact of acute alcoholic hepatitis in the explanted recipient liver on outcome after liver transplantation. Liver Transpl 2007;13:1728–35.

140. Shakil AO, Pinna A, Demetris J, et al. Survival and quality of life after liver transplantation for acute alcoholic hepatitis. Liver Transpl Surg 1997;3:240–4.

141. Immordino G, Gelli M, Ferrante R, et al. Alcohol abstinence and orthotopic liver transplantation in alcoholic liver cirrhosis. Transplant Proc 2009;41:1253–5.

142. Vanlemmens C, Di Martino V, Milan C, et al. Immediate listing for liver transplantation versus standard care for Child-Pugh stage B AC: a randomized trial. Ann Intern Med 2009;150:153–61.

Liver Transplantation in the 21st Century: Expanding the Donor Options

David A. Sass, MD, AGAF[a],*, David J. Reich, MD[b]

KEYWORDS

- Extended criteria donor • Donation after cardiac death
- Living-donor liver transplantation • Cold ischemia time
- Split-liver transplantation • Donor risk index

Liver transplantation has evolved since Dr. Thomas Starzl performed the first orthotopic liver transplant (OLT) over 4 decades ago. Advances in immunosuppressive therapy, medical management, surgical technique, and identification of appropriate indications for OLT have resulted in significant improvements in patients' survival and universal recognition of the procedure as preferred therapy for those suffering from hepatic failure. The number of patients awaiting primary or repeat OLT in the United States has tripled to 18,000 in the last 2 decades.[1,2] Over the same period, organ availability increased from 1700 to 6200 grafts annually[1]; however, the concurrent increase in organ availability has not significantly impacted the rate of wait-list mortality; deaths on the waiting list have increased 5-fold over the same period.[1] The discrepancy between supply and demand and the increasing organ scarcity has motivated select transplant centers to relax customary restrictions to donation, creating the term "extended-criteria" donors (ECD) or "marginal" donors. The precise definitions of these terms remain elusive. There is no consensus as to what makes a graft "marginal" in one center and acceptable in another. The use of these ECD grafts often depends on the judgement of the transplant surgeon and the needs of the recipient.[3–5]

DEFINITIONS

An ECD implies higher risk in comparison with a reference donor. Conceptually, this added risk may manifest as an increased incidence of early failure, namely, delayed

[a] Department of Medicine and Surgery, Division of Gastroenterology and Hepatology, Drexel University College of Medicine, 245 N 15th Street, 12th Floor New College Building, Suite 12324, Philadelphia, PA 19102, USA
[b] Division of Multiorgan Transplantation and Heptobiliary Surgery, Drexel University College of Medicine, 216 N Broad Street, 5th Floor Feinstein Building, Mail Stop 1001, Philadelphia, PA 19102, USA
* Corresponding author.
E-mail address: dsass@drexelmed.edu

Gastroenterol Clin N Am 40 (2011) 641–658
doi:10.1016/j.gtc.2011.06.007
0889-8553/11/$ – see front matter © 2011 Elsevier Inc. All rights reserved.

gastro.theclinics.com

Table 1 Donor factors defining ECD	
Risk of Impaired Graft Function	**Risk of Disease Transmission**
Donor age (>60 years)	Positive hepatitis B and C serologies
Donor obesity	Unexplained cause of death
Steatotic livers (>40% macro)	Known donor malignancy
Donation after cardiac death	"High-risk" lifestyle
Hypernatremia (serum Na > 155 mEq/L)	Active bacterial/viral infections
Hypotension and inotropic support	Elderly donors
Prolonged intensive care stay	
Long ischemia times (CIT > 12 hours)	
Partial liver grafts (split/live donor)	

allograft function or primary nonfunction (PNF), transmission of a donor-derived disease, or, in the case of adult-to-adult living-donor liver transplantation (LDLT), living-donor morbidity. To appreciate the components that define an ECD, it is important to recognize the criteria that define a reference (or ideal) donor: These include age below 40 years, death caused by trauma, donation after brain death (DBD), hemodynamic stability at the time of organ procurement, no steatosis or any other underlying chronic liver disease, and no transmissible disease (infectious or neoplastic).[6]

Durand and colleagues,[7] in a Report of the Paris Consensus Meeting on Expanded Criteria Donors in Liver Transplantation, draw a distinction between an "ideal allograft" and an "ideal donor." They mention that the ideal allograft category may be influenced by variables that are introduced after procurement, such as prolonged cold ischemia time (CIT) or technical variants, such as those occurring with allograft reduction (split-liver allograft). These variables should ideally not be included in the definition of ECD, because the aim is to assess risk at procurement.

ORGAN ALLOCATION AND DISTRIBUTION

Liver allograft allocation and distribution are dependent upon a calculated disease severity score, the Model for End-Stage Liver Disease (MELD) Score,[8] and geographic location of the recipient, with the United States being divided into 11 United Network for Organ Sharing (UNOS) regions. This has resulted in significant discrepancies in waiting list times for OLT and MELD score at the time of transplant. Thus, locations with short candidate wait times, or low MELD at the time of OLT, have the luxury of practicing selective organ donor use. ECD allografts may then be exported out of the vicinity of donor origin, after being declined by all transplant centers within geographic proximity to the donor, either to be prioritized for a higher MELD patient or as an "open offer" for use in an area of donor scarcity.[3] ECD distribution is distinctly different from distribution of optimal organs that remain locally and are allocated by MELD score. ECD recipients are often selected by the transplant center rather than being allocated according to regional wait-list priority.[3]

INDICATORS OF IMPAIRED ALLOGRAFT FUNCTION
Donor Age

Advanced age is a nontechnical and nonmodifiable donor variable that has a significant impact on early allograft function (**Table 1**).[7] Liver weight, liver volume, and blood flow are reduced with aging.[9,10] Older liver allografts have a lower tolerance for preservation. Endothelial injury from cold ischemia occurs earlier in older allografts, increasing the risk for inflammation, thrombosis, and T-cell–mediated rejection.[10] Donor age has steadily increased over recent decades. In 1994, only 20% of deceased donors were 50 years or older. This percentage has increased to 34% by the year 2010.[11] Although early studies suggested that older donors (>50 years) conferred no additional risk to poor outcome compared with younger donors,[12–15] this notion has been refuted by more recent publications using large United States [Scientific Registry for Transplant Recipients (SRTR)] and European (European Liver Transplant Registry) transplant databases.[6,16,17] Feng and colleagues,[6] in a study of donor age correlation with graft failure from UNOS Transplant Registry data of more than 20,000 OLTs, found an increased risk of graft failure, which was significantly higher among donors older than 60 (relative risk of 1.53) and 70 years (relative risk of 1.65) compared with donors younger than 40 years.[6] Donor risk related to age thus represents a continuum. There is, however, no absolute limit of donor age for liver transplantation. Some reports have shown excellent graft survival with octogenarian donors, provided that there are no additional risk factors, such as steatosis or prolonged CIT.[18,19] An important caveat to the utilization of elderly donors is in the setting of hepatitis C virus (HCV). There are convincing data demonstrating early HCV recurrence and decreased survival of patients among HCV recipients of donor allografts older than 60 years,[20–22] and so older donor livers should be used for HCV recipients selectively and with caution.

Donor Gender, Weight, Height, and Race

Some studies have identified donor gender (female gender) as a risk factor for worse post-OLT outcome,[17] whereas others have failed to confirm this.[6] African-American donor race consistently seems to have worse recipient outcome.[6,17] With regard to donor size, less height has been shown to be independently associated with graft failure.[6]

Donor Hypernatremia

Hypernatremia is a frequent clinical finding within the donor population that has a negative impact on function of hepatic allografts.[23] The cause of hypernatremia could be related to derangement of fluid balance and diabetes insipidus in potential donors. The impaired allograft function is postulated to occur owing to a process whereby hepatocytes increase their intracellular osmolality to minimize cellular damage associated with the extracellular hypertonic state.[24] Avolio and colleagues[25] were the first to report a direct correlation between donor serum sodium concentration and peak serum aminotransferase after OLT.[25] Several additional studies have validated this finding,[23,26,27] and in general a donor serum sodium exceeding 155 mEq/dL at procurement is thought to be the threshold for decreased actuarial graft survival. Hypernatremia should preferably be corrected before organ recovery.

Donor Hepatic Steatosis

Steatosis is among the most important factors affecting liver allograft function. With the obesity epidemic in developed countries, it is not uncommon to encounter significant degrees of hepatic steatosis when procuring donor livers. Early functional recovery and regenerative capacity are significantly impaired with steatotic allografts, mostly because of severe ischemia–reperfusion injury.[28] Steatosis has traditionally been classified as microvesicular (which has not correlated with poor allograft function) and macrovesicular. Although the liver is carefully inspected by the surgeon at the time of procurement, a biopsy is the gold standard to obtain an objective assessment on the degree of macrovesicular steatosis,[29] which is subcategorized as mild (<30%), moderate (30%–60%), or severe (>60%). Mild steatosis generally has minimal impact on post-OLT liver function, provided that the CIT is short.[30] When macrovesicular steatosis exceeds 60%, there is consensus that such allografts be discarded because of unacceptably high rates of PNF.[31] Utilizing grafts with moderate macrovesicular steatosis (30%–60%) is a challenging issue because, in this group, the incidence of PNF may reach 15% and the rate of delayed graft function approaches 35%.[31–33] As with other ECD grafts, recipient matching should be based on the number and extent of recipient risk factors and the absence of other negative donor variables, such as advanced donor age and prolonged CIT, to minimize the negative impact on graft and patient outcomes.[34]

CIT

The negative effect of CIT on organ function is intuitive; cold preservation increases anaerobic metabolism and cellular acidosis. Reperfusion after prolonged CIT in human and animal models is associated with inflammatory changes within the allograft, including sinusoidal cell damage, complement activation, small vessel hypercoagulability, and increased levels of interleukin-6 and -8.[35,36] Prolonged CIT is an independent risk factor for the development of both delayed graft function and PNF.[37] There is also an increased incidence of long-term biliary complications.[38] In allografts from otherwise healthy donors younger than 60, the threshold for reduced allograft function secondary to prolonged CIT lies between 14 and 16 hours.[39] Hepatic allografts from steatotic and older age donors (>60 years) are much more sensitive to preservation injury and demonstrate optimal function when CIT is under 8 hours.[12]

Miscellaneous Donor Factors

The role of several other risk factors such as obesity, elevated liver function tests, hypotension, vasopressor use, nutrition, and length of stay in the intensive care unit is less clear and were not found to confer increased risk of graft failure in the most recent study.[6] Certainly, donors at the extremes of these characteristics should be used cautiously.

Donation After Cardiac Death

The last few years has seen a considerable renewal of interest in donation after cardiac death (DCD) donors, formerly known as "non–heart-beating donors," to increase the pool of available organs. The percentage of deceased donors in the United States that are DCD has grown from 1% in 1996 to 10% in 2007,[40] and the number of liver transplants performed using DCD has surged from 0.5% in 1999 to 4.5% in 2008 (**Table 2**),[41] making it the most rapidly expanding component of the donor pool.

DCD has a fundamentally different recovery technique based on cardiopulmonary criteria rather than neurologic criteria for death. Organ retrieval from DCD can be "controlled" or "uncontrolled" based on the Maastricht classification.[42] Controlled DCD undergo circulatory arrest after planned withdrawal of life support with the donor team ready in the operating room to start the procurement process. Uncontrolled DCD are donors who had an unplanned cardiac arrest with failed cardiopulmonary resuscitation, or are dead on arrival to the hospital. Organs from controlled DCD have a better chance of recovery compared with uncontrolled DCD.[43]

The earliest reports of controlled DCD organ transplantation were published 16 years ago by the teams at the University of Pittsburgh[44] and in Madison, Wisconsin.[45]

Table 2
Liver transplants from DCD donors by year of transplantation

Year of Transplant	Total Donors (n)	DCD (n)	DCD, % Donors of Total
1999	4498	23	0.5
2000	4595	39	0.8
2001	4672	69	1.5
2002	4969	79	1.6
2003	5351	111	2.1
2004	5848	185	3.2
2005	6121	271	4.4
2006	6363	289	4.5
2007	6228	307	4.9
2008	6069	276	4.5

Data from Thuluvath PJ, Guidinger MK, Fung JJ, et al. Liver transplantation in the United States, 1999–2008. Am J Transpl 2010;10:1003–19.

In 2000, Reich and colleagues[43] provided the first single-center experience with DCD OLT showing outcomes comparable to those with DBD. In the decade that followed, several other transplant programs have published single-center experiences with controlled DCD showing comparable 1-year patient survivals with DBD OLT (range, 74%–92%).[46–52] DCD 1-year liver graft survival, however, still has a tendency to be lower than with DBD livers (range, 61%–87%).[46–52] Abt and colleagues[50] were the first to report on the high incidence of biliary stricturing and/or bile cast syndrome occurring as a result of the biliary epithelium being extremely vulnerable to ischemia-reperfusion injury. This "ischemic cholangiopathy," the Achilles heel of DCD OLT, has been reported in 9% to 50% of DCD recipients[47–51,53–55] and usually requires frequent biliary manipulations to allow bile drainage, often resulting in allograft loss, retransplantation, or death. Despite many centers showing much poorer outcomes in their DCD versus DBD transplants, a few transplant programs, such as the Mayo, Jacksonville,[46] and Albert Einstein, Philadelphia,[55] groups have reported patient and graft survivals where the DCD cohorts were similar to their DBD counterparts. The Einstein patient and graft survival rates were 90% at 1 year and 85% at 2 years post-OLT. Ischemic cholangiopathy developed in 13% of recipients, causing graft failure in 10%.[55] In the past few years, a number of multicenter pooled registry analyses have emerged highlighting specific criteria for safer use of DCD livers.[56–59] Using younger DCD livers with shorter warm ischemia times and then CITs facilitate the best outcomes.

To date, there has been a lack of standardization with regard to many aspects of DCD, such as precise definitions of terminology, technique, use of vasodilatory drugs, antioxidants, preservation solutions, and the use of anticoagulation.[3] In an effort to standardize procurement protocols and refine reporting of data, updated practice guidelines for organ procurement have been published by UNOS, the Institute of Medicine and the Society of Critical Care Medicine,[60] and in 2009 the American Society of Transplant Surgeons issued recommendations on controlled DCD based on evidence and expert opinion.[61] These American Society of Transplant Surgeons guidelines expound on all aspects of controlled DCD organ procurement including such issues as donor criteria, consent, withdrawal of support, operative technique, biliary concerns, ischemia times, and recipient considerations.[61]

With ischemic cholangiopathy being the Achilles heel of DCD OLT, various authors have proposed recommendations on maneuvers to prevent biliary problems. These include performing an expeditious in situ biliary flush,[55,61] considering arterial revascularization before or simultaneously with portal revascularization,[50,61] use of a T-tube for easy access to the ducts postoperatively for stricture dilation and sludge removal to prevent bile casts,[55,61] and using the bile acid ursodeoxycholic acid posttransplantation. Other suggestions to counter the specter of postoperative ischemic cholangiopathy have included using thrombolytic agents and anticoagulants and replacing the more viscous University of Wisconsin solution with histidine tryptophan ketoglutarate preservation solution.[62] Several transplant groups, including the group at the University of Michigan, use postmortem extracorporeal membrane oxygenation to facilitate restoration of the flow of warm oxygenated blood to the intra-abdominal organs during the interval between death and organ procurement.[63]

Exciting new research endeavors in organ preservation are in development, such as using ex vivo machine perfusion of the liver.[64–67] A technique by Hong and colleagues proposed the novel concept of regulated hepatic reperfusion to modulate ischemia and reperfusion injury during organ revascularization.[68] These and other innovative strategies potentially applicable to DCD are in early development and not yet ready for transfer from bench to bedside.[60]

PREDICTING OUTCOMES: TRANSLATING ECD FACTORS INTO CLINICAL PRACTICE

Investigators have recognized that a combination of multiple factors in ECD donors can substantially increase the risk of graft failure. Thus, as a means to quantify the effect of multiple factors on graft function, several centers have reported a "risk score."[6,69,70] Cameron and colleagues[70] from the University of California, Los Angeles, analyzed 1153 graft–recipient pairs to calculate a donor risk score. Using both univariate and multivariate analyses, significant factors predictive of graft and recipient survival were identified as extended criteria. This study also demonstrated that for each donor risk score, both older and urgent recipients had worse outcomes. In a large, retrospective review of the UNOS SRTR database from more than 20,000 donors, using Cox regression modeling, Feng and colleagues[6] identified 5 donor characteristics that independently predicted a significantly increased risk of graft failure (**Table 3**): Age, race, donor height, donor death (causes of death other than trauma, stroke or anoxia and DCD), and type of graft (partial/split graft). In addition, 2 transplant-related factors (CIT and sharing outside of the local donor service area) were also significantly associated with graft loss (see **Table 3**). All of these factors were used to generate a "donor risk index" (DRI), which is directly related to a predicted rate of graft survival. They found that when the DRI increased from the baseline risk index group (0.0–1.0) to the highest risk index group listed (>2.0), the frequency with which the graft would be discarded was significantly higher, rising from 3.1% to 12.5%.[6] In a similar study from the United Kingdom, Dawwas and colleagues[71] also identified 7 slightly different risk factors for graft loss (see **Table 3**). In the UK setting, the UK donor risk score outperformed the US donor risk score.[24,71] However, both scores need to be externally validated in other populations before firm recommendations about their use can be made.

Transplantation of an ECD organ into a recipient who has a high MELD score may contribute to worsened graft and patient outcomes as compared with transplanting a lower DRI organ. However, high DRI organs still confer a survival benefit to high MELD patients as compared with waiting for lower risk organs. Markov models suggest that

Table 3
Donor and transplant risk factors associated with allograft failure

Risk Factors	5 Donor and 2 Transplant Risk Factors Identified in the United States[6]		6 Donor and 1 Transplant Risk Factor Identified in the UK[71]	
	Risk Factor Reference Value	Increased Risk of Graft Failure, Relative Risk	Risk Factor Reference Value	Increased Risk of Graft Failure, Relative Risk
Donor				
Age	<40	61–70: 1.53 >70: 1.65	Age	Increase by 1.05 per decade
Race	White	African American: 1.19	White	Non-white: 2.17
Size	Height	Increase by 1.07 per 10-cm decrease in height	NR	
Cause of donor death	Cause: trauma	Cardiovascular accident: 1.16 Other: 1.20 DCD: 1.51	NR	
Type of graft	Full graft	Partial/split: 1.52	Full graft	Reduced/split: 1.93
BMI	NS		BMI	Increase by 1.01 per unit increase in BMI
Graft appearance	No data		Normal	Suboptimal: 1.31
Diabetes	NS		No diabetes	Diabetes: 1.41
Transplant				
CIT	CIT	Increase of 1.01 per hour	CIT	Increase of 1.02 per hour
Sharing outside local area	Local area	Same region: 1.11 National: 1.28	NR	

Abbreviations: BMI, body mass index; NR, not reported; NS, not significant.
From Mullhaupt B, Dimitroulis D, Gerlach JT, et al. Hot topics in liver transplantation: organ allocation-extended criteria donor-living donor transplantation. J Hepatol 2008;48:S58–67; with permission.

for patients with a MELD score of greater than 20, immediate transplantation even with grafts that carry a risk as high as 50% for primary graft failure is still associated with a survival benefit.[72] Further reports based on real data and not on modeling approaches are eagerly awaited.[73]

DONOR-TRANSMITTED DISEASE

Donors can transmit both infections and malignancies to OLT recipients during the transplant surgery (see **Table 1**). These also constitute examples of ECD.

HCV-Positive Liver Grafts

About 5% of all potential donors in the United States are positive for antibody to HCV and about half of these donors are HCV RNA positive by polymerase chain reaction.[74]

Utilizing HCV+ allografts for HCV− recipients or HCV+ recipients with an undetectable viral load is usually reserved for extreme circumstances. In contrast, utilization of HCV+ allografts among HCV+ recipients with active viral replication of genotype 1 or 4 is encouraged nowadays in the era of donor scarcity.[3] In fact, current data clearly indicate no difference in HCV recurrence, or graft or patient survival when using HCV+ allografts.[75–78] Provided the donor liver is not fibrotic, survival after transplant can be unimpaired.[79] Recently Peek and Reddy[80] reported preliminary data suggesting that HCV+ grafts may confer an advantage in the HCV+ recipient in terms of recurrence-free graft survival after OLT.[80] Further long-term and multivariate analyses are needed to confirm these findings.

Hepatitis B Core Antibody-Positive Grafts

Donors with past exposure to hepatitis B infection can be used selectively in some recipients. Hepatitis B core antibody-positive (HbcAb+) donors carry a high risk of de novo HBV infection for the HBV naive recipients. However, for patients who are immune to HBV (previous disease or vaccination), it has been found to be safe to use these organs.[81] In the era before prophylaxis, HBV transmission from an HbcAb+ donor to an HbcAb− recipient occurred at rates of 33%–78%, with subsequent accelerated graft loss.[82] The use nucleos(t)ide analog therapy with or without hepatitis B immunoglobulin is now standard of care in the prevention of viral transmission from such HbcAb+ donors.

Transmission of Bacterial and Viral Infections

Bacterial infections in the donor do not represent by themselves a risk factor for liver graft failure. The risk of transmitting a bacterial infection in the case of bacteremia in the donor is low. Early fever and positive cultures in the recipient as well as the presence of yeast justify empiric therapy.[83–85] Donors with documented bacterial meningitis do not preclude transplantation.[86]

There have been scattered reports over the years of transmission of several types of viruses with transplantation, including HIV, West Nile virus (WNV), rabies, and HCV. As a result, UNOS and the Organ Procurement and Transplantation Network established the Disease Transmission Advisory Group in 2005 to monitor such transmissions, provide guidance in these cases, and analyze trends.[87] This was later formalized as the ad hoc Disease Transmission Advisory Committee.[87] There is a policy in the United States mandating the routine screening of potential donors for specific pathogens, including HIV, HBV, HCV, syphilis, cytomegalovirus, tuberculosis, and Epstein–Barr virus.[88]

With regard to WNV infection, current recommendations include excluding potential donors with meningoencephalitic symptoms of undetermined etiology who live in regions of WNV activity, screening with nucleic acid testing (NAT) as close to the time of procurement as possible, and being suspicious when transplant recipients have postoperative fever and/or neurologic symptoms not otherwise explained. Serologic testing of the donor and all recipients from that donor should be performed (as well as lumbar puncture as indicated). At this time there is no specific treatment for WNV.[87]

HIV+ Patients and "High-Risk" Donors

HIV can be readily transmitted through solid organ transplant, but because of improvements in screening protocols there were no reported cases of HIV transmission from 1994 to 2007.[89] In 2007, however, 4 transplant recipients contracted HIV

Box 1
US Centers for Disease Control and Prevention "high-risk" donor classification

1. Men who have had sex with another man in the preceding 5 years.

2. Persons who report nonmedical intravenous, intramuscular, or subcutaneous injection of drugs in the preceding 5 years.

3. Persons with hemophilia or related clotting disorders who have received human-derived clotting factor concentrates.

4. Men and women who have engaged in sex in exchange for drugs or money in the preceding 5 years.

5. Persons who have had sex in the preceding 12 months with any person described in items above or with a person known or suspected to have HIV.

6. Persons who have been exposed in the preceding 12 months to known or suspected HIV-infected blood through percutaneous inoculation or through contact with an open wound, nonintact skin, or mucous membrane.

7. Inmates of correctional systems.

From Rogers MF, Simmonds RJ, Lawton KE, et al. National Center for Infectious Diseases. Guidelines for preventing transmission of HIV through transplantation of human tissues and organs. MMWR 1994;43:1–17.

---

and HCV from a single donor who tested negative by serology.[90] To date, there are no studies examining the transplantation of HIV+ organs into HIV+ recipients. Any potential donor regarded as "high risk" by the US Centers for Disease Control and Prevention standards should undergo NAT.[87] The US Centers for Disease Control and Prevention has provided guidelines for the classification of donors as "high risk," a metric indicating that an organ carries an increased risk of harboring an infectious disease.[91] These donors may fall into any of 7 categories (**Box 1**). Although NAT testing is the superior method of infection detection, it is expensive, time consuming, and difficult to perform relative to antibody testing.[89] There is also a wide variation of NAT practices by organ procurement organizations. In general, NAT for HIV can detect infections 12 to 13 days before ELISA antibody assays.[89] Care should be undertaken when transplanting a "high-risk" donor organ and full disclosure to recipient candidates is imperative.[87] Highly active antiretroviral therapy should be initiated if transmission has occurred.

Transmission of Malignancy

It can be reasonably assumed that the risk of malignancy increases with donor age; thus, transplanting organs from elderly donors may increase the risk of transmitting defined and undefined malignancies.[7] The incidence of cancer in donors is approximately 3%, and the risk of transmitting malignancy by organ transplantation is roughly 0.01%.[92–94] A review on this subject using UNOS data showed a total of 21 donor-related malignancies among 108,062 transplant recipients over 8 years, giving an incidence of tumor transmission to be 0.02%.[95] In general, nonmelanoma skin cancer, low-grade neurologic tumors, and in situ carcinoma seem to be a safe source of solid organs for transplantation,[95] whereas a history of melanoma, choriocarcinoma, lymphoma, or carcinoma of the breast, lung, and colon seem to possess a high rate of cancer transmission, even after long apparent cancer-free survival.[95] Any metastatic malignancy in the donor should exclude donation. Recipients of donors with malignancies should have their immunosuppression modulated because overimmunosuppression reduces immune surveillance that can accelerate tumor growth. The potential benefit from the mammalian target or rapamycin inhibitors, which have both immunosuppressive and antiangiogenic properties, requires further investigation.[96]

USE OF PARTIAL ALLOGRAFTS
Split-Liver Transplantation

Among the numerous efforts to expand the donor pool, OLT with partial allografts has become a viable option for some selected patients with cirrhosis.[97] Split-liver transplantation (SLT) is a technique in which 2 allografts are created from a single cadaver liver. Historically, the principal beneficiaries of SLT have been adult–pediatric recipient pairs; however, with the current scarcity of cadaver organs, there has been renewed interest in expanding these techniques to include 2 adult recipients.[3] The technique was initially reported by Smith in the late 1960s,[98] but successful SLT was not fully realized for nearly 2 decades.[99,100]

The overall success of SLT relies heavily on the severity of the underlying illness in both the donor and recipient. Several groups have developed general selection criteria for both donor and recipient.[101–103] In one of the largest single-center experiences in SLT from University of California, Los Angeles, donors were young, had normal liver function, and short hospitalizations.[104] Even if an optimal donor is selected, SLT is hampered by logistical constraints requiring short CIT and recipient limitations.[7] In general, right allografts have yielded better results than left allografts.[103,105] A recent match pair analysis of patients after whole versus SLT using an extended right liver lobe donor found no difference in either short- or long-term morbidity or mortality.[106] Left grafts remain a technically challenging procedure with a high risk of PNF owing to insufficient parenchymal volume and complex biliary and vascular anastomoses.[107]

Although data emerging from certain high-volume centers in both the United States[108] and Europe[109] revealed equivalent 3-year patient and graft survivals in the SLT group versus whole-graft recipients, multivariate comparison again underscores the importance of both donor and recipient selection as, for example, 3-year survival in healthy, nonurgent recipients approached 90% but fell significantly, to 65%, among urgent split-graft recipients.[108] This notion is supported by Feng's analysis of the large SRTR database where SLT or partial grafts were associated with 52% higher risk of graft failure.[6]

Recently, the American Society of Transplant Surgeons surveyed 83 transplant programs in the United States and Canada to gather preliminary data on applications and outcomes of SLT.[110] With a 93% response rate and data on nearly 400 split grafts, the authors made several interesting observations. In 54% of the donors, the split procedure was performed ex vivo and biliary complications were more frequent among in situ split grafts (17% vs 5%). Among recipients of right trisegment grafts, overall mortality was 15%, with more than 50% of deaths attributable to graft-related complications. The overall incidence of PNF was 4%.[110] Because of the obvious technical difficulties and logistical obstacles, only a small number of high-volume centers in North America routinely undertake SLT. As the in situ technique continues to evolve, this may allow increased organ sharing between centers because the CIT is dramatically reduced and vital anatomic structures may be identified at the time of procurement.[111]

LDLT

Adult-to-adult LDLT is yet another alternative method to overcome the shortage of donor organs and decrease death among patients waiting for OLT. This technique has been widely adopted in Asian countries where brain death is not accepted, although to a lesser extent in Europe and the United States. LDLT developed rapidly in the United States in the latter part of the 1990s. The yearly number peaked in 2001 at 409, encompassing 10% of all adult OLTs that year.[111] LDLT is a unique source of liver graft because it subjects an otherwise healthy individual to a major operative procedure without obvious direct therapeutic benefit. The enthusiasm for this technique has since been tempered owing to the publicized deaths of 4 healthy adult living liver donors at 4 different US centers over the past decade.[112] Since 2001, there has been a steady decline in the number of LDLT being performed annually in the United States, to about 4% of the total volume.

The advantages of LDLT include a significantly reduced waiting time, medical optimization of the recipient before anticipated surgery, and the use of a graft from a healthy donor with minimal ischemia time.[113,114] Disadvantages include receipt of a smaller graft with a high rate of surgical complications in both the donor and recipient. Careful selection of the donor and recipient is crucial to minimize risks and complications and to obtain acceptable outcomes. In US reports, LDLT achieves similar results only after experience has accumulated in centers to overcome a learning curve.[115,116] Liver allografts originating from living donors should be considered extended criteria allografts even though, by definition, living donors are ideal donors, because these partial grafts are associated with more technical complications and an increased risk of graft failure.[114-118]

The Adult-to-Adult Living Donor Liver Transplantation Cohort Study (A2ALL) is a consortium of US liver transplant centers with the primary goal of comparing outcomes of adult-to-adult LDLT with DDLT. In its first detailed report of 385 cases, 90-day and 1-year graft survivals were 87% and 81%, respectively.[117] The outcomes were characterized by frequent biliary complications (30% early, 11% late) and 13% graft failure because of vascular complications, PNF, and sepsis.[117] Foster and colleagues compared the outcomes after adult-to-adult LDLT to those after DDLT using nationwide databases.[111] The 1- and 3-year patient survival rates after LDLT were similar to those after DDLT (89.1% and 80.3% vs 85.7% and 77.7%, respectively). Graft survival rates at 1 and 3 years were also similar (79.3% and 70.1% vs 80.7% and 71.1%, respectively). It should be noted, however, that the severity of illness was substantially lower among the LDLT recipients, whose mean MELD scores are 15.6 versus MELD scores of 22 for the DDLT recipients.[117] Outcomes for LDLT recipients infected with HCV have been a point of some controversy; some centers found no patient and graft survival differences, whereas other centers have reported opposite results. The A2ALL study provides data from the largest studied group of HCV-infected patients undergoing LDLT.[119] In this study, the rate of graft survival was lower in LDLT recipients (65%) than in DLDT (82%; $P = .02$). The effect of the learning curve and surgical experience on LDLT outcomes was particularly important, however.[111] After 20 LDLTs were performed at a center, the graft survival rates for LDLTs and DDLTs were similar (78% vs 82%). Initial enthusiasm for LDLT as being a viable option for patients with hepatocellular carcinoma has been dampened by the A2ALL report showing a higher rate of hepatocellular carcinoma recurrence (29% vs 0%; $P = .002$) within 3 years, than with DDLT (n = 34).[120]

The goal of donor selection and evaluation is to ensure that the potential donor can undergo the hepatectomy without any undue risk and can yield a suitable graft for the recipient.[121] Prospective donor candidates are usually between 18 and 55 years of age, have an identical or compatible blood type to the recipient, and do not have any significant medical comorbidities that could increase the risk associated with surgery. Extensive evaluations are performed including a thorough history, physical examination, psychosocial assessment, laboratory testing, and cross-sectional hepatic imaging to evaluate the liver for parenchymal abnormalities, steatosis, biliary and vascular anatomy, and volumetric assessment of the graft and residual liver. Data from the A2ALL cohort have shed light on the donor evaluation process where an overall acceptance rate of 40% was achieved among more than 1000 potential donor candidates.[122] Because of the altruistic nature of LDLT and to ensure donor safety, it is of vital importance to be able to track donor outcomes, including morbidity, mortality, and effect on quality of life. Unfortunately, there has been no standardized format for reporting these donor complications. Recent data from the retrospective A2ALL study cohort showed that 62% had no complications from the surgery, with only 2% of donors suffering a life-threatening problem or a problem with residual physical effects.[123] Donor death is the most serious potential complication and is estimated to occur in 0.2% of cases.

Although LDLT has decreased in the past several years, it continues to be a valuable source for donor organs, especially for pediatric OLT. However, for LDLT to remain a viable option for OLT, the potential benefits must outweigh the risks for both donor and recipient, and donor safety must be of paramount concern.[124]

CONSENT FOR ECD, DCD, OR "HIGH-RISK" DONOR TRANSPLANTATION

Acceptance of an ECD organ should be consensual for all prospective OLT recipients. After determination of OLT candidacy and successful completion of the OLT evaluation, patients are invited to participate in a process of informed consent that specifically addresses their concerns with respect to the particular donor as well as the transplant procedure. In this meeting, separate consents are signed for the utilization of ECD, DCD, and other "high-risk" donor organs. Details are also provided regarding the option of LDLT. This encounter allows for open dialogue between transplant candidate and surgeon about historical outcome data regarding this ever-increasing organ category. The consent process is repeated again at the time of organ allocation.

SUMMARY

Over the past decade, use of ECD organs for OLT has allowed many transplant programs to afford patients access to an otherwise scarce resource and to maintain center volume. Although overall posttransplant outcomes are inferior to results with optimal, whole-liver grafts, aggressive utilization of ECD and DCD organs significantly lowers median wait-times for OLT, MELD score at OLT, and death while awaiting transplantation. It is incumbent on the transplant community to provide continued scrutiny of the many factors involved in ECD organ utilization, evaluate the degree of risk and benefit such allografts may impart on particular recipients, and thereby provide suitable "matching" to maximize favorable outcomes. Transplant caregivers need to provide patients with evidence-based care decisions, be good stewards of a scarce resource, and maintain threshold survival results for their programs. This requires balancing the urgency with which a transplant is needed and the utility of such a transplant. There is a clear necessity to pursue additional donor research to improve use of these marginal grafts and assess interventions that enhance the safety of ECD livers.

REFERENCES

1. Organ Procurement and Transplantation Network and Scientific Registry of Transplant Recipients. Annual Reports. Available at: www.optn.org. Accessed April 2008.
2. Harper AM, Baker AS. The UNOS OPTN waiting list: 1988–1995. Clin Transpl 1995:69–84.
3. Alkofer B, Samstein B, Guarrera JV, et al. Extended-donor criteria liver allografts. Semin Liver Dis 2006;26:221–33.
4. Renz JF, Kin C, Kinkhabwala M, et al. Utilization of extended donor criteria liver allografts maximizes donor use and patient access to liver transplantation. Ann Surg 2005;242:556–63.
5. Attia M, Silva MA, Mirza DF. The marginal liver donor—an update. Transpl Int 2008;21:713–24.
6. Feng S, Goodrich NP, Bragg-Gresham JL, et al. Characteristics associated with liver graft failure: the concept of a donor risk index. Am J Transplant 2006;6:783–90.
7. Durand F, Renz JF, Alkofer B, et al. Report of the Paris consensus meeting on expanded criteria donors in liver transplantation. Liver Transpl 2008;14:1694–707.
8. Wiesner R, Edwards E, Freeman R, et al. Model for end-stage liver disease (MELD) and allocation of donor livers. Gastroenterology 2003;124:91–6.
9. Wynne HA, Cope LH, Mutch E, et al. The effect of age upon liver volume and apparent liver blood flow in healthy man. Hepatology 1989;9:297–301.
10. Tsukamoto I, Nakata R, Kojo S. Effect of ageing on rat liver regeneration after partial hepatectomy. Biochem Mol Biol Int 1993;30:773–8.
11. Organ Procurement and Transplantation Network and Scientific Registry of Transplant Recipients. Available at: http://optn.transplant.hrsa.gov. Accessed May 2011.
12. Yersiz H, Shaked A, Olthoff K, et al. Correlation between donor age and the pattern of liver graft recovery after transplantation. Transplantation 1995;60:790–4.
13. Emre S, Schwartz ME, Altaca G, et al. Safe use of hepatic allografts from donors older than 70 years. Transplantation 1996;62:62–5.
14. Ikegami T, Nishizaki T, Yanaga K, et al. The impact of donor age on living donor liver transplantation. Transplantation 2000;70:1703–7.
15. Grande L, Rull A, Rimola A, et al. Outcome of patients undergoing orthotopic liver transplantation with elderly donors (over 60 years). Transplant Proc 1997;29:3289–90.
16. Burroughs AK, Sabin CA, Rolles K, et al. 3-month and 12-month mortality after first liver transplant in adults in Europe: predictive models for outcome. Lancet 2006;367:225–32.
17. Ioannou GN. Development and validation of a model predicting graft survival after liver transplantation. Liver Transpl 2006;12:1594–606.
18. Jimenez Romero C, Moreno Gonzalez E, Colina Ruiz F, et al. Use of octogenarian livers safely expands the donor pool. Transplantation 1999;68:572–5.
19. Nardo B, Masetti M, Urbani L, et al. Liver transplantation from donors aged 80 years and over: pushing the limit. Am J Transplant 2004;4:1139–47.
20. Berenguer M, Prieto M, San Juan F, et al. Contribution of donor age to the recent decrease in patient survival among HCV-infected liver transplant recipients. Hepatology 2002;36:202–10.
21. Mutimer DJ, Gunson B, Chen J, et al. Impact of donor age and year of transplantation on graft and patient survival following liver transplantation for hepatitis C virus. Transplantation 2006;81:7–14.
22. Wali M, Harrison RF, Gow PJ, et al. Advancing donor liver age and rapid fibrosis progression following transplantation for hepatitis C. Gut 2002;51:248–52.

23. Gonzalez FX, Rimola A, Grande L, et al. Predictive factors of early postoperative graft function in human liver transplantation. Hepatology 1994;20:565–73.
24. Busuttil RW, Tanaka K. The utility of marginal donors in liver transplantation. Liver Transpl 2003;9:651–63.
25. Avolio AW, Agnes S, Magalini SC, et al. Importance of donor blood chemistry data (AST, serum sodium) in predicting liver transplant outcome. Transplant Proc 1991; 23:2451–2.
26. Figueras J, Busquets J, Grande L, et al. The deleterious effect of donor high plasma sodium and extended preservation in liver transplantation. A multivariate analysis. Transplantation 1996;61:410–3.
27. Markmann JF, Markmann JW, Markmann DA, et al. Preoperative factors associated with outcome and their impact on resource use in 1148 consecutive primary liver transplants. Transplantation 2001;72:1113–22.
28. Verran D, Kusyk T, Painter D, et al. Clinical experience gained from the use of 120 steatotic donor livers for orthotopic liver transplantation. Liver Transpl 2003;9:500–5.
29. Frankel WL, Tranovich JG, Salter L, et al. The optimal number of donor biopsy sites to evaluate liver histology for transplantation. Liver Transpl 2002;8:1044–50.
30. Selzner M, Clavien PA. Fatty liver in liver transplantation and surgery. Semin Liver Dis 2001;21:105–13.
31. Ploeg RJ, D'Alessandro AM, Knechtle SJ, et al. Risk factors for primary dysfunction after liver transplantation—a multivariate analysis. Transplantation 1993;55:807–13.
32. D'Alessandro AM, Kalayoglu M, Sollinger HW, et al. The predictive value of donor liver biopsies on the development of primary nonfunction after orthotopic liver transplantation. Transplant Proc 1991;23:1536–7.
33. Canelo R, Braun F, Sattler B, et al. Is a fatty liver dangerous for transplantation? Transplant Proc 1999;31:414–5.
34. Gordon Burroughs S, Busuttil RW. Optimal utilization of extended hepatic grafts. Surg Today 2009;39:746–51.
35. Schmidt A, Tomasdottir H, Bengtsson A. Influence of cold ischemia time on complement activation, neopterin, and cytokine release in liver transplantation. Transplant Proc 2004;36:2796–8.
36. Shen XD, Gao F, Ke B, et al. Inflammatory responses in a new mouse model of prolonged hepatic cold ischemia followed by arterialized orthotopic liver transplantation. Liver Transpl 2005;11:1273–81.
37. Piratvisuth T, Tredger JM, Hayllar KA, et al. Contribution of true cold and rewarming ischemia times to factors determining outcome after orthotopic liver transplantation. Liver Transpl Surg 1995;1:296–301.
38. Scotte M, Dousset B, Calmus Y, et al. The influence of cold ischemia time on biliary complications following liver transplantation. J Hepatol 1994;21:340–6.
39. Porte RJ, Ploeg RJ, Hansen B, et al. Long-term graft survival after liver transplantation in the UW era: late effects of cold ischemia and primary dysfunction. European Multicentre Study Group. Transpl Int 1998;11(Suppl 1):S164–7.
40. Tuttle-Newhall JE, Krishnan SM, Levy MF, et al. Organ donation and utilization in the United States: 1998–2007. Am J Transplant 2009;9:879–93.
41. Thuluvath PJ, Guidinger MK, Fung JJ, et al. Liver transplantation in the United States, 1999–2008. Am J Transplant 2010;10:1003–19.
42. Reich DJ, Manzarbeitia CY. Nonheart-beating donor liver transplantation. In: Busuttil RW, Klintmalm GB, editors. Transplantation of the liver. Philadelphia: WB Saunders; 2005. p. 529–43.

43. Reich DJ, Munoz SJ, Rothstein KD, et al. Controlled non-heart-beating donor liver transplantation: a successful single center experience, with topic update. Transplantation 2000;70:1159–66.
44. Casavilla A, Ramirez C, Shapiro R, et al. Experience with liver and kidney allografts from non-heart-beating donors. Transplant Proc 1995;27:2898.
45. D'Alessandro AM, Hoffmann RM, Knechtle SJ, et al. Successful extrarenal transplantation from non-heart-beating donors. Transplantation 1995;59:977–82.
46. Grewal HP, Willingham DL, Nguyen J, et al. Liver transplantation using controlled donation after cardiac death donors: an analysis of a large single-center experience. Liver Transpl 2009;15:1028–35.
47. de Vera ME, Lopez-Solis R, Dvorchik I, et al. Liver transplantation using donation after cardiac death donors: long-term follow-up from a single center. Am J Transplant 2009;9:773–81.
48. Fujita S, Mizuno S, Fujikawa T, et al. Liver transplantation from donation after cardiac death: a single center experience. Transplantation 2007;84:46–9.
49. Foley DP, Fernandez LA, Leverson G, et al. Donation after cardiac death: the University of Wisconsin experience with liver transplantation. Ann Surg 2005;242: 724–31.
50. Abt P, Crawford M, Desai N, et al. Liver transplantation from controlled non-heart-beating donors: an increased incidence of biliary complications. Transplantation 2003;75:1659–63.
51. Muiesan P, Girlanda R, Jassem W, et al. Single-center experience with liver transplantation from controlled non-heartbeating donors: a viable source of grafts. Ann Surg 2005;242:732–8.
52. Fukumori T, Kato T, Levi D, et al. Use of older controlled non-heart-beating donors for liver transplantation. Transplantation 2003;75:1171–4.
53. Skaro AI, Jay CL, Baker TB, et al. The impact of ischemic cholangiopathy in liver transplantation using donors after cardiac death: the untold story. Surgery 2009; 146:543–52.
54. Maheshwari A, Maley W, Li Z, et al. Biliary complications and outcomes of liver transplantation from donors after cardiac death. Liver Transpl 2007;13:1645–53.
55. Reich DJ. Nonheartbeating donor organ procurement. In: Humar A, Payne WD, Matas AJ, editors. Atlas of organ transplantation. London: Springer; 2006. p. 23–33.
56. Selck FW, Grossman EB, Ratner LE, et al. Utilization, outcomes, and retransplantation of liver allografts from donation after cardiac death: implications for further expansion of the deceased-donor pool. Ann Surg 2008;248:599–607.
57. Merion RM, Pelletier SJ, Goodrich N, et al. Donation after cardiac death as a strategy to increase deceased donor liver availability. Ann Surg 2006;244:555–62.
58. Lee KW, Simpkins CE, Montgomery RA, et al. Factors affecting graft survival after liver transplantation from donation after cardiac death donors. Transplantation 2006;82:1683–8.
59. Mateo R, Cho Y, Singh G, et al. Risk factors for graft survival after liver transplantation from donation after cardiac death donors: an analysis of OPTN/UNOS data. Am J Transplant 2006;6:791–6.
60. Reich DJ, Hong JC. Current status of donation after cardiac death liver transplantation. Curr Opin Organ Transplant 2010;15:316–21.
61. Reich DJ, Mulligan DC, Abt PL, et al. ASTS recommended practice guidelines for controlled donation after cardiac death organ procurement and transplantation. Am J Transplant 2009;9:2004–11.
62. Fung JJ, Eghtesad B, Patel-Tom K. Using livers from donation after cardiac death donors—a proposal to protect the true Achilles heel. Liver Transpl 2007;13:1633–6.

63. Magliocca JF, Magee JC, Rowe SA, et al. Extracorporeal support for organ donation after cardiac death effectively expands the donor pool. J Trauma 2005;58:1095–101.

64. Guarrera JV, Henry SD, Samstein B, et al. Hypothermic machine preservation in human liver transplantation: the first clinical series. Am J Transplant 2010;10: 372–81.

65. Schreinemachers M, Doorschodt BM, van Gulik TM, et al. Machine perfusion preservation of the liver: a worthwhile clinical activity? Curr Opin Organ Transplant 2007;12:224–30.

66. de Rougemont O, Breitenstein S, Leskosek B, et al. One hour hypothermic oxygenated perfusion (HOPE) protects nonviable liver allografts donated after cardiac death. Ann Surg 2009;250:674–83.

67. Imber CJ, St Peter SD, Lopez de Cenarruzabeitia I, et al. Advantages of normothermic perfusion over cold storage in liver preservation. Transplantation 2002;73: 701–9.

68. Hong JC, Koroleff D, Xia V, et al. Regulated hepatic reperfusion attenuates postreperfusion syndrome and improves survival after prolonged warm ischemia in a swine model (abstract). Am J Transplant 2009;9:S204.

69. Briceno J, Marchal T, Padillo J, et al. Influence of marginal donors on liver preservation injury. Transplantation 2002;74:522–6.

70. Cameron AM, Ghobrial RM, Yersiz H, et al. Optimal utilization of donor grafts with extended criteria: a single-center experience in over 1000 liver transplants. Ann Surg 2006;243:748–53.

71. Dawwas MF, David C, Barber KM, et al . Developing a liver transplantation donor risk index in a national registry (abstract). Hepatology 2007;46:235A.

72. Amin MG, Wolf MP, TenBrook JA Jr, et al. Expanded criteria donor grafts for deceased donor liver transplantation under the MELD system: a decision analysis. Liver Transpl 2004;10:1468–75.

73. Mullhaupt B, Dimitroulis D, Gerlach JT, et al. Hot topics in liver transplantation: organ allocation—extended criteria donor—living donor liver transplantation. J Hepatol 2008;48(Suppl 1):S58–67.

74. Lopez-Navidad A, Caballero F. Extended criteria for organ acceptance. Strategies for achieving organ safety and for increasing organ pool. Clin Transplant 2003;17: 308–24.

75. Testa G, Goldstein RM, Netto G, et al. Long-term outcome of patients transplanted with livers from hepatitis C-positive donors. Transplantation 1998;65:925–9.

76. Marroquin CE, Marino G, Kuo PC, et al. Transplantation of hepatitis C-positive livers in hepatitis C-positive patients is equivalent to transplanting hepatitis C-negative livers. Liver Transpl 2001;7:762–8.

77. Ghobrial RM, Steadman R, Gornbein J, et al. A 10-year experience of liver transplantation for hepatitis C: analysis of factors determining outcome in over 500 patients. Ann Surg 2001;234:384–93.

78. Saab S, Chang AJ, Comulada S, et al. Outcomes of hepatitis C- and hepatitis B core antibody-positive grafts in orthotopic liver transplantation. Liver Transpl 2003;9: 1053–61.

79. Velidedeoglu E, Desai NM, Campos L, et al. The outcome of liver grafts procured from hepatitis C-positive donors. Transplantation 2002;73:582–7.

80. Peek R, Reddy KR. Hepatitis C virus-infected donors in liver transplantation. Gastroenterology 2007;133:381–2.

81. Hartwig MG, Patel V, Palmer SM, et al. Hepatitis B core antibody positive donors as a safe and effective therapeutic option to increase available organs for lung transplantation. Transplantation 2005;80:320–5.

82. Gish RG, Ascher NL. Transmission of hepatitis B virus through allotransplantation. Liver Transpl Surg 1996;2:161–4.
83. Freeman RB, Giatras I, Falagas ME, et al. Outcome of transplantation of organs procured from bacteremic donors. Transplantation 1999;68:1107–11.
84. Cerutti E, Stratta C, Romagnoli R, et al. Bacterial- and fungal-positive cultures in organ donors: clinical impact in liver transplantation. Liver Transpl 2006;12:1253–9.
85. Lumbreras C, Sanz F, Gonzalez A, et al. Clinical significance of donor-unrecognized bacteremia in the outcome of solid-organ transplant recipients. Clin Infect Dis 2001;33:722–6.
86. Lopez-Navidad A, Domingo P, Caballero F, et al. Successful transplantation of organs retrieved from donors with bacterial meningitis. Transplantation 1997;64: 365–8.
87. Teperman L. Donor-transmitted diseases. Liver Transplantation 2010;16:S40–4.
88. Organ Procurement and Transplantation Network. Policy 2: minimum procurement standards for an organ procurement organization (OPO). Rockville (MD): US Department of Health and Human Services; 2009.
89. Singer AL, Kucirka LM, Namuyinga R, et al. The high-risk donor: viral infections in solid organ transplantation. Curr Opin Organ Transplant 2008;13:400–4.
90. Grady D. Four transplant recipients contract HIV. The New York Times November 13, 2007.
91. Rogers MF, Simonds RJ, Lawton KE, et al. National Center for Infectious Diseases. Guidelines for preventing transmission of human immunodeficiency virus through transplantation of human tissue and organs. MMWR 1994;43:1–17. Available at: http://www.cdc.gov/MMWR.
92. Kauffman HM, McBride MA, Cherikh WS, et al. Transplant tumor registry: donors with central nervous system tumors. Transplantation 27 2002;73:579–82.
93. Kauffman HM, McBride MA, Delmonico FL. First report of the United Network for Organ Sharing Transplant Tumor Registry: donors with a history of cancer. Transplantation 2000;70:1747–51.
94. Buell JF, Alloway RR, Steve Woodle E. How can donors with a previous malignancy be evaluated? J Hepatol 2006;45:503–7.
95. Morath C, Schwenger V, Schmidt J, et al. Transmission of malignancy with solid organ transplants (Abs.). Transplantation 2005;80:S164.
96. Vignot S, Faivre S, Aguirre D, et al. mTOR-targeted therapy of cancer with rapamycin derivatives. Ann Oncol 2005;16:525–37.
97. Yersiz H, Cameron AM, Carmody I, et al. Split liver transplantation. Transplant Proc 2006;38:602–3.
98. Smith B. Segmental liver transplantation from a living donor. J Pediatr Surg 1969;4: 126–32.
99. Pichlmayr R, Ringe B, Gubernatis, G, et al. Transplantation of a donor liver to 2 recipients (splitting transplantation): a new method in the further development of segmental liver transplantation. Langenbecks Arch Chir 1989;373:127–30.
100. Bismuth H, Morino M, Castaing D, et al. Emergency orthotopic liver transplantation in two patients using one donor liver. Br J Surg 1989;76:722–4.
101. Renz JF, Yersiz H, Reichert PR, et al. Split-liver transplantation: a review. Am J Transplant 2003;3:1323–35.
102. Azoulay D, Astarcioglu I, Bismuth H, et al. Split-liver transplantation. The Paul Brousse policy. Ann Surg 1996;224:737–46.
103. Humar A, Ramcharan T, Sielaff TD, et al. Split liver transplantation for two adult recipients: an initial experience. Am J Transplant 2001;1:366–72.

104. Yersiz H, Renz JF, Farmer DG, et al. One hundred in situ split-liver transplantations: a single-center experience. Ann Surg 2003;238:496–505.
105. Sommacale D, Farges O, Ettorre GM, et al. In situ split liver transplantation for two adult recipients. Transplantation 2000;69:1005–7.
106. Wilms C, Walter J, Kaptein M, et al. Long-term outcome of split liver transplantation using right extended grafts in adulthood: a matched pair analysis. Ann Surg 2006; 244:865–72.
107. Azoulay D, Castaing D, Adam R, et al. Split-liver transplantation for two adult recipients: feasibility and long-term outcomes. Ann Surg 2001;233:565–74.
108. Ghobrial RM, Yersiz H, Farmer DG, et al. Predictors of survival after In vivo split liver transplantation: analysis of 110 consecutive patients. Ann Surg 2000;232:312–23.
109. Cardillo M, De Fazio N, Pedotti P, et al. Split and whole liver transplantation outcomes: a comparative cohort study. Liver Transpl 2006;12:402–10.
110. Renz JF, Emond JC, Yersiz H, et al. Split-liver transplantation in the United States: outcomes of a national survey. Ann Surg 2004;239:172–81.
111. Foster R, Zimmerman M, Trotter JF. Expanding donor options: marginal, living, and split donors. Clin Liver Dis 2007;11:417–29.
112. Available at: http://www.kdvr.com/news/kdvr-liver-transplant-death.txt,o,3369112. Story. Accessed May 13, 2011.
113. Schiano TD, Kim-Schluger L, Gondolesi G, et al. Adult living donor liver transplantation: the hepatologist's perspective. Hepatology 2001;33:3–9.
114. Trotter JF, Wachs M, Everson GT, et al. Adult-to-adult transplantation of the right hepatic lobe from a living donor. N Engl J Med 2002;346:1074–82.
115. Berg CL, Gillespie BW, Merion RM, et al. Improvement in survival associated with adult-to-adult living donor liver transplantation. Gastroenterology 2007;133:1806–13.
116. Freeman RB Jr, Steffick DE, Guidinger MK, et al. Liver and intestine transplantation in the United States, 1997-2006. Am J Transplant 2008;8:958–76.
117. Olthoff KM, Merion RM, Ghobrial RM, et al. Outcomes of 385 adult-to-adult living donor liver transplant recipients: a report from the A2ALL Consortium. Ann Surg 2005;242:314–23.
118. Pomposelli JJ, Verbesey J, Simpson MA, et al. Improved survival after live donor adult liver transplantation (LDALT) using right lobe grafts: program experience and lessons learned. Am J Transplant 2006;6:589–98.
119. Terrault NA, Shiffman ML, Lok AS, et al. Outcomes in hepatitis C virus-infected recipients of living donor vs. deceased donor liver transplantation. Liver Transpl 2007;13:122–9.
120. Fisher RA, Kulik LM, Freise CE, et al. Hepatocellular carcinoma recurrence and death following living and deceased donor liver transplantation. Am J Transplant 2007;7: 1601–8.
121. Trotter JF. Selection of donors and recipients for living donor liver transplantation. Liver Transpl 2000;6(6 Suppl 2):S52–8.
122. Trotter JF, Wisniewski KA, Terrault NA, et al. Outcomes of donor evaluation in adult-to-adult living donor liver transplantation. Hepatology 2007;46:1476–84.
123. Ghobrial RM, Freise CE, Trotter JF, et al. Donor morbidity after living donation for liver transplantation. Gastroenterology 2008;135:468–76.
124. Mascarenhas RG, Guraker A. Recent advances in liver transplantation for the practicing gastroenterologist. Gastroenterol Hepatol 2009;5:443–50.

Long-Term Management of the Liver Transplant Recipient: Pearls for the Practicing Gastroenterologist

David H. Oustecky, MD[a], Andres R. Riera, MD[b],
Kenneth D. Rothstein, MD[a],*

KEYWORDS
- Liver transplantation • De novo malignancy
- Cardiovascular disease • Metabolic syndrome • Obesity

According to the United States Department of Health and Human Services, from 1988 to 2010, the number of annual liver transplants has increased from 1713 to 6291. Patient survival rates have ranged from 66% to 71% at 7 years and graft survival rates have ranged from 58% to 61% at 7 years.[1] Both the increase in frequency of liver transplantation and the improved survival of transplant recipients are great achievements of modern medicine. With this increase in the number of successful outcomes, there are more liver transplant recipients living both longer and with an improved quality of life.[2] The responsibility for the long-term care for these patients often falls on the shoulders of the practicing gastroenterologist. The identification and treatment of long-term comorbidities such as hypertension, cardiovascular disease, dyslipidemia, obesity, diabetes mellitus, osteoporosis, renal injury, malignancy, rejection, and drug interactions has become a vital element of the management of these patients.[3–8] One pearl to always remember when initiating treatment for any of these comorbidities is that all medications (prescribed or over the counter) need to be approved by the transplant team.

RENAL DYSFUNCTION

Renal injury is a common complication after liver transplantation. The glomerular filtration rate (GFR) can fall as low as 60% of the preoperative GFR measured in the

[a] Drexel University College of Medicine, Department of Gastroenterology and Hepatology, Mail Stop 913, 219 N. Broad Street, 5th Floor, Philadelphia, PA 19107, USA
[b] Drexel University College of Medicine, Department of Medicine, Division of General Internal Medicine, Mail Stop 427, 245 N. Broad Street, Philadelphia, PA 19102, USA
* Corresponding author.
E-mail address: Kenneth.Rothstein@DrexelMed.edu

Gastroenterol Clin N Am 40 (2011) 659–681
doi:10.1016/j.gtc.2011.06.006
0889-8553/11/$ – see front matter © 2011 Elsevier Inc. All rights reserved.

first 6 weeks posttransplantation.[9] It is well known that kidney injury after surgery and long-term chronic renal failure can decrease patient survival.[10] Measurement of the GFR before transplantation is not accurate owing to abnormalities in the fluid status.[11] Creatinine levels may also be inaccurate because they depend on the patient's muscle mass.[12] Likewise, renal function at the moment of the transplant is not a predictor of postoperative renal function.[13,14]

The incidence of acute kidney injury after liver transplantation ranges between 48% and 98%.[15–19] It is very likely that the wide range is secondary to the fact that these studies used different definitions for acute kidney injury.[10] Cabezuelo and colleagues[15] classified acute renal failure after transplantation into early (0–7 days posttransplantation) and late (8–28 days posttransplantation). The most frequent etiologies for early acute renal failure were ischemic acute tubular necrosis and pre-renal azotemia. Sepsis and the use of calcineurin inhibitors were the most common etiologies for patients who developed late acute renal failure.[15]

With the increase in patient survival posttransplantation, chronic kidney disease has become a more common long-term complication. The incidence of chronic kidney disease has been reported as high as 27% at 5 years after transplantation.[11] The most common causes of chronic kidney disease include diabetic nephropathy[20] and calcineurin inhibitor toxicity, with cyclosporine implicated more often than tacrolimus.[21] Focal segmental glomerulosclerosis, acute tubular necrosis, and persistent hepatorenal syndrome have also been implicated.[13] The renal function of all patients after liver transplantation should be monitored regularly. This can be done by screening them for microalbuminuria and measuring GFR regularly. Attention must be given to management of other comorbidities like hypertension, diabetes mellitus, and the use of nephrotoxic drugs.[22]

OSTEOPOROSIS

Osteoporosis after transplantation is related to pretransplant and posttransplant factors. Patients with end-stage liver disease are at a higher risk for abnormal bone mineral metabolism, osteoporosis, and fractures.[5,23,24] Hepatic osteodystrophy is commonly seen and is related to irregular bone metabolism in patients with advanced liver disease.[25] The prevalence of osteoporosis at the spine or hip ranges between 11% and 52% in patients awaiting liver transplantation.[26–30] The main posttransplant complications are avascular necrosis, fracture, and osteoporosis.[12] In the first 6 to 12 months after transplantation, the rates of fractures and bone loss significantly increases.[5] Fracture rates range from 17% to 65% of patients with increased bone loss and most commonly affect the spine and ribs.

Guichelaar and colleagues[28] confirmed that there is a higher risk for bone loss in patients with advanced primary sclerosing cholangitis and primary biliary cirrhosis. They also found a direct correlation between corticosteroid use and decreased bone mass. The main effect of steroids in the bone is suppression of bone formation itself.[31] Bone loss and fractures owing to steroid therapy are more frequent during the first 6 months of treatment.[31,32] It has also been suggested that there may be a rapid decline of this fracture risk after discontinuing therapy with steroids.[33] The use of calcineurin inhibitors may also contribute to osteoporosis.[34]

Even before transplantation, an assessment of bone health should be obtained. All patients should have a dual-emission x-ray absorptiometry scan as part of the pretransplant evaluation as well as serum tests to measure calcium, phosphate, parathyroid hormone, and serum 25-hydroxyvitamin D levels.[12] Patients should follow a healthy diet with good calcium intake, maintain a normal body weight, and participate in physical exercise. Alendronate started after transplantation along with calcium and vitamin D supplementation has been shown to reduce bone loss in patients with osteopenia and osteoporosis.[35]

CARDIOVASCULAR DISEASE

It has been estimated that approximately 26% of patients undergoing workup for liver transplantation have asymptomatic coronary artery disease (CAD).[36] The Framingham score demonstrates a higher 10-year probability of coronary heart disease in liver transplant recipients (11%) when compared with the general population (7%).[37] Patients with mild to moderate CAD have significantly higher rates of complications after transplantation,[38,39] with markedly increased morbidity and mortality.[40] Risk factors for cardiovascular disease include male gender, smoking tobacco, arterial hypertension, obesity, family history of CAD, diabetes mellitus, and hyperlipidemia.[36] More often than in the regular population, 2 or more of these risk factors are present in the liver transplant patient. Nonalcoholic fatty liver disease is also a strong predictor of diffuse arterial disease; therefore, these patients should be carefully screened before liver transplantation.[41,42]

The management of risk factors for cardiovascular disease should be proactive and should involve a multidisciplinary team of physicians. An important piece of this team should be the gastroenterologist, who should be familiar with the most recent guidelines for the approach and management of these risk factors. The risk factors for CAD and the approach to their management are discussed.

THE METABOLIC SYNDROME

Patients with cirrhosis become malnourished as part of the natural course of the disease. If the outcomes after liver transplantation are favorable, these patients will recover their original nutritional state and, in some cases, they may cross the limits of a healthy nutrition state.[43] With the increased survival rates after transplantation, metabolic complications are becoming more common. They often lead to an increased morbidity and mortality in this population.[44]

The metabolic syndrome is a combination of metabolic complications that include arterial hypertension, diabetes mellitus, dyslipidemia (high triglycerides and low levels of high-density lipoprotein cholesterol), and obesity.[45] The prevalence of posttransplant metabolic syndrome has been reported to be found in as many as 58% of posttransplant patients.[46] It is known that many of the immunosuppressive agents used after transplant can predispose to the development of metabolic disorders.[47] These factors, combined with others, increase the risk of developing metabolic complications after liver transplantation. Fortunately, most of these factors are modifiable.

Risk factors for the development of metabolic syndrome after liver transplant include advanced age at transplant, increased body mass index (BMI) after transplantation, presence of diabetes before transplantation, smoking history, the use of steroids or cyclosporine, and indication for liver transplant (hepatitis C, alcohol, or cryptogenic cirrhosis).[44,46]

Despite some differences in prevalence, studies have confirmed the deleterious effect of metabolic syndrome after liver transplantation. Laryea and colleagues[46] showed a higher risk of vascular events in those patients with metabolic syndrome after liver transplantation. These vascular events included acute coronary syndrome, stroke, myocardial infarction, cardiac death, and transient ischemic attacks. There is a higher risk for the development of cirrhosis after transplantation among those patients with both the metabolic syndrome and hepatitis C.[48] After a liver transplant, all patients should be monitored regularly for the development of obesity, dyslipidemia, diabetes, and hypertension. Patients should be encouraged to participate in programs that include diet modifications and exercise.[43]

OBESITY

The World Health Organization uses the BMI to define obesity. A person with a BMI greater than or equal to 30 kg/m^2 is considered obese.[49] The incidence of obesity during the first year after transplantation has been reported between 15% and 41%.[50,51] Obesity is a well-known, major risk factor for cardiovascular problems, diabetes mellitus, the metabolic syndrome, sleep apnea, and many other chronic diseases including nonalcoholic steatohepatitis. Weight gain after transplantation is an important marker of recovery after surgery; however, many patients gain more weight than needed.[50] Generally, patients who are overweight or obese before liver transplantation will maintain the same body habitus after transplantation, and one third of patients with normal weight before the surgery will become overweight or obese posttransplantation.[52]

Factors that influence the development of obesity after liver transplantation include genetic factors, decreased physical activity, altered dietary habits, and side effects of medications, especially immunosuppressive drugs.[3] The role of corticosteroid use is controversial; in some studies, their use of was associated with obesity,[52,53] whereas other studies did not show a correlation.[50,51,54] Cyclosporine seems to be related to weight gain more than tacrolimus, but this could be because patients on cyclosporine had higher caloric intakes than those on tacrolimus.[52,55]

Obesity is a preventable risk factor. A BMI should be calculated at every visit to the transplant center and this should be plotted in tables to evaluate progress.[3] The management of obese and overweight patients must be proactive and should include dietary education, an exercise program, and counseling. In some cases, pharmacologic agents or bariatric surgery could be considered for appropriate candidates. A study with tetrahydrolipstatin (Orlistat) on 15 patients, showed some benefit at 3 and 6 months, but it seemed to interfere with tacrolimus levels.[56] Minimizing the use of steroids in the immunosuppressive regimen may also help to prevent weight gain. Bariatric surgery may be useful in selected cases, but this has not been formally evaluated.

DIABETES

According to the American Diabetes Association, diabetes is defined as an abnormality of one of the following 4 measurements: Hemoglobin A1C, fasting plasma glucose, random elevated glucose with symptoms, or an abnormal glucose tolerance test.[57] New-onset diabetes mellitus is a well-known complication after solid organ transplantation. Its incidence ranges between 2.5% and 25% of liver transplant recipients.[58] Diabetes mellitus can result in reduced patient and graft survival after transplantation.[59]

Risk factors for the development of diabetes after transplant include African-American and Hispanic ethnicities, obesity, age (>40 years), first-degree relatives with diabetes type 2, high triglycerides, low levels of high-density lipoprotein cholesterol, hypertension, and immunosuppressive therapy with corticosteroids, tacrolimus and, to a lesser degree, cyclosporine.[43] Hepatitis C virus (HCV) infection is also recognized as a risk factor for the development of diabetes.[60]

To improve posttransplant patient and graft survivals, blood glucose levels should be monitored regularly in all patients.[12,61] If a patient is diagnosed with new-onset diabetes after transplantation, specific testing must occur. Hemoglobin A1C should be checked every 3 months as wells as periodic screening for diabetic complications including tests for microalbuminuria, ophthalmologic examinations and foot care annually.[62] The approach to the treatment of these patients should include life-style modifications and when not sufficient, antidiabetic agents.[3] Further interventions include adjustment of immunosuppressive therapy to achieve a target hemoglobin A1C of less than 7%.[42,62] The use of the antiglycemic agents should follow the conventional approach recommended by organizations like the American Diabetes Association. However, it is important to remember that most of the oral medications available are metabolized by the liver. Their use should be limited to patients with stable graft function.

HYPERTENSION

Hypertension is commonly defined as a blood pressure higher than 140/90 mmHg. The prevalence after liver transplantation has been reported as high as 77%.[63] Elevation of systemic vascular resistance is felt to be one of the causes of hypertension after liver transplantation.[64] Calcineurin inhibitors can amplify this increase in the systemic vascular resistance by potentiating the release of vasoconstricting agents and reducing the expression of vasodilatory agents.[65] Some studies have reported a lesser prevalence of hypertension in patients treated with tacrolimus when compared with those treated with cyclosporine.[37,66] Another factor contributing to the elevation of blood pressure is the use of corticosteroids, which cause retention of salt and water while suppressing nitric oxide production.[67]

Currently, hypertension guidelines do not have specific recommendations for the management of hypertension in liver transplant patients.[67] As with other risk factor for cardiovascular disease, the management of hypertension in the liver transplant patient must start with lifestyle modifications, including weight control, dietary restrictions, regular exercise, and smoking cessation. The goal is a blood pressure lower than 140/90 mmHg and lower than 130/80 for those patients with additional cardiovascular risk factors.[3] If these measures are insufficient, pharmacologic therapy should be initiated. Because of their potent vasodilatory effect, calcium channel blockers are commonly used in transplant patients.[68] Nifedipine, amlodipine, or isradipine may interact less with the cytochrome P450 system resulting in reduced effect on the immunosuppressive levels.[67] Another group of medications that has been used is selective β-blockers. These medications are especially useful in those patients with reflex tachycardia owing to calcium channel blockers or in those patients with a high cardiac output state after transplantation.[69] If monotherapy with any of these drugs is not successful, they can be combined with a thiazide diuretic.

Another important consideration is the role of steroids as a possible cause of the hypertension. Stegall and colleagues[70] demonstrated that hypertensive medications could be stopped in some patients after steroid withdrawal. Angiotensin-converting enzyme inhibitors, angiotensin receptor blockers, and spironolactone can be used, but patients should be monitored closely because of the tendency of these agents to cause hyperkalemia.

DYSLIPIDEMIA

Most patients with end-stage liver disease have abnormal lipid metabolism. The prevalence of dyslipidemia after liver transplantation ranges from 66% to 85%, with hypertriglyceridemia being the most common.[44] Predictive factors include greater weight gain after transplantation[43] and the immunosuppressive regimen used. There are some reports that the use of tacrolimus may have a lower incidence of dyslipidemia when compared with cyclosporine.[71] Tarantino and colleagues[72] followed 29 kidney transplant patients taking tacrolimus over 6 years after transplantation and described significant changes in plasma lipid concentration only during the first 6 months of therapy. Although steroids may produce dyslipidemia, a steroid-free immunosuppression regimen posttransplantation has not been shown to reduce the rates of dyslipidemia.[73]

Dyslipidemia after transplantation often persists despite dietary modifications.[74] A fasting lipid profile should be performed every year in all liver transplant patients. Life-style modifications should be encouraged when the low-density lipoprotein cholesterol level is above 100 mg/dL, and if there is little improvement, pharmacologic therapy should be initiated. In those patients with a baseline low-density lipoprotein cholesterol level of 130 mg/dL or the presence of diabetes mellitus, pharmacologic therapy is indicated.[3]

Despite multiple concerns, statins remain the drug of choice for transplant patients. Statins have been used in solid organ transplant recipients for several years and are usually well tolerated.[75] Low initial doses with titration as needed and close follow-up should be considered.[42] For a patient with pure hypertriglyceridemia, fish oil can be used with minimal side effects.[76]

MEDICATION INTERACTIONS

Tacrolimus, cyclosporine, mycophenolate mofetil, and sirolimus are among the most commonly prescribed immunosuppressive agents in the liver transplant population. Additional medications that are administered to the patient may alter the serum levels of these agents and thus the level of immunosupression. **Tables 1** and **2** include many commonly prescribed medications that may alter the serum levels of these common immunosuppressive agents. All patients should be instructed to discuss any new medications with their health care provider.

ALCOHOL ABUSE

Despite being a controversial indication for liver transplantation, end-stage liver disease secondary to alcohol abuse is a common disease condition that leads to transplantation. Because alcoholics may be responsible for their condition, some have suggested that these individuals be given lower priority for organ allocation.[77] Survival after transplantation owing to alcoholic liver disease is similar to that of other causes, but it will be compromised if there is recidivism after surgery.[78,79] Even though the majority of patients transplanted because of alcoholic liver disease will have a positive outcome, some of them will resume alcohol consumption.[80]

Factors linked with recurrence of alcohol abuse after liver transplantation include pretransplant abstinence duration (<1 year), presence of dependence versus abuse, presence of other psychiatric illnesses (mainly depression and anxiety), coexistent drug abuse, and quality of social support.[80,81] Refining patient selection based on risk factors for alcohol abuse recurrence might improve survival after transplantation. Vigilant monitoring for recurrent alcoholism should be undertaken after transplantation is complete.

TOBACCO ABUSE

With the improvement of immunosuppressive regimens, the main causes of long-term morbidity and mortality after liver transplantation are cardiovascular diseases, metabolic disturbances, and malignancies.[82,83] Smoking is a well-recognized risk factor

Table 1
Pharmacologic agents associated with decreased immunosuppression levels

Tacrolimus	Sirolimus	Cyclosporine	Mycophenolate Mofetil
Antiseizure			
Phenytoin	Phenytoin	Phenytoin	
Phenobarbital	Phenobarbital	Phenobarbital	
Carbamazepine	Carbamazepine	Carbamazepine	
Other gastrointestinal			
		Octreotide	Aluminum hydroxide-magnesium hydroxide
			Cholestyramine
Antifungals			
Caspofungin			
Antibacterials			
		Nafcillin	Metronidazole
		Co-trimoxazole	
Antituberculosis Rifampin			
Rifampin	Rifampin	Rifampin	
Rifabutin	Rifabutin		
Antidepressants			
St. John's wort	St. John's wort		
Quinolones			
			Ciprofloxacin
			Norfloxacin
Immunosuppressants			
Sirolimus			Cyclosporine
Penicillins			
			Amoxicillin-clavulanate
Antiplatelets			
		Ticlopidine	
Phosphate binders			
			Sevelamer
			Proton pump inhibitors

for cardiovascular diseases and some malignancies. Up to 20% of transplant centers consider smoking as a contraindication for liver transplantation.[84]

Addiction to both alcohol and tobacco combined has been reported in about 90% of alcoholics.[85] DiMartini and colleagues[86] reported that among those patients transplanted for alcoholic liver disease, 50% were smoking at 3 months after the surgery. They also reported that the number of cigarettes per day increased throughout the first 12 months after transplantation.

A study published by Marrero and colleagues[87] reported the association between smoking and the development of hepatocellular carcinoma (HCC) in patients with cirrhosis. They recommended closer evaluation of smoking history of patients undergoing workup for liver transplantation. It is reasonable to predict that transplant recipients who continue smoking after surgery might have increased prevalence of medical problems.[88]

Table 2
Pharmacologic agents associated with increased immunosuppression levels

Tacrolimus	Sirolimus	Cyclosporine	Mycophenolate Mofetil
CCBs			
Verapamil	Verapamil	Verapamil	
Nicardipine	Nicardipine	Nicardipine	
Diltiazem	Diltiazem	Diltiazem	
Nifedipine			
Antivirals			
			Ganciclovir
			Acyclovir
			Valganciclovir
			Valacyclovir
Corticosteroids			
Methylprednisolone		Methyl-prednisolone	
Macrolides			
Clarithromycin		Clarithromycin	
Erythromycin		Erythromycin	
Other Gastrointestinal			
Metoclopramide	Metoclopramide	Metoclopramide	
Aluminum hydroxide-magnesium hydroxide	Cisapride		
Anti-inflammatory			
			Salicylates
Antifungals			
Fluconazole	Fluconazole	Fluconazole	
Ketoconazole	Ketoconazole	Ketoconazole	
Itraconazole	Itraconazole	Itraconazole	
Clotrimazole	Clotrimazole		
Voriconazole			
Anti-Parkinsons			
Bromocriptine	Bromocriptine	Bromocriptine	
GYN			
Danazol	Danazol	Danazol	
Ethinyl estradiol			
H-2 blockers			
Cimetidine	Cimetidine		
Anti-gout			
		Allopurinol	Probenecid
HIV			
Protease inhibitors	Protease inhibitors		
Proton pump inhibitors			
Omeprazole			

(continued on next page)

Table 2 (continued)			
Tacrolimus	Sirolimus	Cyclosporine	Mycophenolate Mofetil
Immunosuppressants			
Cyclosporine			
Antidepressants			
Nefazodone			
Other antibacterials			
Chloramphenicol			

Abbreviation: CCB, calcium channel blockers.

Tobacco addiction is a relapsing disorder that requires an active approach to decrease its prevalence and prevent relapse.[88] Intervention programs to reduce smoking should be aimed at active smokers as well as former smokers, and these programs should continue posttransplantation.[89] Diagnosis of smoking abuse and the need to comply with cessation therapies must be reinforced during all physician–patient encounters.

PREGNANCY

Patients often recover their ability to conceive after liver transplantation. Contraception should be initiated before this occurs. Liver transplant recipients and their infants are at an increased risk of obstetric complications. A recent study of 206 liver transplant recipients demonstrated higher rates of fetal mortality, antepartum admissions, and maternal and fetal complications.[90] These patients also suffered from an increased rate of both gestational hypertension and postpartum hemorrhage. The most favorable timing of conception after liver transplantation remains controversial. Current recommendations suggest waiting for at least 2 years after transplantation.[91] The favored means of contraception in this population is the barrier method. Hormonal contraception may also be considered; data regarding the use of intrauterine devices after transplantation are lacking.[92] The United states Food and Drug Administration classifies calcineurin inhibitors as pregnancy category C (animal reproduction studies have shown an adverse effect on the fetus and there are no adequate and well-controlled studies in humans, but potential benefits may warrant use of the drug in pregnant women despite potential risks). Mycophenolate mofetil is classified as a pregnancy category D drug (there is positive evidence of human fetal risk based on adverse reaction data from investigational or marketing experience or studies in humans, but potential benefits may warrant use of the drug in pregnant women despite potential risks). Given the increased risks associated with the use of mycophenolate mofetil, 2 methods of contraception are recommended in those patients receiving this medication.[92] Any transplant patient who becomes pregnant should be considered as a "high-risk" pregnancy because both the mother and the infant are at risk for complications. Their management should be undertaken by a multidisciplinary team including physicians from the division of maternal fetal medicine.

RECURRENT LIVER DISEASE

Certain liver diseases may recur even after a successful transplantation. The recurrence of these disease states influences both graft and patient survival. Metabolic

Table 3 Common characteristics of rejection			
	Early Acute	Late Acute	Chronic
Time of presentation	1–30 days	Within 1st year	Months to years
Incidence	20%–40%	20%–40%	<2%
Histologic features	Portal, bile duct, and venous inflammation. Ballooning and bilirrubinostasis are common. Fibrosis not seen.	Portal, bile duct, and venous inflammation. Histologic features are less classical than early acute rejection. Ballooning and bilirrubinostasis are uncommon. Typically mild fibrosis.	In early stages, inflammatory and degenerative changes in bile ducts. After progression, ductopenia (loss of bile ducts) and obliterative arteriopathy are present. Ballooning and bilirrubinostasis are common. Pattern of fibrosis is variable and progresses with time
Differential diagnosis	Biliary obstruction, reperfusion injury	Autoimmune hepatitis (recurrence and de novo), recurrent viral hepatitis	Recurrent primary biliary sclerosis and primary sclerosing cholangitis
Response to treatment	Reversible	Reversible	Irreversible

diseases and congenital anatomic anomalies often do not recur after liver transplantation. Unfortunately, infectious hepatitis, autoimmune hepatitis, primary biliary cirrhosis, hemochromatosis, primary sclerosing cholangitis, nonalcoholic fatty liver disease, and alcohol-associated liver disease can all recur.[93] Recurrent disease should be considered whenever evaluating a transplant patient with elevated liver enzymes. Special attention should be paid to those individuals with HCV, because viremia and histologic injury after transplantation are almost universal.[94]

ALLOGRAFT REJECTION

The incidence of rejection after liver transplantation has been significantly decreased by advances in immunosuppression. Allograft rejection is usually classified based on time of presentation after transplantation (early vs late), response to immunosuppression (reversible vs irreversible), and histologic features.[95] The "gold standard" for diagnosis of rejection is the liver biopsy. Recurrence of hepatitis C continues to be a challenge when diagnosing rejection, even when a liver biopsy is performed.[96] **Table 3** describes the most common characteristics of the different types of rejection.

BILIARY COMPLICATIONS

Biliary complications remain a major cause of morbidity and mortality after liver transplantation. The incidence ranges between 5% and 32%.[97] The most common complications include strictures, bile leaks, sphincter of Oddi dysfunction, and stone formation.[97,98] The patency of the hepatic artery must be confirmed whenever biliary complications, such as strictures or bilomas occur, because the hepatic artery supplies blood to the bile ducts after liver transplantation.

One of the most important risk factors is the type of anastomosis performed during the transplant. Duct-to-duct choledochocholechostomy or roux-en-Y choledochoje-junostomy are frequently performed. An advantage of the duct-to-duct reconstruction is the capability of preserving the sphincter of Oddi as well as easy access to the biliary tree by endoscopy.[99,100] Reperfusion injury, primary sclerosing cholangitis, cytomegalovirus infection, the use of donation after death, and ABO incompatibility are additional risk factors that predispose a patient to postoperative biliary complications.[97,98,100-105]

The clinical manifestations of biliary complications vary. Bile leaks are more common in the immediate postoperative period, whereas strictures usually present weeks to months after the surgery.[97] Patients can be asymptomatic and found to have an elevation of their liver function tests or they can present with nonspecific symptoms like abdominal pain, fever, or anorexia.[97,98,105] If there is suspicion of biliary complications, an abdominal Doppler ultrasonography can offer pertinent information about the biliary tree as well as the hepatic vasculature. Unfortunately, ultrasound has a low sensitivity to detect common bile duct obstruction. If the ultrasound is nondiagnostic and complications cannot be ruled out, magnetic resonance cholangiopancreatography or endoscopic retrograde cholangiopancreatography should be considered. Magnetic resonance cholangiopancreatography offers a sensitivity of 93% to 100%, and specificity of 92% to 98%[98] for diagnosis of biliary complications. It also has less risk of complication than endoscopic retrograde cholangiopancreatography,[97] but does not offer the possibility of therapeutic intervention.

Biliary strictures are one of the most common complications. The incidence ranges between 4% and 16% for deceased donors.[97,98] Strictures can be divided by time into early strictures (0-4 weeks after surgery) and late strictures (>4 weeks after surgery). Early strictures are more commonly secondary to surgical technical problems. Late strictures are usually the consequence of ischemia owing to vascular insults. Strictures have also been classified based on their location into either anastomotic or nonanastomotic strictures.[98,105] The treatment of anastomotic strictures includes a combination of endoscopic balloon dilatation and the use of plastic stents.[106-109] In patients who have undergone roux-en-Y reconstruction, percutaneous transhepatic cholangiogram with dilatation and the placement of a percutaneous transhepatic catheter is recommended.[98] If these approaches are not successful, the next step to consider is surgical repair. Nonanastomotic lesions are most likely secondary to ischemia. Their incidence is lower than anastomotic lesions (0.5%-9.6%).[110] The treatment is same approach used for anastomotic lesions but the time to response is usually longer.[111]

Bilomas are the result of bile rupture with extravasation of the bile in the abdomen or the liver. Small bilomas communicating with the biliary tree usually resolve spontaneously. Some bilomas may require the placement of a biliary stent in the extrahepatic bile duct. If there is no communication with the biliary tree, percutaneous drainage is usually required along with the administration of antibiotics.[97,98] Surgical drainage should be reserved for bilomas that do not respond to the above mentioned treatment.

The most common cause of common bile duct filling defects is gallstones.[112] Sludge, migrated stents, and blood clots can also cause filling defects in the common bile duct. Previous strictures, bacterial infection, and obstruction can predispose to stones and sludge.[105,113] Endoscopic retrograde cholangiopancreatography with sphincterotomy is the recommended intervention but sometimes repeated sessions may be necessary.[97] Casts can also produce filling defects. Their management can require basket extraction, stent placement, and lithotripsy.[114]

VASCULAR COMPLICATIONS

Hepatic artery thrombosis (HAT) after liver transplantation is one of the most significant causes of morbidity and mortality.[115] Its incidence has been reported between 2.5% and 9%.[115–117] HAT can be classified into early (0–4 weeks after transplantation) or late HAT (>4 weeks after transplantation). Early HAT has a more aggressive course compared with late HAT, which has a slower progression.[115,118]

The incidence of early HAT has been reported to be between 1.2% and 6%.[115,119,120] The mortality rate ranges between 11% and 56%, whereas the rate of retransplantation has been reported as high as 83%.[115,117,121] Its presentation varies, including fulminant graft failure, sepsis, abscess, or bile duct injury, including leaks, strictures, or cholangitis.[115] It can be diagnosed by Doppler ultrasonography, contrast-enhanced computed tomography, and angiography.[115,122,123]

Common factors implicated in the development of HAT include operative complications, older age of donors, hypercoagulable states, increased transfusion requirements during transplantation, number of episodes of rejection, cytomegalovirus infection, recipient hepatitis C–related liver disease, and smoking.[116,124–132] Abou and colleagues[116] reported a decreased incidence of HAT for patients who received prophylactic anticoagulation therapy after the surgery.

The management of early HAT is mostly surgical, including operative exploration, thrombectomy, and revision of the anastomosis.[115,121,130] Many of these patients require retransplantation and can be listed as United Network for Organ Sharing status 1 if HAT occurs within 1 week of the original transplant. In those patients without symptoms, nonoperative approaches can be attempted. Angiography with thrombolysis, with or without stenting, can be successful in some asymptomatic patients.[133]

Late HAT has a more insidious course when compared with early HAT. Its incidence ranges between 2% and 25%.[118] The clinical presentation includes fever, hepatic abscesses, biliary leaks, and jaundice. It can be diagnosed by Doppler ultrasonography of the abdomen and may be discovered during routine follow-up imaging. Management usually includes broad spectrum antibiotics, drainage of abscesses if present, treatment of sepsis, and treatment of any biliary tract complications. Depending on the grafts response to HAT, retransplantation can be considered once sepsis has resolved and if no other therapy has been successful.[115]

Additional vascular complications after liver transplantation include portal vein thrombosis (PVT) and Budd–Chiari syndrome. In a study of 4234 liver transplant recipients, the incidence of PVT after transplant was found to be 2%.[134] Patients with PVT may present with elevated transaminases, ascites, and portal hypertension with gastrointestinal bleeding. Techniques used for management of PVT have included reexploration and thrombectomy, portosystemic shunting, catheter-directed therapy, anticoagulation without surgical therapy, and primary retransplantation, with varying levels of success.

Budd–Chiari syndrome is often defined as any process that leads to a disruption or reduction of the normal blood flow out of the liver. In a study of 776 liver transplant patients, 1.2% were found to have venous outflow obstruction after transplantation.[135] Typical presentation includes new-onset ascites, hepatomegaly, or an elevation in liver function tests. Treatment in this population had included percutaneous transluminal angioplasty or metallic stent placement. When interventional therapy fails liver retransplantation can be considered.[135]

MALIGNANCY

The development of malignancy must be recognized whenever managing a liver transplant recipient. The probability of de novo malignancy in this population has been reported to be as high as 13% at 5 years post liver transplantation and 26% at 8 years post liver transplantation.[136] Many different types of malignancies have been described in the posttransplant population. Among them, dermatologic, gastrointestinal, lymphoproliferative, and head and neck neoplasms, as well as recurrent HCC, have been described most often.[137–143] Unexplained weight loss and any other signs or symptoms related to these malignancies should be thoroughly investigated. Risk factors for the development of malignancy include immunosuppression intensity and agents, HCV infection, smoking, a history of sun exposure, and alcoholic cirrhosis.[144]

Multiple investigations have failed to show a significant increase in the incidence of colorectal cancer after liver transplantation compared with controls.[137,145–147] Special attention, however, must be paid to those individuals who have received a liver transplantation as a result of to primary sclerosing cholangitis. Inflammatory bowel disease can be found in up to 75% of primary sclerosing cholangitis patients.[148] It has been shown that patients transplanted for primary sclerosing cholangitis do have an increased risk of developing colorectal cancer compared with patients transplanted for other causes.[149] Similarly, it has been demonstrated that liver transplant patients with ulcerative colitis have a higher standardized incidence ratio of colon cancer compared with those patients those without ulcerative colitis.[123] The American Society for Gastrointestinal Endoscopy currently recommends that patients with ulcerative colitis or extensive Crohn's colitis begin surveillance colonoscopy with multiple biopsies every 1 to 2 years after 8 years of disease.[150] Finkenstedt and colleagues[151] have shown that a screening colonoscopy performed 3 years after liver transplantation for any cause can decrease mortality. It remains unclear whether liver transplantation patients require increased screening for colorectal cancer, but one must surely be aware of any alarm symptoms that develop in this population and have a low threshold for a comprehensive investigation.

Head and neck cancer has been described in the posttransplant population. Risk factors include prior smoking and alcohol history,[144] as well as transplantation performed for treatment of alcoholic cirrhosis.[138] The incidence has been reported to be as high as 2%.[152] The mean time to diagnosis has been reported to be as early as 34.3 months after liver transplantation.[153] Patients should be counseled to abstain from both alcohol consumption and tobacco use. Examination of the head, neck, and oral mucosa is recommended as part of the annual evaluation.

Gynecologic malignancies in patients who have undergone liver transplantation have been described rarely in the literature. Ovarian,[154] cervical,[155,156] vulvar,[156] and endometrial[157] neoplasms may develop. In a review of the literature, Oruc and colleagues[158] described the development of 21 de novo breast cancers among 5330 liver transplant recipients. The mean age at the time of diagnosis was 54.5 years. The mean interval from the time of the transplant was 58.9 months, but there was a wide range of 3 months to 13 years. Despite the infrequent occurrence of gynecologic malignancies seen after transplantation, vigilant screening still must be undertaken. The American Cancer Society recommends yearly gynecologic examinations and Papanicolaou smears for those women who are receiving chronic immunosuppression. Women in their 20s and 30s should have a clinical breast examination as part of a periodic health examination by a health professional every 3 years. Starting at age

40, women should have a clinical breast examination by a health professional yearly. Patients should be encouraged to begin a yearly mammography after the age of 40 for the detection of breast cancer.

Posttransplant lymphoproliferative disorder (PTLD) is a potentially fatal complication among liver transplantation recipients that may lead to death more than 50% of the time.[159] PTLD is often due to either a polyclonal or monoclonal proliferation of B-cells. The incidence of PTLD has been reported to be as high as 2.6%.[152] Risk factors for the disease include a negative Epstein–Barr virus serostatus of the transplant recipient and the type of immunosuppression administered, specifically high-dose steroids and OKT3.[160,161] Additional risk factors include liver transplantation for HCV-related and alcoholic cirrhosis as well as an age greater than 50 years.[159] Clinical manifestations of the disease include lymphadenopathy and infiltration of organs, including the central nervous system, stomach, intestines, lungs, skin, and the allograft itself.[162] Treatment of PTLD has included reduction of immunosuppression and the use of chemotherapy, rituximab, and antiviral agents.[163]

Dermatologic malignancies are the most common malignancies seen after solid organ transplantation. Melanomas, squamous cell carcinomas, actinic keratoses, and basal cell carcinomas have been described in liver transplant recipients.[164] The overall incidence of skin cancer after liver transplantation has been reported to be as high as 3.2% in 1 study.[152] Known risk factors include sunlight exposure, skin-type, tobacco consumption, and immunosuppression.[139,165] The use of azathioprine or corticosteroids, but not cyclosporine, has been shown to confer an increased risk of cutaneous squamous cell carcinoma.[166] Although immunosuppressive regimens may be difficult to alter, patients must be counseled to limit sun exposure and wear sunscreen at all times.[164] Self-skin examination and a regular dermatologic evaluation, preferably by a dermatologist, are recommended for screening purposes.[167] If any suspicious lesions are detected, early referral to a dermatologist is suggested.

With the development and institution of the Milan Criteria, rates of recurrent HCC in the liver transplantation population have been reduced. Even so, HCC can recur in 4% to 10% of patients.[168] In patients transplanted for HCC and HCV, predictors of HCC recurrence are posttransplant Hepatitis Activity Index of 4 or greater at 4 months, alanine aminotransferase level of 100 U/L or higher at 4 months, and vascular invasion in the explanted liver.[143] Measurement of serum α-fetoprotein levels every 6 months and annual liver computed tomography or magnetic resonance imaging have been recommended as a posttransplant screening regimen for the detection of recurrent HCC.

The development of lung cancer in liver transplantation recipients is higher than in the general population. The incidence has been reported to be as high as 2.1%.[169] The mean time to the development of lung cancer ranges from 42 to 86 months after transplantation.[153,169] Patients who develop lung cancer after liver transplantation either smoked tobacco before transplantation or continued thereafter. Those individuals transplanted for alcoholic cirrhosis are also at a higher risk for the development of lung cancer,[169] but it is difficult to know if the use of alcohol has direct carcinogenic effects or if it is a marker for tobacco use, because most heavy drinkers tend to also be heavy smokers. Patients should strongly advised to stop any tobacco consumption. Finkenstedt and colleagues[151] have used either an annual computed tomography or chest x-ray to screen for lung cancer. Currently, there are no accepted screening guidelines for the early detection of lung cancer. Screening high-risk individuals should be performed at the physicians' discretion.

VACCINATIONS

The effectiveness of vaccines may be reduced in organ transplant recipients owing to the use of immunosuppressive agents. Even so, there are many immunizations that should be provided to liver transplant recipients. Recommended immunizations include vaccines for hepatitis A and B, meningococcus, pneumococcus, influenza, and tetanus-diphtheria. The US Centers for Disease Control recommends an annual influenza vaccine and a tetanus vaccine every 10 years. The human papilloma virus vaccination should be provided to individuals under the age of 26 years and preferably before they become sexually active. Live or attenuated vaccines are contraindicated in liver transplantation patients because of the risk of bacterial or viral reactivation. Notably, varicella, herpes zoster, and measles, mumps, and rubella vaccinations are contraindicated in the liver transplantation recipient.[170] In addition, household contacts of liver transplantation patients, including children or grandchildren, must receive inactivated vaccines to avoid shedding potentially infectious pathogens. Varicella immune status should be documented so that prophylactic therapy can be administered in the event of exposure to susceptible patients.[171]

SUMMARY

Liver transplantation is becoming more common and patients are surviving longer after transplantation. Special care must be paid to the long-term management of these patients because they are at increased risk for medical problems, malignancies, and adverse effects from immunosuppression. A stable and continuing relationship must be developed between the physician and the patient to optimize the long-term outcomes for these individuals.

REFERENCES

1. Goh A. An analysis of liver transplant survival rates from the UNOS registry. Clin Transpl 2008:19–34.
2. Desai R, Jamieson NV, Gimson AE, et al. Quality of life up to 30 years following liver transplantation. Liver Transpl Oct 2008;14:1473–9.
3. Munoz SJ, Elgenaidi H. Cardiovascular risk factors after liver transplantation. Liver Transpl 2005;11(Suppl 2):S52–6.
4. Vallejo GH, Romero CJ, de Vicente JC. Incidence and risk factors for cancer after liver transplantation. Crit Rev Oncol Hematol 2005;56:87–99.
5. Stein E, Ebeling P, Shane E. Post-transplantation osteoporosis. Endocrinol Metab Clin North Am 2007;36:937–63.
6. Biancofiore G, Davis CL. Renal dysfunction in the perioperative liver transplant period. Curr Opin Organ Transplant 2008;13:291–7.
7. Kadayifci A. Metabolic syndrome and liver transplantation. Panminerva Med 2009; 51:205–13.
8. Munoz LE, Nanez H, Rositas F, et al. Long-term complications and survival of patients after orthotopic liver transplantation. Transplant Proc 2010;42:2381–2.
9. Gonwa TA, Morris CA, Goldstein RM, et al. Long-term survival and renal function following liver transplantation in patients with and without hepatorenal syndrome — experience in 300 patients. Transplantation 1991;51:428–30.
10. Yalavarthy R, Edelstein CL, Teitelbaum I. Acute renal failure and chronic kidney disease following liver transplantation. Hemodial Int 2007;11(Suppl 3):S7–12.
11. Cohen AJ, Stegall MD, Rosen CB, et al. Chronic renal dysfunction late after liver transplantation. Liver Transpl 2002;8:916–21.

12. Liu LU, Schiano TD. Long-term care of the liver transplant recipient. Clin Liver Dis 2007;11:397–416.
13. Gonwa TA, Mai ML, Melton LB, et al. End-stage renal disease (ESRD) after ortho-topic liver transplantation (OLTX) using calcineurin-based immunotherapy: risk of development and treatment. Transplantation 2001;72:1934–9.
14. Nair S, Verma S, Thuluvath PJ. Pretransplant renal function predicts survival in patients undergoing orthotopic liver transplantation. Hepatology 2002;35:1179–85.
15. Cabezuelo JB, Ramirez P, Rios A, et al. Risk factors of acute renal failure after liver transplantation. Kidney Int 2006;69:1073–80.
16. Ishitani M, Wilkowski M, Stevenson W, et al. Outcome of patients requiring hemo-dialysis after liver transplantation. Transplant Proc 1993;25:1762–3.
17. McCauley J, Van Thiel DH, et al. Acute and chronic renal failure in liver transplanta-tion. Nephron 1990;55:121–8.
18. Nuno J, Cuervas-Mons V, Vicente E, et al. Renal failure after liver transplantation: analysis of risk factors in 139 liver transplant recipients. Transplant Proc 1995;27: 2319–20.
19. Rimola A, Gavaler JS, Schade RR, et al. Effects of renal impairment on liver transplantation. Gastroenterology 1987;93:148–56.
20. Pillebout E, Nochy D, Hill G, et al. Renal histopathological lesions after orthotopic liver transplantation (OLT). Am J Transplant 2005;5:1120–9.
21. Ojo AO, Held PJ, Port FK, et al. Chronic renal failure after transplantation of a nonrenal organ. N Engl J Med 2003;349:931–40.
22. O'Riordan A, Wong V, McCormick PA, et al. Chronic kidney disease post-liver transplantation. Nephrol Dial Transplant 2006;21:2630–6.
23. Hay JE. Osteoporosis in liver diseases and after liver transplantation. J Hepatol 2003;38:856–65.
24. Maalouf NM, Shane E. Osteoporosis after solid organ transplantation. J Clin Endo-crinol Metab 2005;90:2456–65.
25. Goel V, Kar P. Hepatic osteodystrophy. Trop Gastroenterol 2010;31:82–6.
26. Carey EJ, Balan V, Kremers WK, et al. Osteopenia and osteoporosis in patients with end-stage liver disease caused by hepatitis C and alcoholic liver disease: not just a cholestatic problem. Liver Transpl 2003;9:1166–73.
27. Cohen A, Shane E. Osteoporosis after solid organ and bone marrow transplantation. Osteoporos Int 2003;14:617–30.
28. Guichelaar MM, Kendall R, Malinchoc M, et al. Bone mineral density before and after OLT: long-term follow-up and predictive factors. Liver Transpl 2006;12:1390–402.
29. Monegal A, Navasa M, Guanabens N, et al. Bone disease after liver transplantation: a long-term prospective study of bone mass changes, hormonal status and histo-morphometric characteristics. Osteoporos Int 2001;12:484–92.
30. Sokhi RP, Anantharaju A, Kondaveeti R, et al. Bone mineral density among cirrhotic patients awaiting liver transplantation. Liver Transpl 2004;10:648–53.
31. Lichtenstein GR, Sands BE, Pazianas M. Prevention and treatment of osteoporosis in inflammatory bowel disease. Inflamm Bowel Dis 2006;12:797–813.
32. Sambrook P, Birmingham J, Kempler S, et al. Corticosteroid effects on proximal femur bone loss. J Bone Miner Res 1990;5:1211–6.
33. Van Staa TP, Leufkens HG, Abenhaim L, et al. Use of oral corticosteroids and risk of fractures. J Bone Miner Res 2005;20:1487–94.
34. Cvetkovic M, Mann GN, Romero DF, et al. The deleterious effects of long-term cyclosporine A, cyclosporine G, and FK506 on bone mineral metabolism in vivo. Transplantation 1994;57:1231–7.

35. Millonig G, Graziadei IW, Eichler D, et al. Alendronate in combination with calcium and vitamin D prevents bone loss after orthotopic liver transplantation: a prospective single-center study. Liver Transpl 2005;11:960–6.
36. Tiukinhoy-Laing SD, Rossi JS, Bayram M, et al. Cardiac hemodynamic and coronary angiographic characteristics of patients being evaluated for liver transplantation. Am J Cardiol 2006;98:178–81.
37. Neal DA, Gimson AE, Gibbs P, Alexander GJ. Beneficial effects of converting liver transplant recipients from cyclosporine to tacrolimus on blood pressure, serum lipids, and weight. Liver Transpl 2001;7:533–9.
38. Carey WD, Dumot JA, Pimentel RR, et al. The prevalence of coronary artery disease in liver transplant candidates over age 50. Transplantation 1995;59:859–64.
39. Diedrich DA, Findlay JY, Harrison BA, et al. Influence of coronary artery disease on outcomes after liver transplantation. Transplant Proc 2008;40:3554–7.
40. Johnston SD, Morris JK, Cramb R, et al. Cardiovascular morbidity and mortality after orthotopic liver transplantation. Transplantation 2002;73:901–6.
41. Gastaldelli A, Kozakova M, Hojlund K, et al. Fatty liver is associated with insulin resistance, risk of coronary heart disease, and early atherosclerosis in a large European population. Hepatology 2009;49:1537–44.
42. Watt KD, Charlton MR. Metabolic syndrome and liver transplantation: a review and guide to management. J Hepatol 2010;53:199–206.
43. Anastacio LR, Lima AS, Toulson Davisson Correia MI. Metabolic syndrome and its components after liver transplantation: incidence, prevalence, risk factors, and implications. Clin Nutr 2010;29:175–9.
44. Pagadala M, Dasarathy S, Eghtesad B, et al. Posttransplant metabolic syndrome: an epidemic waiting to happen. Liver Transpl 2009;15:1662–70.
45. Alberti KG, Eckel RH, Grundy SM, et al. Harmonizing the metabolic syndrome: a joint interim statement of the International Diabetes Federation Task Force on Epidemiology and Prevention; National Heart, Lung, and Blood Institute; American Heart Association; World Heart Federation; International Atherosclerosis Society; and International Association for the Study of Obesity. Circulation 2009;120:1640–5.
46. Laryea M, Watt KD, Molinari M, et al. Metabolic syndrome in liver transplant recipients: prevalence and association with major vascular events. Liver Transpl 2007;13:1109–14.
47. McPartland KJ, Pomposelli JJ. Update on immunosuppressive drugs used in solid-organ transplantation and their nutrition implications. Nutr Clin Pract 2007;22:467–73.
48. Hanouneh IA, Feldstein AE, McCullough AJ, et al. The significance of metabolic syndrome in the setting of recurrent hepatitis C after liver transplantation. Liver Transpl 2008;14:1287–93.
49. Obesity: preventing and managing the global epidemic. Report of a WHO consultation. World Health Organ Tech Rep Ser 2000;894:i–xii, 1–253.
50. Richards J, Gunson B, Johnson J, et al. Weight gain and obesity after liver transplantation. Transpl Int 2005;18:461–6.
51. Stegall MD, Everson G, Schroter G, et al. Metabolic complications after liver transplantation. Diabetes, hypercholesterolemia, hypertension, and obesity. Transplantation 1995;60:1057–60.
52. Everhart JE, Lombardero M, Lake JR, et al. Weight change and obesity after liver transplantation: incidence and risk factors. Liver Transpl Surg 1998;4:285–96.
53. Canzanello VJ, Schwartz L, Taler SJ, et al. Evolution of cardiovascular risk after liver transplantation: a comparison of cyclosporine A and tacrolimus (FK506). Liver Transpl Surg 1997;3:1–9.

54. Richardson RA, Garden OJ, Davidson HI. Reduction in energy expenditure after liver transplantation. Nutrition 2001;17:585–9.
55. MI TDC, Rego LO, Lima AS. Post-liver transplant obesity and diabetes. Curr Opin Clin Nutr Metab Care 2003;6:457–60.
56. Cassiman D, Roelants M, Vandenplas G, et al. Orlistat treatment is safe in overweight and obese liver transplant recipients: a prospective, open label trial. Transpl Int 2006;19:1000–5.
57. Diagnosis and classification of diabetes mellitus. Diabetes Care 2010;33(Suppl 1):S62–9.
58. Montori VM, Basu A, Erwin PJ, et al. Posttransplantation diabetes: a systematic review of the literature. Diabetes Care 2002;25:583–92.
59. Yoo HY, Thuluvath PJ. The effect of insulin-dependent diabetes mellitus on outcome of liver transplantation. Transplantation 2002;74:1007–12.
60. Allison ME, Wreghitt T, Palmer CR, et al. Evidence for a link between hepatitis C virus infection and diabetes mellitus in a cirrhotic population. J Hepatol 1994;21:1135–9.
61. Davidson J, Wilkinson A, Dantal J, et al. New-onset diabetes after transplantation: 2003 International consensus guidelines. Proceedings of an international expert panel meeting. Barcelona, Spain, 19 February 2003. Transplantation 2003;75(10 Suppl):SS3–24.
62. Standards of medical care in diabetes—2011. Diabetes Care 2011;34(Suppl 1): S11–61.
63. Neal DA, Tom BD, Luan J, et al. Is there disparity between risk and incidence of cardiovascular disease after liver transplant? Transplantation 2004;77:93–9.
64. Shirakami G, Murakawa M, Shingu K, et al. Perioperative plasma concentrations of endothelin and natriuretic peptides in children undergoing living-related liver transplantation. Anesth Analg 1996;82:235–40.
65. Calo L, Semplicini A, Davis PA, et al. Cyclosporin-induced endothelial dysfunction and hypertension: are nitric oxide system abnormality and oxidative stress involved? Transpl Int 2000;13(Suppl 1):S413–8.
66. Dikow R, Degenhard M, Kraus T, et al. Blood pressure profile and treatment quality in liver allograft recipients-benefit of tacrolimus versus cyclosporine. Transplant Proc 2004;36:1512–5.
67. Najeed SA, Saghir S, Hein B, et al. Management of hypertension in liver transplant patients. Int J Cardiol 2011 Jan 5 [Epub ahead of print].
68. Curtis JJ, Luke RG, Jones P, et al. Hypertension in cyclosporine-treated renal transplant recipients is sodium dependent. Am J Med 1988;85:134–8.
69. Textor SC, Taler SJ, Canzanello VJ, et al. Posttransplantation hypertension related to calcineurin inhibitors. Liver Transpl 2000;6:521–30.
70. Stegall MD, Everson GT, Schroter G, et al. Prednisone withdrawal late after adult liver transplantation reduces diabetes, hypertension, and hypercholesterolemia without causing graft loss. Hepatology 1997;25:173–7.
71. Steinmuller TM, Graf KJ, Schleicher J, et al. The effect of FK506 versus cyclosporine on glucose and lipid metabolism—a randomized trial. Transplantation 1994;58:669–74.
72. Tarantino G, Palmiero G, Polichetti G, et al. Long-term assessment of plasma lipids in transplant recipients treated with tacrolimus in relation to fatty liver. Int J Immunopathol Pharmacol 2010;23:1303–8.
73. Klintmalm GB, Washburn WK, Rudich SM, et al. Corticosteroid-free immunosuppression with daclizumab in HCV(+) liver transplant recipients: 1-year interim results of the HCV-3 study. Liver Transpl 2007;13:1521–31.

74. Kobashigawa JA, Kasiske BL. Hyperlipidemia in solid organ transplantation. Transplantation 1997;63:331–8.
75. Martin JE, Cavanaugh TM, Trumbull L, et al. Incidence of adverse events with HMG-CoA reductase inhibitors in liver transplant patients. Clin Transplant 2008;22: 113–9.
76. McKenney JM, Sica D. Role of prescription omega-3 fatty acids in the treatment of hypertriglyceridemia. Pharmacotherapy 2007;27:715–28.
77. Glannon W. Responsibility, alcoholism, and liver transplantation. J Med Philos 1998;23:31–49.
78. Cuadrado A, Fabrega E, Casafont F, et al. Alcohol recidivism impairs long-term patient survival after orthotopic liver transplantation for alcoholic liver disease. Liver Transpl 2005;11:420–6.
79. Pfitzmann R, Schwenzer J, Rayes N, et al. Long-term survival and predictors of relapse after orthotopic liver transplantation for alcoholic liver disease. Liver Transpl 2007;13:197–205.
80. Gedaly R, McHugh PP, Johnston TD, et al. Predictors of relapse to alcohol and illicit drugs after liver transplantation for alcoholic liver disease. Transplantation 2008;86: 1090–5.
81. Dom G, Francque S, Michielsen P. Risk for relapse of alcohol use after liver transplantation for alcoholic liver disease: a review and proposal of a set of risk assessment criteria. Acta Gastroenterol Belg 2010;73:247–51.
82. Borg MA, van der Wouden EJ, Sluiter WJ, et al. Vascular events after liver transplantation: a long-term follow-up study. Transpl Int 2008;21:74–80.
83. Reich D, Rothstein K, Manzarbeitia C, et al. Common medical diseases after liver transplantation. Semin Gastrointest Dis 1998;9:110–25.
84. Olbrisch ME, Benedict SM, Haller DL, et al. Psychosocial assessment of living organ donors: clinical and ethical considerations. Prog Transplant 2001;11:40–9.
85. Batel P, Pessione F, Maitre C, et al. Relationship between alcohol and tobacco dependencies among alcoholics who smoke. Addiction 1995;90:977–80.
86. DiMartini A, Javed L, Russell S, et al. Tobacco use following liver transplantation for alcoholic liver disease: an underestimated problem. Liver Transpl 2005;11:679–83.
87. Marrero JA, Fontana RJ, Fu S, et al. Alcohol, tobacco and obesity are synergistic risk factors for hepatocellular carcinoma. J Hepatol 2005;42:218–24.
88. Munoz SJ. Tobacco use by liver transplant recipients: grappling with a smoking gun. Liver Transpl 2005;11:606–9.
89. van der Heide F, Dijkstra G, Porte RJ, et al. Smoking behavior in liver transplant recipients. Liver Transpl 2009;15:648–55.
90. Coffin CS, Shaheen AA, Burak KW, et al. Pregnancy outcomes among liver transplant recipients in the United States: a nationwide case-control analysis. Liver Transpl 2010;16:56–63.
91. Nagy S, Bush MC, Berkowitz R, et al. Pregnancy outcome in liver transplant recipients. Obstet Gynecol 2003;102:121–8.
92. Surti B, Tan J, Saab S. Pregnancy and liver transplantation. Liver Int 2008;28: 1200–6.
93. El-Masry M, Gilbert CP, Saab S. Recurrence of non-viral liver disease after orthotopic liver transplantation. Liver Int 2011;31:291–302.
94. Ponziani FR, Gasbarrini A, Pompili M, et al. Management of hepatitis C virus infection recurrence after liver transplantation: an overview. Transplant Proc 2011;43:291–5.
95. Neil DA, Hubscher SG. Current views on rejection pathology in liver transplantation. Transpl Int 2010;23:971–83.
96. Hubscher SG. Transplantation pathology. Semin Liver Dis 2009;29:74–90.

97. Ayoub WS, Esquivel CO, Martin P. Biliary complications following liver transplantation. Dig Dis Sci 2010;55:1540–6.
98. Londono MC, Balderramo D, Cardenas A. Management of biliary complications after orthotopic liver transplantation: the role of endoscopy. World J Gastroenterol 2008; 14:493–7.
99. Pascher A, Neuhaus P. Biliary complications after deceased-donor orthotopic liver transplantation. J Hepatobiliary Pancreat Surg 2006;13:487–96.
100. Scatton O, Meunier B, Cherqui D, et al. Randomized trial of choledochocholedochostomy with or without a T tube in orthotopic liver transplantation. Ann Surg 2001;233:432–7.
101. Graziadei IW, Schwaighofer H, Koch R, et al. Long-term outcome of endoscopic treatment of biliary strictures after liver transplantation. Liver Transpl 2006;12: 718–25.
102. Sanchez-Urdazpal L, Batts KP, Gores GJ, et al. Increased bile duct complications in liver transplantation across the ABO barrier. Ann Surg 1993;218:152–8.
103. Sanchez-Urdazpal L, Gores GJ, Ward EM, et al. Diagnostic features and clinical outcome of ischemic-type biliary complications after liver transplantation. Hepatology 1993;17:605–9.
104. Sanchez-Urdazpal L, Gores GJ, Ward EM, et al. Ischemic-type biliary complications after orthotopic liver transplantation. Hepatology 1992;16:49–53.
105. Thuluvath PJ, Pfau PR, Kimmey MB, et al. Biliary complications after liver transplantation: the role of endoscopy. Endoscopy 2005;37:857–63.
106. Alazmi WM, Fogel EL, Watkins JL, et al. Recurrence rate of anastomotic biliary strictures in patients who have had previous successful endoscopic therapy for anastomotic narrowing after orthotopic liver transplantation. Endoscopy 2006;38: 571–4.
107. Pasha SF, Harrison ME, Das A, et al. Endoscopic treatment of anastomotic biliary strictures after deceased donor liver transplantation: outcomes after maximal stent therapy. Gastrointest Endosc 2007;66:44–51.
108. Verdonk RC, Buis CI, Porte RJ, et al. Anastomotic biliary strictures after liver transplantation: causes and consequences. Liver Transpl 2006;12:726–35.
109. Zoepf T, Maldonado-Lopez EJ, Hilgard P, et al. Balloon dilatation vs. balloon dilatation plus bile duct endoprostheses for treatment of anastomotic biliary strictures after liver transplantation. Liver Transpl 2006;12:88–94.
110. Sharma S, Gurakar A, Jabbour N. Biliary strictures following liver transplantation: past, present and preventive strategies. Liver Transpl 2008;14:759–69.
111. Rizk RS, McVicar JP, Emond MJ, et al. Endoscopic management of biliary strictures in liver transplant recipients: effect on patient and graft survival. Gastrointest Endosc 1998;47:128–35.
112. Thuluvath PJ, Atassi T, Lee J. An endoscopic approach to biliary complications following orthotopic liver transplantation. Liver Int 2003;23:156–62.
113. Verdonk RC, Buis CI, Porte RJ, et al. Biliary complications after liver transplantation: a review. Scand J Gastroenterol Suppl 2006;243:89–101.
114. Shah JN, Haigh WG, Lee SP, et al. Biliary casts after orthotopic liver transplantation: clinical factors, treatment, biochemical analysis. Am J Gastroenterol 2003;98: 1861–7.
115. Warner P, Fusai G, Glantzounis GK, et al. Risk factors associated with early hepatic artery thrombosis after orthotopic liver transplantation— univariable and multivariable analysis. Transpl Int 2011;24:401–8.

116. Abou El-Ella K, Al Sebayel M, Ramirez C, et al. Outcome and risk factors of hepatic artery thrombosis after orthotopic liver transplantation in adults. Transplant Proc 2001;33:2712–3.
117. Stange BJ, Glanemann M, Nuessler NC, et al. Hepatic artery thrombosis after adult liver transplantation. Liver Transpl 2003;9:612–20.
118. Valente JF, Alonso MH, Weber FL, et al. Late hepatic artery thrombosis in liver allograft recipients is associated with intrahepatic biliary necrosis. Transplantation 1996;61:61–5.
119. Del Gaudio M, Grazi GL, Ercolani G, et al. Outcome of hepatic artery reconstruction in liver transplantation with an iliac arterial interposition graft. Clin Transplant 2005; 19:399–405.
120. Jain A, Costa G, Marsh W, et al. Thrombotic and nonthrombotic hepatic artery complications in adults and children following primary liver transplantation with long-term follow-up in 1000 consecutive patients. Transpl Int 2006;19:27–37.
121. Pinna AD, Smith CV, Furukawa H, et al. Urgent revascularization of liver allografts after early hepatic artery thrombosis. Transplantation 1996;62:1584–7.
122. Berstad AE, Brabrand K, Foss A. Clinical utility of microbubble contrast-enhanced ultrasound in the diagnosis of hepatic artery occlusion after liver transplantation. Transpl Int 2009;22:954–60.
123. Oo YH, Gunson BK, Lancashire RJ, et al. Incidence of cancers following orthotopic liver transplantation in a single center: comparison with national cancer incidence rates for England and Wales. Transplantation 2005;80:759–64.
124. Drazan K, Shaked A, Olthoff KM, et al. Etiology and management of symptomatic adult hepatic artery thrombosis after orthotopic liver transplantation (OLT). Am Surg 1996;62:237–40.
125. Lisman T, Porte RJ. Hepatic artery thrombosis after liver transplantation: more than just a surgical complication? Transpl Int 2009;22:162–4.
126. Madalosso C, de Souza NF Jr, Ilstrup DM, et al. Cytomegalovirus and its association with hepatic artery thrombosis after liver transplantation. Transplantation 1998;66: 294–7.
127. Oh CK, Pelletier SJ, Sawyer RG, et al. Uni- and multi-variate analysis of risk factors for early and late hepatic artery thrombosis after liver transplantation. Transplantation 2001;71:767–72.
128. Pastacaldi S, Teixeira R, Montalto P, et al. Hepatic artery thrombosis after orthotopic liver transplantation: a review of nonsurgical causes. Liver Transpl 2001;7:75–81.
129. Varotti G, Grazi GL, Vetrone G, et al. Causes of early acute graft failure after liver transplantation: analysis of a 17-year single-centre experience. Clin Transplant 2005;19:492–500.
130. Vivarelli M, Cucchetti A, La Barba G, et al. Ischemic arterial complications after liver transplantation in the adult: multivariate analysis of risk factors. Arch Surg 2004;139: 1069–74.
131. Vivarelli M, La Barba G, Legnani C, et al. Repeated graft loss caused by recurrent hepatic artery thrombosis after liver transplantation. Liver Transpl 2003;9:629–31.
132. Pungpapong S, Manzarbeitia C, Ortiz J, et al. Cigarette smoking is associated with an increased incidence of vascular complications after liver transplantation. Liver Transpl 2002;8:582–7.
133. Singhal A, Stokes K, Sebastian A, et al. Endovascular treatment of hepatic artery thrombosis following liver transplantation. Transpl Int 2010;23:245–56.
134. Duffy JP, Hong JC, Farmer DG, et al. Vascular complications of orthotopic liver transplantation: experience in more than 4,200 patients. J Am Coll Surg 2009;208: 896–903.

135. Ma Y, He XS, Zhu XF, et al. [The cause and management of postoperative venous outflow obstruction after orthotopic liver transplantation]. Zhonghua Wai Ke Za Zhi 2008;46:1133–5.

136. Xiol X, Guardiola J, Menendez S, et al. Risk factors for development of de novo neoplasia after liver transplantation. Liver Transpl 2001;7:971–5.

137. Albright JB, Bonatti H, Stauffer J, et al. Colorectal and anal neoplasms following liver transplantation. Colorectal Dis 2010;12:657–66.

138. Duvoux C, Delacroix I, Richardet JP, et al. Increased incidence of oropharyngeal squamous cell carcinomas after liver transplantation for alcoholic cirrhosis. Transplantation 1999;67:418–21.

139. Jimenez-Romero C, Manrique Municio A, Marques Medina E, et al. Incidence of de novo nonmelanoma skin tumors after liver transplantation for alcoholic and nonalcoholic liver diseases. Transplant Proc 2006;38:2505–7.

140. Marques E, Jimenez C, Manrique A, et al. Development of lymphoproliferative disease after liver transplantation. Transplant Proc 2008;40:2988–9.

141. Perera GK, Child FJ, Heaton N, et al. Skin lesions in adult liver transplant recipients: a study of 100 consecutive patients. Br J Dermatol 2006;154:868–72.

142. Presser SJ, Schumacher G, Neuhaus R, et al. De novo esophageal neoplasia after liver transplantation. Liver Transpl 2007;13:443–50.

143. Zendejas-Ruiz I, Hemming AW, Chen C, et al. Recurrent Hepatocellular Carcinoma in Liver Transplant Recipients with Hepatitis C. J Gastrointest Cancer 2010 Nov 23 [Epub ahead of print].

144. Chak E, Saab S. Risk factors and incidence of de novo malignancy in liver transplant recipients: a systematic review. Liver Int 2010;30:1247–58.

145. Aigner F, Boeckle E, Albright J, et al. Malignancies of the colorectum and anus in solid organ recipients. Transpl Int 2007;20:497–504.

146. Rudraraju M, Osowo AT, Singh V, et al. Do patients need more frequent colonoscopic surveillance after liver transplantation? Transplant Proc 2008;40:1522–4.

147. Silva MA, Jambulingam PS, Mirza DF. Colorectal cancer after orthotopic liver transplantation. Crit Rev Oncol Hematol 2005;56:147–53.

148. Chapman RW. The colon and PSC: new liver, new danger? Gut. 1998;43:595–6.

149. Vera A, Gunson BK, Ussatoff V, et al. Colorectal cancer in patients with inflammatory bowel disease after liver transplantation for primary sclerosing cholangitis. Transplantation 2003;75:1983–8.

150. Leighton JA, Shen B, Baron TH, et al. ASGE guideline: endoscopy in the diagnosis and treatment of inflammatory bowel disease. Gastrointest Endosc 2006;63:558–65.

151. Finkenstedt A, Graziadei IW, Oberaigner W, et al. Extensive surveillance promotes early diagnosis and improved survival of de novo malignancies in liver transplant recipients. Am J Transplant 2009;9:2355–61.

152. Jimenez C, Rodriguez D, Marques E, et al. De novo tumors after orthotopic liver transplantation. Transplant Proc 2002;34:297–8.

153. Jain AB, Yee LD, Nalesnik MA, et al. Comparative incidence of de novo nonlymphoid malignancies after liver transplantation under tacrolimus using surveillance epidemiologic end result data. Transplantation 1998;66:1193–200.

154. Tanaka H, Sato H, Konishi Y, et al. Endometrial adenocarcinoma after liver transplantation. J Obstet Gynaecol Res 2005;31:224–6.

155. Nagarsheth NP, Kalir T, Rahaman J. Post-transplant lymphoproliferative disorder of the cervix. Gynecol Oncol 2005;97:271–5.

156. Penn I. Posttransplantation de novo tumors in liver allograft recipients. Liver Transpl Surg 1996;2:52–9.

157. Molmenti EP, Molmenti H, Weinstein J, et al. Syndromic incidence of ovarian carcinoma after liver transplantation, with special reference to anteceding breast cancer. Dig Dis Sci 2003;48:187–9.
158. Oruc MT, Soran A, Jain AK, et al. De novo breast cancer in patients with liver transplantation: University of Pittsburgh's experience and review of the literature. Liver Transpl 2004;10:1–6.
159. Duvoux C, Pageaux GP, Vanlemmens C, et al. Risk factors for lymphoproliferative disorders after liver transplantation in adults: an analysis of 480 patients. Transplantation 2002;74:1103–9.
160. Aucejo F, Rofaiel G, Miller C. Who is at risk for post-transplant lymphoproliferative disorders (PTLD) after liver transplantation? J Hepatol 2006;44:19–23.
161. Kremers WK, Devarbhavi HC, Wiesner RH, et al. Post-transplant lymphoproliferative disorders following liver transplantation: incidence, risk factors and survival. Am J Transplant 2006;6:1017–24.
162. Ben-Ari Z, Amlot P, Lachmanan SR, Tur-et al. Posttransplantation lymphoproliferative disorder in liver recipients: characteristics, management, and outcome. Liver Transpl Surg 1999;5:184–91.
163. Evens AM, Roy R, Sterrenberg D, et al. Post-transplantation lymphoproliferative disorders: diagnosis, prognosis, and current approaches to therapy. Curr Oncol Rep 2010;12:383–94.
164. Ulrich C, Jurgensen JS, Degen A, et al. Prevention of non-melanoma skin cancer in organ transplant patients by regular use of a sunscreen: a 24 months, prospective, case-control study. Br J Dermatol 2009;161(Suppl 3):78–84.
165. Herrero JI, Espana A, Quiroga J, et al. Nonmelanoma skin cancer after liver transplantation. Study of risk factors. Liver Transpl 2005;11:1100–6.
166. Ingvar A, Smedby KE, Lindelof B, et al. Immunosuppressive treatment after solid organ transplantation and risk of post-transplant cutaneous squamous cell carcinoma. Nephrol Dial Transplant 2010;25:2764–71.
167. Kovach BT, Stasko T. Skin cancer after transplantation. Transplant Rev (Orlando) 2009;23:178–89.
168. Mazzaferro V, Regalia E, Doci R, et al. Liver transplantation for the treatment of small hepatocellular carcinomas in patients with cirrhosis. N Engl J Med 1996;334:693–9.
169. Jimenez C, Manrique A, Marques E, et al. Incidence and risk factors for the development of lung tumors after liver transplantation. Transpl Int 2007;20:57–63.
170. Recommended adult immunization schedule—United States, 2011. MMWR Morb Mortal Wkly Rep 2011;60:1–4.
171. Munoz SJ, Rothstein KD, Reich D, et al. Long-term care of the liver transplant recipient. Clin Liver Dis 2000;4:691–710.

Index

Note: Page numbers of article titles are in **bold face** type.

A

A2ALL study, of liver transplantation, 651–652
ABIC (age-bilirubin-INR-creatinine) score, for alcoholic hepatitis, 612, 614, 618
Abstinence, in alcoholic hepatitis, 619
Academic Medical Center of Amsterdam, bioartificial liver, 531–532
Acamprosate, for alcoholic hepatitis, 619
N-Acetylcysteine
  for acute liver failure, 530
  for alcoholic hepatitis, 629
Acoustic radiation force imaging, for hepatic fibrosis, 515–516
Acute liver failure, **523–539**
  N-acetylcysteine for, 530
  brain edema in, 524–527
  cardiovascular support for, 529
  coagulopathy in, 527–528
  definition of, 523
  diagnosis of, 523–524
  epidemiology of, 523
  hepatocyte transplantation for, 532–533
  infections in, 528–529
  initial management of, 523–524
  kidney failure in, 529
  liver transplantation for, 532
  liver-assist devices for, 530–532
  metabolic issues in, 529
  respiratory support for, 529
  systemic inflammatory response syndrome in, 528
Adefovir, for hepatitis B, 497–500
Adrenal insufficiency, in acute liver failure, 529
Adult-to-adult living liver transplantation, 651–652
ADVANCE study, for hepatitis C, 488, 490
Age considerations, in liver donation, 642–643
Age-bilirubin-INR-creatinine (ABIC) score, for alcoholic hepatitis, 612, 614, 618
Alanine aminotransferase
  as hepatitis B treatment endpoint, 497–498
  in fibrosis, 509
Albumin, for hepatorenal syndrome, 590–591, 593
Albumin dialysis, for acute liver failure, 530–531
Alcohol abuse, after liver transplantation, 664

Gastroenterol Clin N Am 40 (2011) 683–694
doi:10.1016/S0889-8553(11)00072-0
0889-8553/11/$ – see front matter © 2011 Elsevier Inc. All rights reserved.

gastro.theclinics.com

Alcoholic hepatitis, **611–639**
  severity scores for, 611–619
  treatment of, 618, 620–632
Alcoholics Anonymous, 619
Alpha-adrenergic receptor agonists, for hepatorenal syndrome, 588–590
American Society of Transplant Surgeons guidelines, 645–646
Ammonia accumulation, in acute liver failure, 524
Angiogenesis, as target for hepatocellular carcinoma treatment, 604–605
Angiotensin receptor blockers, for varices, 569
Angiotensin-converting enzyme inhibitors, for varices, 569
Anti-angiogenesis agents, as target for hepatocellular carcinoma treatment, 604–605
Antibiotics, for alcoholic hepatitis, 629
Antioxidants, for alcoholic hepatitis, 629
Antithrombin deficiency, in acute liver failure, 528
Arterial vasodilatation, in hepatorenal syndrome, 583
Ascites, in alcoholic hepatitis, 620–621
Aspartate aminotransferase
  as hepatitis B treatment endpoint, 497–498
  in fibrosis, 509
AST to platelet count ratio index, in fibrosis, 509–510, 513

B

Baclofen, for alcoholic hepatitis, 619
BAL Support System, for acute liver failure, 532
Balloon placement, for nonalcoholic fatty liver disease, 550–551
Banding, for esophageal varices, 569–571, 574
Barbiturates, for cerebral edema, in acute liver failure, 527
Bariatric surgery, for nonalcoholic fatty liver disease, 551–554
Beads, for chemoembolization, for hepatocellular carcinoma, 602–603
Benzodiazepines, for alcohol withdrawal, 620
Beta blockers, nonselective, for varices, 562–566
Betaine, for nonalcoholic fatty liver disease, 548–549
Bevacizumab, for hepatocellular carcinoma, 605
Biliary complications, after liver transplantation, 668–670
Biliopancreatic diversion, for nonalcoholic fatty liver disease, 551–553
Bilirubin, early change in, in alcoholic hepatitis, 614
Bioartificial liver support, for acute liver failure, 531–532
Biochemical endpoint, in hepatitis C treatment, 497–498
Bioenterics intragastric balloon, for nonalcoholic fatty liver disease, 550–551
Biopsy, liver
  as treatment endpoint, 496–497
  before transplantation, 644
  for fibrosis, 509, 512, 518
Bleeding disorders, in acute liver failure, 527–528
BMS-650032, for hepatitis C, 492
BMS-790052, for hepatitis C, 492
Boceprevir, for hepatitis C, 483–486, 489–490
Brain, edema of, in acute liver failure, 524–527
Breast cancer, after liver transplantation, 672
Budd-Chiari syndrome, after liver transplantation, 670–671

C

Cancer. *See also* Hepatocellular carcinoma.
   after liver transplantation, 671–672
   in liver donor, 649–650
Cardiac death, liver donation after, 644–646
Cardiac output
   in acute liver failure, 529
   in hepatorenal syndrome, 585
Cardiovascular disease, after liver transplantation, 661
Carvedilol, for varices, 567, 569
Cerebral blood flow, in acute liver failure, 524–525
Cerebral edema, in acute liver failure, 524–527
Chemoembolization, for hepatocellular carcinoma, 602–603
Child-Turcotte-Pugh score, for alcoholic hepatitis, 612–613, 615–619
Cholangiopathy, ischemic, in liver transplantation, 645–646
Cirrhosis
   hepatorenal syndrome in. *See* Hepatorenal syndrome.
   in alcoholic hepatitis, 620–621
Clofibrate, for nonalcoholic fatty liver disease, 549–550
Coagulopathy, in acute liver failure, 527–528
Cold ischemia time, before liver transplantation, 644
Colorectal cancer, after liver transplantation, 671
Computed tomography, xenon-enhanced, for cerebral blood flow measurement, 525
Coronary artery disease, after liver transplantation, 661
Corticosteroids, for alcoholic hepatitis, 620–626
Cryoprecipitate, in acute liver failure, 528
Cyclosporine, drug interactions with, 664–667

D

Death, cardiac, liver donation after, 644–646
Delirium tremens, 620
Detoxification devices, for acute liver failure, 530–531
Diabetes mellitus, after liver transplantation, 662–663
Dialysis, albumin, for acute liver failure, 530–531
Diet, for alcoholic hepatitis, 620
Discriminant function index, for alcoholic hepatitis, 611–612, 615–618
Distal splenorenal shunt, for varices, 572
DNA analysis, for hepatitis B virus, as treatment endpoint, 498–500
Donors, for liver transplantation. *See* Liver transplantation, extended-criteria donors for.
Dopamine, for acute liver failure, 529
Doppler ultrasonography, transcranial, for cerebral blood flow measurement, 525
Doxorubicin beads, for hepatocellular carcinoma, 602–603
Drug resistance, in hepatitis C virus, 483
Duodenal switch operation, for nonalcoholic fatty liver disease, 551–552
Dyslipidemia, after liver transplantation, 663–664

E

Early change in bilirubin level score, for alcoholic hepatitis, 614
Edema, cerebral, in acute liver failure, 524–527

Effective arterial blood volume, in hepatorenal syndrome, 583–584
Elastography, for hepatic fibrosis, 512–515, 518
Electroencephalography, for cerebral blood flow measurement, 525
Electrolyte abnormalities, in acute liver failure, 529
Embolization, for hepatocellular carcinoma, 602–604
Encephalopathy, hepatic
    in acute liver failure, 524–527
    in alcoholic hepatitis, 620–621
Endoscopic treatment, for nonalcoholic fatty liver disease, 550–551
Endoscopic variceal ligation, 569–571, 574
Entecavir, for hepatitis B, 497–500
Enteral feeding, for alcoholic hepatitis, 620
Erlotinib, for hepatocellular carcinoma, 605
Esophageal varices, **561–579**
    banding of, 569–571, 574
    in alcoholic hepatitis, 620–621
    pharmacologic treatment of, 561–569, 571, 574
    prevention of, 563–566, 570–571, 573, 575
    recurrent, 565, 571
    shunts for, 572–575
Etanercept, for alcoholic hepatitis, 628–629
Ethanol injection, for hepatocellular carcinoma, 601
Ethical issues, in liver transplantation, 630
European Liver Fibrosis panel, 511–512
Everolimus, for hepatocellular carcinoma, 605
EVOLVE-1 study, of hepatocellular carcinoma, 605
Extracorporeal liver support, for acute liver failure, 530–531

F

Fatty liver disease, nonalcoholic. See Nonalcoholic fatty liver disease.
FIB-4 index, for fibrosis, 511
Fibrinogen deficiency, in acute liver failure, 528
Fibroblasts, activation of, fibrosis in, 508
FibroScan, 512–514
Fibrosis, hepatic. See Hepatic fibrosis.
FIBROSpect panel, 511–512
FibroSure test, 511–512
FibroTest, 510–513
Fluid therapy, for acute liver failure, 529
Forns index, for fibrosis, 511
Fresh frozen plasma, in acute liver failure, 528
Fulminant liver failure. See Acute liver failure.

G

GAHS (Glasgow Alcoholic Hepatitis Score), 612–616, 618–619
Gallstones, after liver transplantation, 669
Gastric banding, for nonalcoholic fatty liver disease, 551–552
Gastric bypass, for nonalcoholic fatty liver disease, 551–552
Gender considerations, in liver donation, 643

Glasgow Alcoholic Hepatitis Score, 612–616, 618–619
Granulocytapheresis, for alcoholic hepatitis, 629–630
Gynecologic cancer, after liver transplantation, 671–672

H

HALT-C (Hepatitis C Antiviral Long-term Treatment against Cirrhosis) trial, 512
Head and neck cancer, after liver transplantation, 671
HeBeAg, monitoring of, in hepatitis B, 500–501
HeBsAg, monitoring of, in hepatitis B, 500–501
Height, of liver donor, 643
Hemodynamics, in acute liver failure, 529
Hemorrhage, variceal. See Esophageal varices.
Hepascore, for fibrosis, 511
HepatAssist device, for acute liver failure, 531
Hepatic artery thrombosis, after liver transplantation, 670
Hepatic encephalopathy
    in acute liver failure, 524–527
    in alcoholic hepatitis, 620–621
Hepatic fibrosis, **507–521**
    biopsy for, 509, 518
    clinical implications of, 508–509
    diseases with, 508–509
    in hepatitis B, 496–497
    noninvasive assessment of
        clinical applications of, 516–518
        serum markers, 509–512
        techniques for, 512–516
    pathogenesis of, 508
    staging of, 509
Hepatic venous pressure gradient, in varices, 561–562, 565
Hepatitis
    alcoholic, **611–639**
    in fatty liver disease. See Nonalcoholic fatty liver disease.
    radiation-induced, 603
Hepatitis B
    in liver donor, 648
    treatment of, **495–505**
        biochemical endpoint in, 497–498
        goals of, 495–496
        histologic end point in, 496–497
        serologic end points in, 500–501
        virologic end point in, 498–500
Hepatitis C, **481–494**
    drug resistance in, 483
    epidemiology of, 481
    fibrosis in, 507–517
    in liver donor, 647–648

treatment of
  combination therapy for, 491–492
  N53/4A protease inhibitors in, 483–490
  NS5B RNA polymerase inhibitors in, 491
virology of, 482–483
Hepatitis C Antiviral Long-term Treatment against Cirrhosis (HALT-C) trial, 512
Hepatocellular carcinoma, **599–610**
  after liver transplantation, 672
  epidemiology of, 599
  locoregional therapies for
    ablation, 601–602
    chemoembolization, 602–603
    radioembolization, 603–604
  molecular targeted therapies for, 604–605
  screening for, 599
  surgery for, 600–601
Hepatocyte transplantation, for acute liver failure, 532–533
Hepatorenal syndrome, **581–598**
  diagnosis of, 581
  in alcoholic hepatitis, 620–621
  incidence of, 581
  liver transplantation for, 593–594
  pathogenesis of, 582–585
  precipitants of, 581
  prognosis for, 594
  types of, 581–582
  vasoconstrictors for
    basis for, 585
    efficacy of, 591–593
    TIPS with, 593
    types of, 585–591
Histologic end point, in hepatitis C treatment, 496–497
Human immunodeficiency virus infection, in liver donor, 648–649
Hypernatremia, in liver donor, 643
Hypertension
  intracranial, in acute liver failure, 524–527
  portal, varices in. See Esophageal varices.
  systemic, after liver transplantation, 663
Hypertonic saline solution, for cerebral edema, in acute liver failure, 527
Hypertriglyceridemia, after liver transplantation, 663–664
Hyperventilation, for cerebral edema, in acute liver failure, 526
Hypoglycemia, in acute liver failure, 529
Hypothermia therapy, for cerebral edema, in acute liver failure, 526–527

I

ILLUMINATE study, for hepatitis C, 488–489
Immunosuppressive drugs, drug interactions with, 664–667
Infections
  in acute liver failure, 528
  in liver donor, 648

Infliximab, for alcoholic hepatitis, 628
INFORM study, for hepatitis C, 491–492
Interleukin(s), for alcoholic hepatitis, 630
Intracranial hypertension, in acute liver failure, 524–527
Intragastric balloon, for nonalcoholic fatty liver disease, 550–551
Ischemic cholangiopathy, in liver transplantation, 645
Isosorbide-5-mononitrate, for esophageal varices, 564–566

J

Jugular bulb catheter, for cerebral blood flow measurement, 525

K

Kidney
    acute injury of, in liver transplantation, 659–660
    chronic disease of, after liver transplantation, 659–660
    dysfunctional autoregulation of, in hepatorenal syndrome, 584
    failure of. *See also* Hepatorenal syndrome.
       in acute liver failure, 529
    transplantation of, for hepatorenal syndrome, 593–594

L

Lamivudine, for hepatitis B, 497–501
Laparoscopic adjustable gastric banding, for nonalcoholic fatty liver disease,
    551–553
Lille score, for alcoholic hepatitis, 612, 614, 619
Liver
    biopsy of
       as treatment endpoint, 496–497
       before transplantation, 644
       for fibrosis, 509, 512, 518
    resection of, for hepatocellular carcinoma, 600
Liver disorders. *See also* Hepatitis.
    acute liver failure, **523–539**
    fibrosis, 496–497, **507–521**
    hepatocellular carcinoma, **599–610,** 672
    hepatorenal syndrome, **581–598,** 620–621
    nonalcoholic fatty liver disease, 507–517, **541–559,** 620–621
    transplantation for. *See* Liver transplantation.
    varices, **561–579,** 620–621
Liver transplantation
    adult-to-adult living transplantation, 651–652
    complication management after, **659–681**
       alcohol abuse, 664
       biliary, 668–670
       cardiovascular disease, 661
       diabetes mellitus, 662–663
       dyslipidemia, 663–664
       hypertension, 663
       kidney dysfunction, 659–660

malignancy, 671–672
medication interactions, 664–667
metabolic syndrome, 661–662
obesity, 662
osteoporosis, 660–661
pregnancy, 667
recurrent liver disease, 667–668
rejection, 668
tobacco abuse, 664–665, 667
vaccinations and, 673
vascular, 670–671
ethical issues in, 630
extended-criteria donors for, **641–658**
consent for, 652
definitions of, 641–642
disease transmission from, 647–650
impaired allograft function indicators, 642–646
organ allocation and distribution and, 642
outcomes of, 646–647
partial allografts in, 650–652
for acute liver failure, 532
for alcoholic hepatitis, 630–632
for hepatocellular carcinoma, 600–601
for hepatorenal syndrome, 593–594
for nonalcoholic fatty liver disease, 554–555
recidivism after, 631
six months abstinence rule for, 631–632
split-liver, 650
Liver-assist devices, for acute liver failure, 530–532
Lorazepam, for alcohol withdrawal, 620
Lung cancer, after liver transplantation, 672
Lung injury, in acute liver failure, 529

M

Magnetic resonance elastography, for hepatic fibrosis, 514–515, 518
Magnetic resonance imaging, for hepatic fibrosis, 516
Magnetic resonance spectroscopy, for hepatic fibrosis, 516
Malnutrition, in alcoholic hepatitis, 620
Mannitol, for cerebral edema, in acute liver failure, 526
Mechanical ventilation, for acute liver failure, 529
MELD score
for alcoholic hepatitis, 612–613, 615–619
for liver transplantation, 642, 646–647
Metabolic disorders, in acute liver failure, 529
Metabolic syndrome, after liver transplantation, 661–662
Metformin, for nonalcoholic fatty liver disease, 545–547
Methyl prednisolone, for alcoholic hepatitis, 623–624
Microwave ablation, for hepatocellular carcinoma, 601–602
Midodrine, for hepatorenal syndrome, 588–589, 593
Milan criteria, for hepatocellular carcinoma, 600–601

Model for End-Stage Liver Disease (MELD) score
    for alcoholic hepatitis, 612–613, 615–619
    for liver transplantation, 642, 646–647
Modified discriminant function, for alcoholic hepatitis, 611–612, 619
Molecular adsorbent recirculating system, for acute liver failure, 530–531
Mycophenolate mofetil, drug interactions with, 664–667
Myofibroblasts, in fibrosis, 508

N

N53/4A protease inhibitors, for hepatitis C, 483–490
Nadolol, for varices, 562–566
Naltrexone, for alcoholic hepatitis, 619
Nitroglycerin, for varices, 568
Nonalcoholic fatty liver disease, **541–559**
    endoscopic treatment of, 550–551
    fibrosis in, 507–517
    histology of, 541–542
    natural history of, 541
    pathogenesis of, 541–542
    pharmacologic treatment of, 542–550
    spectrum of, 541
    surgical treatment of, 551–555
Nonalcoholic steatohepatitis. *See also* Nonalcoholic fatty liver disease.
    fibrosis in, 507–517
Norepinephrine
    for acute liver failure, 529
    for hepatorenal syndrome, 589–590
NS5B RNA polymerase inhibitors, for hepatitis C, 491
Nucleoside inhibitors, for hepatitis C, 491
Nucleotide analog agents, for hepatitis B, 495, 497
Nutrition, for alcoholic hepatitis, 620

O

Obesity
    after liver transplantation, 662
    fatty liver disease in. *See* Nonalcoholic fatty liver disease.
Octreotide
    for hepatorenal syndrome, 590, 593
    for varices, 567–568
Osteoporosis, after liver transplantation, 660–661
Oxandrolone, for alcoholic hepatitis, 620
Oxazepam, for alcohol withdrawal, 620
Oxidative stress, in alcoholic hepatitis, 629

P

Paris Consensus Meeting on Expanded Criteria Donors in Liver Transplantation, 642
Peginterferon, for hepatitis B, 498–501
Pentobarbital, for alcohol withdrawal, 620
Pentoxifylline

for alcoholic hepatitis, 626–628
    for nonalcoholic fatty liver disease, 547–548
Peritonitis, spontaneous bacterial, in alcoholic hepatitis, 620–621
Phenobarbital, for alcohol withdrawal, 620
Pioglitazone, for nonalcoholic fatty liver disease, 542–543
PIVENS trial, for nonalcoholic fatty liver disease, 543
Portal hypertension, varices in. See Esophageal varices.
Portal vein thrombosis, after liver transplantation, 670
Portocaval H-graft shunt, for varices, 572
Posttransplant lymphoproliferative disorder, after liver transplantation, 672
Prazosin, for esophageal varices, 565–566
PRECISION study, of chemoembolization, 602–603
Prednisolone, for alcoholic hepatitis, 620, 623–625
Prednisone, for alcoholic hepatitis, 623–624
Pregnancy, after liver transplantation, 667
Probiotics, for alcoholic hepatitis, 629
Probucol, for nonalcoholic fatty liver disease, 547
Propofol, for alcohol withdrawal, 620
Propranolol, for varices, 562–566
Protease inhibitors, for hepatitis C, 483–490
PROVE (Protease inhibition for Viral Evaluation) trials, for hepatitis C, 486–488

R

Race, of liver donor, 643
Radioembolization, for hepatocellular carcinoma, 603–604
Radiofrequency ablation, for hepatocellular carcinoma, 601–602
Rapamycin inhibitors, for hepatocellular carcinoma, 605
REALIZE study, for hepatitis C, 489–490
Recidivism, after liver transplantation, 631
Rejection, in liver transplantation, 668
Resistance, drug, in hepatitis C virus, 483
Respiratory support, for acute liver failure, 529
RESPOND trials, for hepatitis C, 485–486, 490
Rifaximin, for alcoholic hepatitis, 629
Rosiglitazone, for nonalcoholic fatty liver disease, 543–544
Roux-en-Y gastric bypass, for nonalcoholic fatty liver disease, 551–553

S

Saline solution, hypertonic, for cerebral edema, in acute liver failure, 527
Sclerotherapy, for varices, 566, 570
Serine Protease Inhibitor Therapy (SPRINT) trials, 483–485
Serologic end points, in hepatitis B treatment, 500–501
Serum markers, for fibrosis, 509–512, 518
SHARP trial, for hepatocellular carcinoma, 604–605
Shunts, for varices, 571–575
Sildenafil, for varices, 569
Simvastatin, for varices, 569
Sirolimus, drug interactions with, 664–667
Six months abstinence rule, for liver transplantation, 631–632

Skin cancer, after liver transplantation, 672
Sleeve gastrectomy, for nonalcoholic fatty liver disease, 551
Smoking, liver transplantation and, 664–665, 667
Somatostatin, for varices, 567–568
Sorafenib, for hepatocellular carcinoma, 604–605
Sphincter of Oddi, injury of, in liver transplantation, 668–669
Splanchnic vasodilatation, in hepatorenal syndrome, 583
Split-liver transplantation, 650
SPRINT (Serine Protease Inhibitor Therapy) trials, 483–485, 490
Statins, for dyslipidemia, 664
Steatosis
    hepatic. See Nonalcoholic fatty liver disease.
    in liver donor, 643–644
Stellate cells, activation of, fibrosis in, 508
Strictures, biliary, after liver transplantation, 669
Sunitinib, for hepatocellular carcinoma, 604–605
Systemic inflammatory response syndrome, in acute liver failure, 528

T

Tacrolimus, drug interactions with, 664–667
Telaprevir, for hepatitis C, 486–490
Telbivudine, for hepatitis B, 497–499
Tenofovir, for hepatitis B, 497–499
Terlipressin
    for acute liver failure, 529
    for hepatorenal syndrome, 586–588, 591–592
    for varices, 566–568
Thiazolidinediones, for nonalcoholic fatty liver disease, 542–544
TIPS (transjugular intrahepatic portosystemic shunt), for varices, 571–575
Tobacco use, liver transplantation and, 664–665, 667
Transarterial chemoembolization, for hepatocellular carcinoma, 602–603
Transcranial Doppler ultrasonography, for cerebral blood flow measurement, 525
Transient elastography, for hepatic fibrosis, 512–514, 518
Transjugular intrahepatic portosystemic shunt, for varices, 571–575
Transplantation
    hepatocyte, for acute liver failure, 532–533
    liver. See Liver transplantation.
Tumor necrosis factor inhibitors, for alcoholic hepatitis, 628–629

U

Ultrasonography, for cerebral blood flow measurement, 525
Ultrasound-based transient elastography, for hepatic fibrosis, 512–514, 518
United Network for Organ Sharing regions, 642
United States Acute Liver failure Study Group, 524
Ursodeoxycholic acid, for nonalcoholic fatty liver disease, 549–550

V

Vaccinations, after liver transplantation, 673
Vapreotide, for varices, 567–568

Varices. *See* Esophageal varices.
Vascular complications, after liver transplantation, 670–671
Vasoconstrictors, for varices, 566–567
Vasopressin, for varices, 566–567
Vasopressin analogs, for hepatorenal syndrome, 585–588
Vertical banded gastroplasty, for nonalcoholic fatty liver disease, 551–553
Viral infections, in liver donor, 648
Virologic end point, in hepatitis C treatment, 498–500
Vitamin E, for nonalcoholic fatty liver disease, 544–545

W

Weight, of liver donor, 643
West Nile virus infection, in liver donor, 648
Withdrawal, alcohol, 620

Y

Yttrium-90 microspheres, for hepatocellular carcinoma, 603–604

Printed and bound by CPI Group (UK) Ltd, Croydon, CR0 4YY

03/10/2024

01040457-0005